W9-AKC-524

For Reference

Not to be taken from this room

Death and Dying
SOURCEBOOK

FOURTH EDITION

Health Reference Series

Death and Dying
SOURCEBOOK

FOURTH EDITION

Basic Consumer Health Information about End-of-Life Care and Related Perspectives, Including End-of-Life Symptoms and Treatments, Pain Management, Quality-of-Life Concerns, Patients' Rights and Privacy Issues, Advance Directives, Physician-Assisted Suicide, Caregiving, Organ Donation, Funeral Arrangements, and Grief

Along with Statistical Data, Information about the Leading Causes of Death, a Glossary, and Directories of Support Groups and Other Resources

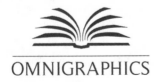

OMNIGRAPHICS

615 Griswold St., Ste. 520, Detroit, MI 48226

Bibliographic Note
Because this page cannot legibly accommodate all the copyright notices, the Bibliographic
Note portion of the Preface constitutes an extension of the copyright notice.

* * *

OMNIGRAPHICS

Angela L. Williams, *Managing Editor*

* * *

Copyright © 2020 Omnigraphics

ISBN 978-0-7808-1731-9

E-ISBN 978-0-7808-1732-6

Library of Congress Cataloging-in-Publication Data

Names: Omnigraphics, Inc. | Williams, Angela, 1963- editor.

Title: Death and dying sourcebook / Angela L. Williams.

Description: Fourth edition. | Detroit, MI : Omnigraphics, Inc., 2019. | Series: Health
reference series | Includes index. | Summary: "Provides basic consumer health
information about management of end-of-life symptoms, caregiving and facility
evaluation, and legal and economic issues associated with end-of-life. Includes index,
glossary of related terms, and other resources"-- Provided by publisher.

Identifiers: LCCN 2019030309 (print) | LCCN 2019030310 (ebook) | ISBN
9780780817319 (library binding) | ISBN 9780780817326 (ebook)

Subjects: LCSH: Death. | Terminal care.

Classification: LCC R726.8 .D3785 2019 (print) | LCC R726.8 (ebook) | DDC
616.02/9--dc23

LC record available at https://lccn.loc.gov/2019030309

LC ebook record available at https://lccn.loc.gov/2019030310

Table of Contents

Preface xi

Part I: End-of-Life Perspectives

Chapter 1 — Providing Care and Comfort at
the End of Life 3

Chapter 2 — Making End-of-Life Healthcare
Decisions 11

Chapter 3 — Cultural Response to Death 19

Chapter 4 — Spirituality in End-of-Life Care 21

Chapter 5 — Chronic Illness in Old Age 37

Chapter 6 — Fact Sheet on End of Life 43

Chapter 7 — Research Findings about End-of-Life
Care and Outcomes 47

Section 7.1 — The BEACON Study on
End-of-Life Care 48

Section 7.2 — Telephone-Based Rehab
Program for Cancer
Patients 52

Section 7.3 — Family Involvement
Improves End-of-Life Care 56

Part II: Medical Management of End-of-Life Symptoms

Chapter 8 — Palliative Care 59

    Section 8.1 — What Is Palliative Care? 60

    Section 8.2 — Palliative Wound Care 64

    Section 8.3 — Palliative Care in Cancer 69

Chapter 9 — Chronic Illnesses and End-of-Life Care 73

Chapter 10 — Pain Management and Assessment 75

    Section 10.1 — Pain: An Overview 76

    Section 10.2 — Cancer Pain Control 80

    Section 10.3 — Pain Assessment in
                  Patients with Dementia 93

Chapter 11 — Managing and Treating Fatigue 97

    Section 11.1 — Fatigue: More Than Being
                  Tired 98

    Section 11.2 — Cancer and Fatigue 101

    Section 11.3 — Coping with Fatigue after
                  Cancer Treatment 114

Chapter 12 — Acute Respiratory Distress Syndrome 117

Chapter 13 — Artificial Hydration and Nutrition 125

Chapter 14 — Nutrition in Cancer Care 129

Chapter 15 — Delirium 149

    Section 15.1 — What Is Delirium? 150

    Section 15.2 — Delirium among Cancer
                  Patients 155

Part III: Medical Decisions Surrounding the End of Life

Chapter 16 — Preferences for Care at the End of Life 159

Chapter 17 — End-of-Life Care for Dementia 167

Chapter 18 — End-of-Life Care for Advanced Cancer 171

Chapter 19 — HIV/AIDS and End-of-Life Issues 181

Chapter 20 — Ethics and Legal Issues in Palliative Care 191

Chapter 21 — Last Days of Life 195

Chapter 22—Termination of Life-Sustaining
            Treatments.. 205

Chapter 23—Organ Donation of the Deceased and
            Transplantation 213

Chapter 24—Physician-Assisted Suicide and
            Euthanasia.. 221

Part IV: End-of-Life Care Facilities

Chapter 25—Long-Term Care.. 227

        Section 25.1—What Is Long-Term Care?........ 228

        Section 25.2—Long-Term Care; Making
                    the Right Decision 235

        Section 25.3—Choosing a Nursing Home 236

Chapter 26—Home Care for Critically Ill Patients 239

        Section 26.1—Home Care for Cancer
                    Patients 240

        Section 26.2—Home Healthcare for
                    Critically Ill and Older
                    Adults... 251

        Section 26.3—Assistive Devices and
                    Rehabilitative Technologies
                    for Patients with Chronic
                    Conditions 254

Chapter 27—Palliative Care and Hospice Care:
            Comforting the Terminally Ill............................. 257

Chapter 28—End-of-Life Care Settings................................... 261

Chapter 29—Insurance for End-of-Life Care 265

        Section 29.1—Insurance Coverage for
                    Hospice 266

        Section 29.2—Long-Term-Care Insurance...... 270

Part V: End-of-Life Caregiving

Chapter 30—Communications among Patients,
            Families, and Providers...................................... 279

        Section 30.1—Effective Communication
                    for Effective Care...................... 280

Section 30.2—Talk about End-of-Life
Wishes 281

Section 30.3—Communication in
Cancer Care 283

Chapter 31—Long-Distance Caregiving 289

Chapter 32—Take Care of Yourself While Caring
for Others 295

Section 32.1—How to Share Caregiving
Responsibilities with
Family Members 296

Section 32.2—Tips for Caregiver
Self-Care 299

Section 32.3—Coping with Caregiving 301

Chapter 33—Things to Look out for as Death
Approaches 305

Chapter 34—What to Do When Death Occurs 309

Part VI: Death and Children: Information for Parents

Chapter 35—When a Child Has Cancer 315

Chapter 36—Pediatric Palliative Care 325

Chapter 37—Sudden Infant Death Syndrome 333

Chapter 38—Stillbirth, Miscarriage, and Infant
Death 339

Section 38.1—Stillbirth 340

Section 38.2—Miscarriage 344

Section 38.3—Infant Death 349

Chapter 39—Helping Children Cope with Death 355

Section 39.1—Grief and Developmental
Stages 356

Section 39.2—Guiding Children through
Grief 361

Chapter 40—Collaborative Pediatric Critical Care
Research Network 365

Part VII: Legal and Economic Issues at the End of Life

Chapter 41—Getting Your Affairs in Order 375

Chapter 42—Patients' Rights 381

    Section 42.1—Informed Consent 382

    Section 42.2—Health Information
                Privacy Rights 389

    Section 42.3—Informed Consent for
                Clinical Trials 391

Chapter 43—Advance Directives 397

Chapter 44—Financial Assistance for Long-Term
               or End-of-Life Care 407

Chapter 45—Social Security Benefits 413

Chapter 46—Duties of a Personal Representative
               (Executor) 417

Chapter 47—Understanding the Family and
               Medical Leave Act (FMLA) 421

Part VIII: Final Arrangements

Chapter 48—Funeral Services: An Overview 429

Chapter 49—Planning a Funeral 441

Chapter 50—Military Funeral Planning 445

Chapter 51—Cremation Explained 449

Chapter 52—Medical Certification of Death 451

Chapter 53—If Death Occurs While Traveling 457

Chapter 54—Grief, Bereavement, and Coping
               with Loss 461

Chapter 55—Mourning the Death of a Spouse 469

Part IX: Mortality Statistics

Chapter 56—Life Expectancy: Global Trends 477

Chapter 57—Mortality Trends in the United States 483

Chapter 58—Leading Causes of Death in the
United States 491

Chapter 59—Life Expectancy at Birth 499

Chapter 60—Infant and Maternal Mortality
Trends and Disparities 503

Chapter 61—Work-Related Fatalities 509

Chapter 62—Childhood Risk of Injury-Related Death 513

Chapter 63—Suicide Facts and Statistics 517

Chapter 64—Alcohol-Attributable Deaths 521

Chapter 65—Deaths from Stroke 527

Part X: Additional Help and Information

Chapter 66—Glossary of End-of-Life Terms 531

Chapter 67—Support Groups for End-of-Life Issues 543

Chapter 68—Resources for Information about
Death and Dying 545

Index 557

Preface

About This Book

Although death is considered a taboo subject, it is inevitable. Some people die suddenly while others pass away after long-term struggles with chronic disabilities or diseases. Considering the dying process in advance allows people to talk about their choices concerning end-of-life medical preferences. Discussing these topics can be difficult, but appropriate planning allows people to remain in charge of their healthcare even after they are no longer able to make decisions. Additionally, knowledge about loved ones' wishes can help friends and families cope with the shock and grief of death.

Death and Dying Sourcebook, Fourth Edition provides information about end-of-life perspectives and the medical management of symptoms that can occur as death draws near. It discusses palliative care and describes the issues surrounding end-of-life care and the process of organ donation. The book also addresses caregiver concerns and provides information about children and death. Facts about legal and economic issues at the end of life, funerals and other final arrangements, and grief are also included, along with statistical data, a glossary, and directories of support groups and other resources.

How to Use This Book

This book is divided into parts and chapters. Parts focus on broad areas of interest. Chapters are devoted to single topics within a part.

Part I: End-of-Life Perspectives begins by defining end-of-life care and discusses the importance of end-of-life planning. Cultural and spiritual concerns that impact end-of-life decisions are discussed, and research findings about end-of-life care are also described.

Part II: Medical Management of End-of-Life Symptoms begins with an explanation of palliative and end-of-life care. Pain management and assessment is discussed in detail, and information on managing and treating fatigue is also provided. Specific information for cancer and dementia patients is also included.

Part III: Medical Decisions Surrounding the End of Life presents facts about care in the last days of life, organ donation, and physician-assisted suicide. It also provides specific information for commonly experienced end-of-life issues related to dementia, advanced cancer, and human immunodeficiency virus/acquired immune deficiency syndrome (HIV/AIDS).

Part IV: End-of-Life Care Facilities offers guidelines for evaluating care facilities and selecting options based on the needs of patients and caregivers. Hospice care, long-term care, home care, and other alternatives are described.

Part V: End-of-Life Caregiving has practical information for caregivers about coordinating communications among patients, families, and healthcare and support service providers. Topics include how to help at the end of life, what to do when death occurs, and self-care tips for caregivers.

Part VI: Death and Children: Information for Parents provides advice about caring for terminally ill children and grieving the death of a child. Guidance for helping children cope with death, funerals, and grief is also presented.

Part VII: Legal and Economic Issues at the End of Life presents guidelines for advance directives, financial assistance, taxes, and Social Security issues. It also describes patients' legal rights, the Family and Medical Leave Act (FMLA), and the duties of an executor.

Part VIII: Final Arrangements offers practical information about planning funerals or memorial services, certification of death, and how to facilitate arrangements if death occurs while traveling. Chapters on grief which address bereavement, how to help grieving people, and tips for working through grief are also included.

Part IX: Mortality Statistics includes global and national mortality trends and statistics on the leading causes of death in the United

States, life expectancy at birth, and common causes of fatalities. Disparities in deaths from suicide, alcohol, and stroke are also discussed.

Part X: Additional Help and Information includes a glossary of end-of-life terms, a directory of support groups for end-of-life concerns, and a directory of organizations able to provide more information about death and dying.

Bibliographic Note

This volume contains documents and excerpts from publications issued by the following U.S. government agencies: Administration for Community Living (ACL); Agency for Healthcare Research and Quality (AHRQ); Benefits.gov; Centers for Disease Control and Prevention (CDC); Centers for Medicare & Medicaid Services (CMS); *Eunice Kennedy Shriver* National Institute of Child Health and Human Development (NICHD); Federal Trade Commission (FTC); Health Resources and Services Administration (HRSA); Internal Revenue Service (IRS); National Cancer Institute (NCI); National Heart, Lung, and Blood Institute (NHLBI); National Institute of Nursing Research (NINR); National Institute on Aging (NIA); National Institute on Alcohol Abuse and Alcoholism (NIAAA); National Institutes of Health (NIH); *NIH News in Health*; Rehabilitation Research & Development Service (RR&D); U.S. Bureau of Labor Statistics (BLS); U.S. Department of Education (ED); U.S. Department of Health and Human Services (HHS); U.S. Department of Labor (DOL); U.S. Department of Veterans Affairs (VA); U.S. Environmental Protection Agency (EPA); U.S. Food and Drug Administration (FDA); and U.S. Social Security Administration (SSA).

It may also contain original material produced by Omnigraphics and reviewed by medical consultants.

About the Health Reference Series

The *Health Reference Series* is designed to provide basic medical information for patients, families, caregivers, and the general public. Each volume takes a particular topic and provides comprehensive coverage. This is especially important for people who may be dealing with a newly diagnosed disease or a chronic disorder in themselves or in a family member. People looking for preventive guidance, information about disease warning signs, medical statistics, and risk factors for health problems will also find answers to their questions in the *Health Reference Series*. The *Series*, however, is not intended to serve as a tool for diagnosing illness, in prescribing treatments, or as a substitute for the physician/patient relationship. All people concerned about medical symptoms or the possibility of disease are encouraged to seek professional care from an appropriate healthcare provider.

A Note about Spelling and Style

Health Reference Series editors use *Stedman's Medical Dictionary* as an authority for questions related to the spelling of medical terms and *The Chicago Manual of Style* for questions related to grammatical structures, punctuation, and other editorial concerns. Consistent adherence is not always possible, however, because the individual volumes within the *Series* include many documents from a wide variety of different producers, and the editor's primary goal is to present material from each source as accurately as is possible. This sometimes means that information in different chapters or sections may follow other guidelines and alternate spelling authorities. For example, occasionally a copyright holder may require that eponymous terms be shown in possessive forms (Crohn's disease vs. Crohn disease) or that British spelling norms be retained (leukaemia vs. leukemia).

Medical Review

Omnigraphics contracts with a team of qualified, senior medical professionals who serve as medical consultants for the *Health Reference Series*. As necessary, medical consultants review reprinted and originally written material for currency and accuracy. Citations including the phrase "Reviewed (month, year)" indicate material reviewed by this team. Medical consultation services are provided to the *Health Reference Series* editors by:
Dr. Vijayalakshmi, MBBS, DGO, MD
Dr. Senthil Selvan, MBBS, DCH, MD
Dr. K. Sivanandham, MBBS, DCH, MS (Research), PhD

Our Advisory Board

We would like to thank the following board members for providing initial guidance on the development of this series:

- Dr. Lynda Baker, Associate Professor of Library and Information Science, Wayne State University, Detroit, MI

- Nancy Bulgarelli, William Beaumont Hospital Library, Royal Oak, MI

- Karen Imarisio, Bloomfield Township Public Library, Bloomfield Township, MI
- Karen Morgan, Mardigian Library, University of Michigan-Dearborn, Dearborn, MI
- Rosemary Orlando, St. Clair Shores Public Library, St. Clair Shores, MI

Health Reference Series *Update Policy*

The inaugural book in the *Health Reference Series* was the first edition of *Cancer Sourcebook* published in 1989. Since then, the *Series* has been enthusiastically received by librarians and in the medical community. In order to maintain the standard of providing high-quality health information for the layperson the editorial staff at Omnigraphics felt it was necessary to implement a policy of updating volumes when warranted.

Medical researchers have been making tremendous strides, and it is the purpose of the *Health Reference Series* to stay current with the most recent advances. Each decision to update a volume is made on an individual basis. Some of the considerations include how much new information is available and the feedback we receive from people who use the books. If there is a topic you would like to see added to the update list, or an area of medical concern you feel has not been adequately addressed, please write to:

Managing Editor
Health Reference Series
Omnigraphics
615 Griswold St., Ste. 520
Detroit, MI 48226

Part One

End-of-Life Perspectives

Chapter 1

Providing Care and Comfort at the End of Life

Comfort care is an essential part of medical care at the end of life. It is care that helps or soothes a person who is dying. The goals are to prevent or relieve suffering as much as possible and to improve the quality of life (QOL) while respecting the dying person's wishes.

You are probably reading this because someone close to you is dying. You wonder what will happen. You want to know how to give comfort, what to say, what to do. You might like to know how to make dying easier—how to help ensure a peaceful death, with treatment consistent with the dying person's wishes.

A peaceful death might mean something different to you than to someone else. Your sister might want to know when death is near so she can have a few last words with the people she loves and take care of personal matters. Perhaps your mother has said she would like to be at home when she dies, while your father wants to be in a hospital where he can receive treatment for his illness until the very end.

Some people want to be surrounded by family and friends; others want to be alone. Of course, often one does not get to choose. But, avoiding suffering, having your end-of-life wishes followed, and being treated with respect while dying are common hopes.

This chapter includes text excerpted from "Providing Care and Comfort at the End of Life," National Institute on Aging (NIA), National Institutes of Health (NIH), May 17, 2017.

Generally speaking, people who are dying need care in four areas—physical comfort, mental and emotional needs, spiritual issues, and practical tasks. Their families need support as well. In this chapter, you will find a number of ways you can help someone who is dying. Always remember to check with the healthcare team to make sure these suggestions are appropriate for your situation.

What Is End-of-Life Care?

"End-of-life care" is the term used to describe the support and medical care given during the time surrounding death. Such care does not happen only in the moments before breathing ceases and the heart stops beating. Older people often live with one or more chronic illnesses and need a lot of care for days, weeks, and even months before death.

When a doctor says something like, "I am afraid the news is not good. There are no other treatments for us to try. I am sorry," it may close the door to the possibility of a cure, but it does not end the need for medical support. Nor does it end the involvement of family and friends.

There are many ways to provide care for an older person who is dying. Such care often involves a team. If you are reading this, then you might be part of such a team.

Being a caregiver for someone at the end of life can be physically and emotionally exhausting. In the end, accept that there may be no perfect death, just the best you can do for the one you love. And, the pain of losing someone close to you may be softened a little because, when you were needed, you did what you could.

End of Life: Providing Physical Comfort

There are ways to get rid of pain when a person is dying. Discomfort can come from a variety of problems. For each, there are things you or a healthcare provider can do, depending on the cause. For example, a dying person can be uncomfortable because of:

Pain

Watching someone you love die is hard enough, but thinking that person is also in pain makes it worse. Not everyone who is dying experiences pain, but there are things you can do to help someone who does. Experts believe that care for someone who is dying should focus on relieving pain without worrying about possible long-term problems of drug dependence or abuse.

4

Do not be afraid of giving as much pain medicine as is prescribed by the doctor. Pain is easier to prevent than to relieve, and severe pain is hard to manage. Try to make sure that the level of pain does not get ahead of pain-relieving medicines. If the pain does not stay controlled, inform the doctor or nurse. Medicines can be increased or changed. If this does not help, then ask for a consultation with a palliative medical specialist who has experience in pain management for seriously ill patients.

Struggling with severe pain can be draining. It can make it hard for families to be together in a meaningful way. Pain can affect mood— being in pain can make someone seem angry or short-tempered. Although understandable, irritability resulting from pain might make it hard to talk, hard to share thoughts and feelings.

What about Morphine and Other Painkillers?

Morphine is an opiate, a strong drug used to treat serious pain. Sometimes, morphine is also given to ease the feeling of shortness of breath. Pain medication can make people confused or drowsy. You might have heard that giving morphine leads to a quicker death. Is that true? Most experts think this is unlikely, especially if increasing the dose is done carefully. Successfully reducing pain and/or concerns about breathing can provide needed comfort to someone who is close to dying.

Breathing Problems

Shortness of breath or the feeling that breathing is difficult is a common experience at the end of life. The doctor might call this dyspnea. Worrying about the next breath can make it hard for important conversations or connections. Try raising the head of the bed, opening a window, using a humidifier, or having a fan circulating air in the room. Sometimes, morphine or other pain medications can help relieve the sense of breathlessness.

People very near death might have noisy breathing, sometimes called a "death rattle." This is caused by fluids collecting in the throat or by the throat muscles relaxing. It might help to try turning the person to rest on one side. There is also a medicine that can be prescribed that may help clear this up. Not all noisy breathing is a death rattle. It may help to know that this noisy breathing is usually not upsetting to the dying person, even if it is to family and friends.

5

Skin Irritation

Skin problems can be very uncomfortable. With age, the skin naturally becomes drier and more fragile, so it is important to take extra care with an older person's skin. Gently applying alcohol-free lotion can relieve dry skin and be soothing.

Dryness on parts of the face, such as the lips and eyes, can be a common cause of discomfort near death. A lip balm could keep this from getting worse. A damp cloth placed over closed eyes might relieve dryness. If the inside of the mouth seems dry, giving ice chips (if the person is conscious) or wiping the inside of the mouth with a damp cloth, cotton ball, or specially treated swab might help.

Sitting or lying in one position puts constant pressure on sensitive skin, which can lead to painful bed sores (sometimes called "pressure ulcers"). When a bedsore first forms, the skin gets discolored or darker. Watch carefully for these discolored spots, especially on the heels, hips, lower back, and back of the head.

Turning the person from side to back and to the other side every few hours may help prevent bedsores. Try putting a foam pad under an area such as a heel or elbow to raise it off the bed and reduce pressure. Ask if a special mattress or chair cushion might also help. Keeping the skin clean and moisturized is always important.

Digestive Problems

Nausea, vomiting, constipation, and loss of appetite are common issues at the end of life. The causes and treatments for these symptoms are varied, so talk to a doctor or nurse right away. There are medicines that can control nausea or vomiting or relieve constipation, a common side effect of strong pain medications.

If someone near death wants to eat but is too tired or weak, you can help with feeding. To address the loss of appetite, try gently offering favorite foods in small amounts. Or, try serving frequent, smaller meals rather than three big ones.

You do not have to force a person to eat. Going without food and/or water is generally not painful, and eating can add to the discomfort. Losing one's appetite is a common and normal part of dying. Swallowing may also be a problem, especially for people with dementia. A conscious decision to give up food can be part of a person's acceptance that death is near.

Temperature Sensitivity

People who are dying may not be able to tell you that they are too hot or too cold, so watch for clues. For example, someone who is too

6

warm might repeatedly try to remove a blanket. You can take off the blanket and try a cool cloth on her or his head.

If a person is hunching her or his shoulders, pulling the covers up, or even shivering—those could be signs of cold. Make sure there is no draft, raise the heat, and add another blanket. Avoid electric blankets because they can get too hot.

Fatigue

It is common for people nearing the end of life to feel tired and have little or no energy. Keep activities simple. For example, a bedside commode can be used instead of walking to the bathroom. A shower stool can save a person's energy, as can switching to sponging off in bed.

Managing End-of-Life Mental and Emotional Needs

Complete end-of-life care also includes helping the dying person manage mental and emotional distress. Someone who is alert near the end of life might understandably feel depressed or anxious. It is important to treat emotional pain and suffering. Encouraging conversations about feelings might help. You might want to contact a counselor, possibly one familiar with end-of-life issues. If depression or anxiety is severe, medicine may help.

A dying person may also have some specific fears and concerns. She or he may fear the unknown or worry about those left behind. Some people are afraid of being alone at the very end. This feeling can be made worse by the understandable reactions of family, friends, and even the medical team. For example, when family and friends do not know how to help or what to say, sometimes they stop visiting. Or, someone who is already beginning to grieve may withdraw.

Doctors may feel helpless because they cannot cure their patients. Some seem to avoid a dying patient. This can add to a dying person's sense of isolation. If this is happening, discuss your concerns with the family, friends, or the doctor.

The simple act of physical contact—holding hands, a touch, or a gentle massage—can make a person feel connected to those she or he loves. It can be very soothing. Warm your hands by rubbing them together or running them under warm water.

Try to set a comforting mood. Remember that listening and being present can make a difference. For example, Gordon loved a party, so it was natural for him to want to be around family and friends when he was dying. Ellen always liked spending quiet moments with one or two people at a time, so she was most comfortable with just a few visitors.

Some experts suggest that when death is very near, music at a low volume and soft lighting are soothing. In fact, near the end of life, music therapy might improve mood, help with relaxation, and lessen pain. Listening to music might also evoke memories those present can share. For some people, keeping distracting noises such as televisions and radios to a minimum is important.

Often, just being present with a dying person is enough. It may not be necessary to fill the time with talking or activity. Your quiet presence can be a simple and profound gift for a dying family member or friend.

Managing End-of-Life Spiritual Needs

People nearing the end of life may have spiritual needs as important as their physical concerns. Spiritual needs include finding meaning in one's life and ending disagreements with others, if possible. The dying person might find peace by resolving unsettled issues with friends or family. Visits from a social worker or a counselor may also help.

Many people find solace in their faith. Others may struggle with their faith or spiritual beliefs. Praying, talking with someone from one's religious community (such as a minister, priest, rabbi, or imam), reading religious texts, or listening to religious music may bring comfort.

Family and friends can talk to the dying person about the importance of their relationship. For example, adult children can share how their father has influenced the course of their lives. Grandchildren can let their grandfather know how much he has meant to them. Friends can relate how they value years of support and companionship. Family and friends who cannot be present could send a recording of what they would like to say or a letter to be read out loud.

Sharing memories of good times is another way some people find peace near death. This can be comforting for everyone. Some doctors think it is possible that even if a patient is unconscious, she or he might still be able to hear. It is probably never too late to say how you feel or to talk about fond memories.

Always talk to, not about, the person who is dying. When you come into the room, it is a good idea to identify yourself, saying something like, "Hi, Juan. It is Mary, and I have come to see you." Another good idea is to have someone write down some of the things said at this time—both by and to the person who is dying. In time, these words might serve as a source of comfort to family and friends. People who are looking for ways to help may welcome the chance to aid the family by writing down what is said.

There may come a time when a dying person who has been confused suddenly seems clear-thinking. Take advantage of these moments, but understand that they might be only temporary, not necessarily a sign she or he is getting better. Sometimes, a dying person may appear to see or talk to someone who is not there. Try to resist the temptation to interrupt or say they are imagining things. Give the dying person the space to experience their own reality.

Planning Ahead for End-of-Life Needs

Many practical jobs need to be done at the end of life—both to relieve the person who is dying and to support the caregiver. Everyday tasks can be a source of worry for someone who is dying, and they can overwhelm a caregiver. Taking over small daily chores around the house—such as picking up the mail or newspaper, writing down phone messages, doing a load of laundry, feeding the family pet, taking children to soccer practice, or picking up medicine from the pharmacy—can provide a much-needed break for caregivers.

A person who is dying might be worried about who will take care of things when she or he is gone. Offering reassurance—"I will make sure your African violets are watered," "Jessica has promised to take care of Bandit," "Dad, we want mom to live with us from now on"—might provide a measure of peace. Reminding the dying person that her or his personal affairs are in good hands can also bring comfort.

Everyone may be asking the family, "What can you do for him?" It helps to make a specific offer. Say to the family, "Let me help with" and suggest something, such as bringing meals for the caregivers, paying bills, walking the dog, or babysitting. If you are not sure what to offer, talk to someone who has been through a similar situation. Find out what kind of help was useful.

If you want to help but cannot get away from your own home, you could schedule other friends or family to help with small jobs or bring in meals. This can allow the immediate family to give their full attention to the person who is dying.

If you are the primary caregiver, ask for help when you need it and accept help when it is offered. Do not hesitate to suggest a specific task to someone who offers to help. Friends and family are probably anxious to do something for you and/or the person who is dying, but they may be reluctant to repeatedly offer when you are so busy.

Keeping close friends and family informed can feel overwhelming. Setting up an outgoing voicemail message, a blog, an e-mail list, a private Facebook page, or even a phone tree can reduce the number

9

of calls you have to make. Some families create a blog or website to share news, thoughts, and wishes.

Questions to Ask about Providing End-of-Life Comfort

Family and friends can provide comfort and ease to someone nearing the end of life. Here are some questions you can ask the doctor in charge:

• Since there is no cure, what will happen next?

• Why are you suggesting this test or treatment?

• Will the treatment bring physical comfort?

• Will the treatment speed up or slow down the dying process?

• What can we expect to happen in the coming days or weeks?

Here are some questions you can ask the caregiver:

• How are you doing? Do you need someone to talk to?

• Would you like to go out for an hour or two? I could stay here while you are away.

• Who has offered to help you? Do you want me to work with them to coordinate our efforts?

• Can I help, maybe . . . walk the dog, answer the phone, go to the drug store or grocery store, or watch the children (for example)... for you?

Chapter 2

Making End-of-Life Healthcare Decisions

It can be overwhelming to be asked to make healthcare decisions for someone who is dying and no longer able to make her or his own decisions. It is even more difficult if you do not have written or verbal guidance. How do you decide what type of care is right for someone? Even when you have written documents, some decisions still might not be clear since the documents may not address every situation you could face.

Approaches to Making Healthcare Decisions: "Substituted" and "Best Interests"

Two approaches might be useful. One is to put yourself in the place of the person who is dying and try to choose as she or he would. This is called "substituted judgment." Some experts believe that decisions should be based on substituted judgment whenever possible.

Another approach, known as "best interests," is to decide what would be best for the dying person. This is sometimes combined with substituted judgment.

This chapter includes text excerpted from "Understanding Healthcare Decisions at the End of Life," National Institute on Aging (NIA), National Institutes of Health (NIH), May 17, 2017.

If you are making decisions for someone at the end of life and are trying to use one of these approaches:

- Has the dying person ever talked about what she or he would want at the end of life?

- Has she or he expressed an opinion about how someone else was being treated?

- What were her or his values in life? What gave meaning to life? Maybe it was being close to family—watching them grow and making memories together. Perhaps just being alive was the most important thing.

As a decision-maker without specific guidance from the dying person, you need to ask the doctor:

- What might we expect to happen in the next few hours, days, or weeks if we continue our current course of treatment?

- Why is this new test being suggested?

- Will it change the current treatment plan?

- Will a new treatment help my relative get better?

- How would the new treatment change her or his quality of life?

- Will it give more quality time with family and friends?

- How long will this treatment take to make a difference?

- If we choose to try this treatment, can we stop it at any time? For any reason?

- What are the side effects of the approach you are suggesting?

- If we try this new treatment and it does not work, what then?

- If we do not try this treatment, what will happen?

- Is the improvement we saw today an overall positive sign or just something temporary?

It is a good idea to have someone with you when discussing these issues with the medical staff. Having someone take notes or remember details can be very helpful. If you are unclear about something you are told, do not be afraid to ask the doctor or nurse to repeat it or to say it another way that does make sense to you. Keep asking questions until you have all the information you need to make decisions. Make sure you know how to contact a member of the medical team if you have a question or if the dying person needs something.

Sometimes, the whole family wants to be involved in every decision. Maybe that is the family's cultural tradition. Or, maybe the person dying did not pick one person to make healthcare choices before becoming unable to do so. That is not unusual, but it makes sense to choose one person to be the contact when dealing with medical staff. The doctors and nurses will appreciate having to phone only one person.

Even if one family member is named as the decision-maker, it is a good idea, as much as possible, to have a family agreement about the care plan. If you cannot agree on a care plan, a decision-maker, or even a spokesperson, the family might consider a mediator, someone trained to bring people with different opinions to a common decision.

In any case, as soon as it is clear that the patient is nearing the end of life, the family should try to discuss with the medical team which end-of-life care approach they want for their family members. That way, decision making for crucial situations can be planned and may feel less rushed.

Are You Faced with Making End-of-Life Choices for Someone Close to You?

You have thought about the person's values and opinions, and you have asked the healthcare team to explain the treatment plan and what you can expect to happen. But, there are other issues that are important to understand in case they arise. What if the dying person starts to have trouble breathing and a doctor says a ventilator might be needed? Maybe one family member wants the healthcare team to do everything possible to keep this relative alive. What does that involve? Or, what if family members cannot agree on end-of-life care or they disagree with the doctor? What happens then?

If Someone Says "Do Everything Possible" When Someone Is Dying, What Does That Mean?

This means that if someone is dying, all measures that might keep vital organs working will be tried—for example, using a ventilator to support breathing or starting dialysis for failing kidneys. Such life support can sometimes be a temporary measure that allows the body to heal itself and begin to work normally again. It is not intended to be used indefinitely in someone who is dying.

13

What Can Be Done If Someone's Heart Stops Beating—Experiences Cardiac Arrest?

Cardiopulmonary resuscitation (CPR) can sometimes restart a stopped heart. It is most effective in people who were generally healthy before their heart stopped. During CPR, the doctor repeatedly pushes on the chest with great force and periodically puts air into the lungs. Electric shocks (called "defibrillation") may also be used to correct an abnormal heart rhythm, and some medicines might also be given. Although not usually shown on television, the force required for CPR can cause broken ribs or a collapsed lung. Often, CPR does not succeed in older adults who have multiple chronic illnesses or who are already frail.

What If Someone Needs Help Breathing or Has Completely Stopped Breathing—Experiences Respiratory Arrest?

If a patient has very severe breathing problems or has stopped breathing, a ventilator may be needed. A ventilator forces the lungs to work. Initially, this involves intubation, putting a tube attached to a ventilator down the throat into the trachea or windpipe. Because this tube can be quite uncomfortable, people are often sedated with very strong intravenous medicines. Restraints may be used to prevent them from pulling out the tube. If the person needs ventilator support for more than a few days, the doctor might suggest a tracheotomy, sometimes called a "trach" (rhymes with "make"). This tube is then attached to the ventilator. This is more comfortable than a tube down the throat and may not require sedation. Inserting the tube into the trachea is a bedside surgery. A tracheotomy can carry risks, including a collapsed lung, a plugged tracheostomy tube, or bleeding.

How Can I Be Sure the Medical Staff Know the Patient Has a Do-Not-Resuscitate Order?

Tell the doctor in charge as soon as the patient or person making healthcare decisions decides that CPR or other life-support procedures should not be performed. The doctor will then write this on the patient's chart using terms, such as "DNR" (Do Not Resuscitate), "DNAR" (Do Not Attempt to Resuscitate), "AND" (Allow Natural Death), or "DNI" (Do Not Intubate). DNR forms vary by state and are usually available online.

14

If end-of-life care is given at home, a special nonhospital DNR, signed by a doctor, is needed. This ensures that if emergency medical technicians (EMTs) are called to the house, they will respect your wishes. Make sure it is kept in a prominent place so EMTs can see it. Without a nonhospital DNR, in many states, EMTs are required to perform CPR and similar techniques. Hospice staff can help determine whether a medical condition is part of the normal dying process or something that needs the attention of EMTs.

Do Not Resuscitate orders do not stop all treatment. They only mean that CPR and a ventilator will not be used. These orders are not permanent—they can be changed if the situation changes.

Should Pacemakers (or Similar Devices) Be Turned Off When Someone Is Dying?

A pacemaker is a device implanted under the skin on the chest that keeps a heartbeat regular. It will not keep a dying person alive. Some people have an implantable cardioverter-defibrillator (ICD) under the skin. An ICD shocks the heart back into regular rhythm when needed. The ICD should be turned off at the point when life support is no longer wanted. This can be done at the bedside without surgery.

What Does It Mean If the Doctor Suggests a Feeding Tube?

If a patient cannot or would not eat or drink, the doctor might suggest a feeding tube. While a patient recovers from an illness, getting nutrition temporarily through a feeding tube can be helpful. But, at the end of life, a feeding tube might cause more discomfort than not eating. For people with dementia, tube feeding does not prolong life or prevent aspiration.

As death approaches, loss of appetite is common. Body systems start shutting down, and fluids and food are not needed as before. Some experts believe that at this point few nutrients are absorbed from any type of nutrition, including those received through a feeding tube. Further, after a feeding tube is inserted, the family might need to make a difficult decision about when, or if, to remove it.

If tube feeding will be tried, there are two methods that could be used. In the first, a feeding tube, known as a "nasogastric" or "NG tube," is threaded through the nose down to the stomach to give nutrition for a short time. Sometimes, the tube is uncomfortable. Someone with an NG tube might try to remove it. This usually means the person has to be restrained, which could mean binding her or his hands to the bed.

If tube feeding is required for an extended time, then a gastric or G tube is put directly into the stomach through an opening made in the side or abdomen. This second method is sometimes called a "percutaneous endoscopic gastrostomy" (PEG) tube. It carries risks of infection, pneumonia, and nausea.

Hand-feeding (sometimes called "assisted oral feeding") is an alternative to tube feeding. This approach may have fewer risks, especially for people with dementia.

Should Someone Who Is Dying Be Sedated?

Sometimes, for patients very near the end of life, the doctor might suggest sedation to manage symptoms that are not responding to other treatments and are still making the patient uncomfortable. This means using medicines to put the patient in a sleep-like state. Many doctors suggest continuing to use comfort care measures such as pain medicine even if the dying person is sedated. Sedatives can be stopped at any time. A person who is sedated may still be able to hear what you are saying—so try to keep speaking directly to, not about, her or him. Do not say things you would not want the patient to hear.

Are Antibiotics Helpful When Someone Is Dying?

Antibiotics are medicines that fight infections caused by bacteria. Lower respiratory infections (such as pneumonia) and urinary tract infections are often caused by bacteria and are common in older people who are dying. Many antibiotics have side effects, so the value of trying to treat an infection in a dying person should be weighed against any unpleasant side effects. If someone is already dying when the infection began, giving antibiotics is probably not going to prevent death but might make the person feel more comfortable.

Do Patients Have the Right to Refuse Treatment?

Choosing to stop treatment that is not curing or controlling an illness, or deciding not to start a new treatment, is completely legal—whether the choice is made by the person who is dying or by the person making healthcare decisions. Some people think this is like allowing death to happen. The law does not consider refusing such treatment to be either suicide or euthanasia, sometimes called "mercy killing."

What Happens If the Doctor and I Have Different Opinions about Care for Someone Who Is Dying?

Sometimes medical staff, the patient, and family members disagree about a medical care decision. This can be especially problematic when the dying person cannot tell the doctors what kind of end-of-life care she or he wants. For example, the family might want more active treatment, such as chemotherapy, than the doctors think will be helpful. If there is an advance directive explaining the patient's preferences, those guidelines should determine care.

Without the guidance of an advance directive, if there is a disagreement about medical care, it may be necessary to get a second opinion from a different doctor or to consult the ethics committee or patient representative, also known as an "ombudsman," of the hospital or facility. Palliative care consultation may also be helpful. An arbitrator (mediator) can sometimes assist people with different views to agree on a plan.

If the Doctor Is Unfamiliar with Our Views about Dying What Should We Do?

America is a rich melting pot of religions, races, and cultures. Ingrained in each tradition are expectations about what should happen as life nears its end. It is important for everyone involved in a patient's care to understand how each family background may influence expectations, needs, and choices.

Your background may be different from that of the doctor with whom you are working. Or, you might be used to a different approach to making healthcare decisions at the end of life than your medical team. For example, many healthcare providers look to a single person—the dying person or her or his chosen representative—for important healthcare decisions at the end of life. But, in some cultures, the entire immediate family takes on that role.

It is helpful to discuss your personal and family traditions with your doctors and nurses. If there are religious or cultural customs surrounding death that are important to you, make sure to tell your healthcare providers.

Knowing that these practices will be honored could comfort the dying person. Telling the medical staff ahead of time may also help

17

avoid confusion and misunderstanding when death occurs. Make sure you understand how the available medical options presented by the healthcare team fit into your family's desires for end-of-life care.

Questions to Ask When Making Healthcare Decisions

Here are some questions you might want to ask the medical staff:

- What is the care plan? What are the benefits and risks?
- How often should we reassess the care plan?
- If we try using a ventilator to help with breathing and decide to stop, how will that be done?
- If my family member is dying, why does she or he have to be connected to all those tubes and machines? Why do we need more tests?
- What is the best way for our family to work with the care staff?
- How can I make sure I get a daily update on my family member's condition?
- Will you call me if there is a change in her or his condition?

Communicating with Your Healthcare Team

Make sure the healthcare team knows what is important to your family surrounding the end of life. You might say:

- In my religion, we . . . (then describe your religious traditions regarding death)
- Where we come from . . . (tell what customs are important to you at the time of death)
- In our family when someone is dying, we prefer . . . (describe what you hope to have happened)

Chapter 3

Cultural Response to Death

Cultures have different ways of coping with death.

The grief felt for the loss of loved ones occurs in people of all ages and cultures. Different cultures, however, have different myths and mysteries about death that affect the attitudes, beliefs, and practices of the bereaved.

Individual, personal experiences of grief are similar in different cultures.

The ways in which people of all cultures feel grief personally are similar. This has been found to be true even though different cultures have different mourning ceremonies and traditions to express grief.

Cultural issues that affect people who are dealing with the loss of a loved one include rituals, beliefs, and roles.

Helping family members cope with the death of a loved one includes showing respect for the family's culture and the ways they honor death. The following questions may help caregivers learn what is needed by the person's culture:

- What are the cultural rituals for coping with dying, the deceased person's body, and honoring the death?

- What are the family's beliefs about what happens after death?

This chapter includes text excerpted from "Grief, Bereavement, and Coping with Loss (PDQ®)—Patient Version," National Cancer Institute (NCI), March 6, 2013. Reviewed September 2019.

- What does the family feel is a normal expression of grief and the acceptance of the loss?

- What does the family consider to be the roles of each family member in handling the death?

- Are certain types of death, less acceptable (for example, suicide), or are certain types of death especially hard for that culture (for example, the death of a child)?

Death, grief, and mourning are normal life events. All cultures have practices that best meet their needs for dealing with death. Caregivers who understand the ways different cultures respond to death can help patients of these cultures work through their own normal grieving process.

Chapter 4

Spirituality in End-of-Life Care

National surveys consistently support the idea that religion and spirituality are important to most individuals in the general population. More than 90 percent of adults express a belief in God, and slightly more than 70 percent of individuals surveyed identified religion as one of the most important influences in their lives. Yet even widely held beliefs, such as survival of the soul after death or a belief in miracles, vary substantially by gender, education, and ethnicity.

Research indicates that both patients and family caregivers commonly rely on spirituality and religion to help them deal with serious physical illnesses, expressing a desire to have specific spiritual and religious needs and concerns acknowledged or addressed by medical staff. These needs, although widespread, may take different forms between and within cultural and religious traditions.

A survey of hospital inpatients found that 77 percent of patients reported that physicians should take patients' spiritual needs into consideration, and 37 percent wanted physicians to address religious beliefs more frequently.

This chapter includes text excerpted from "Spirituality in Cancer Care (PDQ®)—Health Professional Version," National Cancer Institute (NCI), April 19, 2017.

Paying attention to the religious or spiritual beliefs of seriously ill patients has a long tradition within inpatient medical environments. Addressing such issues has been viewed as the domain of hospital chaplains or a patient's own religious leader. In this context, systematic assessment has usually been limited to identifying a patient's religious preference; responsibility for the management of apparent spiritual distress has been focused on referring patients to the chaplain service. Although healthcare providers may address such concerns themselves, they are generally very ambivalent about doing so, and there has been relatively little systematic investigation addressing the physician's role. These issues, however, are being increasingly addressed in medical training.

Interest in and recognition of the function of religious and spiritual coping in adjustment to serious illness has been growing. New ways to assess and address religious and spiritual concerns as part of the overall quality of life are being developed and tested. Limited data support the possibility that spiritual coping is one of the most powerful means by which patients draw on their own resources to deal with a serious illness; however, patients and their family-member caregivers may be reluctant to raise religious and spiritual concerns with their professional healthcare providers. Increased spiritual well-being in a seriously ill population may be linked with lower anxiety about death, but greater religious involvement may also be linked to an increased likelihood of desire for extreme measures at the end of life. Given the importance of religion and spirituality to patients, integrating the systematic assessment of such needs into medical care, including outpatient care, is crucial. The development of better assessment tools will make it easier to discern which aspects of religious and spiritual coping may be important in a particular patient's adjustment to illness.

Of equal importance is the consideration of how and when to address religion and spirituality with patients and the best ways to do so in different medical environments. Although addressing spiritual concerns is often considered an end-of-life issue, such concerns may arise at any time after diagnosis. Acknowledging the importance of these concerns and addressing them, even briefly, at diagnosis may facilitate better adjustment throughout the course of treatment and create a context for richer dialogue later in the illness.

In this chapter, unless otherwise stated, evidence and practice issues as they relate to adults are discussed. The evidence and application to practice related to children may differ significantly from information related to adults.

Spirituality Definitions

Specific religious beliefs and practices should be distinguished from the idea of a universal capacity for spiritual and religious experiences. Although this distinction may not be salient or important on a personal basis, it is important conceptually for understanding various aspects of evaluation and the role of different beliefs, practices, and experiences in coping with illness.

The most useful general distinction to make in this context is between "religion" and "spirituality." There is no general agreement on definitions of either term, but there is general agreement on the usefulness of this distinction. A number of reviews address matters of definition.

- Religion can be viewed as a specific set of beliefs and practices associated with a recognized religion or denomination.

- Spirituality is generally recognized as encompassing experiential aspects, whether related to engaging in religious practices or acknowledging a general sense of peace and connectedness. The concept of spirituality is found in all cultures and is often considered to encompass a search for ultimate meaning through religion or other paths.

In healthcare, concerns about spiritual or religious well-being have sometimes been viewed as an aspect of complementary and alternative medicine (CAM), but this perception may be more characteristic of providers than of patients. In one study, virtually no patients but about 20 percent of providers said that CAM services were sought to assist with spiritual or religious issues.

Religion is highly culturally determined; spirituality is considered a universal human capacity, usually—but not necessarily—associated with and expressed in religious practice. Most individuals consider themselves both spiritual and religious. Some may consider themselves religious but not spiritual; others, including some atheists (people who do not believe in the existence of God) or agnostics (people who believe that God cannot be shown to exist), may consider themselves spiritual but not religious.

One effort to characterize individuals by types of spiritual and religious experience identified the following three groups, using cluster analytic techniques:

1. Religious individuals who highly value religious faith, spiritual well-being, and the meaning of life.

23

2. Existential individuals who highly value spiritual well-being but not religious faith.

3. Nonspiritual individuals who have little value for religiousness, spirituality, or a sense of the meaning of life.

Individuals in the third group were far more distressed about their illness and were experiencing worse adjustment. There is as yet no consensus on the number or types of underlying dimensions of spirituality or religious engagement.

From the perspective of both the research and clinical literature on the relationships between religion, spirituality, and health, it is important to consider how these concepts are defined and used by investigators and authors. Much of the epidemiological literature that has indicated a relationship between religion and health has been based on definitions of religious involvement such as:

• Membership in a religious group

• Frequency of church attendance

Assessing specific beliefs or religious practices, such as belief in God, frequency of prayer, or reading religious material is somewhat more complex. Individuals may engage in such practices or believe in God without necessarily attending church services. Terminology also carries certain connotations. The term "religiosity," for example, has a history of implying fervor and perhaps undue investment in particular religious practices or beliefs. The term "religiousness" may be a more neutral way to refer to the dimension of religious practice.

Spirituality and spiritual well-being are more challenging to define. Some definitions limit spirituality to mean profound mystical experiences; however, in considerations of effects on health and psychological well-being, the more helpful definitions focus on accessible feelings, such as:

• A sense of inner peace

• Existential meaning

• Awe when walking in nature

For the purposes of this discussion, it is assumed that there is a continuum of meaningful spiritual experiences, from the common and accessible to the extraordinary and transformative. Both the type and intensity of experience may vary. Other aspects of spirituality that have been identified by those working with medical patients include the following:

- A sense of meaning and peace

- A sense of faith

- A sense of connectedness to others or to God

Low levels of these experiences may be associated with poorer coping.

The definition of acute spiritual distress must be considered separately. Spiritual distress may result from the belief that a life-threatening illness reflects punishment by God or may accompany a preoccupation with the question "Why me?" A patient may also suffer a loss of faith. Although many individuals may have such thoughts at some time after diagnosis, only a few individuals become obsessed with these thoughts or score high on a general measure of religious and spiritual distress (such as the Negative subscale of the Religious Coping Scale (the RCOPE–Negative)). High levels of spiritual distress may contribute to poorer health and psychosocial outcomes.

Religion and spirituality have been shown to be significantly associated with measures of adjustment and with the management of symptoms in patients. Religious and spiritual coping have been associated with lower levels of patient discomfort as well as reduced hostility, anxiety, and social isolation in patients and in family caregivers. Specific characteristics of strong religious beliefs, including hope, optimism, freedom from regret, and life satisfaction, have also been associated with improved adjustment in individuals diagnosed with cancer or any life-threatening illness.

A large national survey of 361 paired U.S. survivors and caregivers (caregivers included spouses and adult children) found that for both survivors and caregivers, the peace factor of the Functional Assessment of Chronic Illness Therapy-Spiritual Well-Being (FACIT-Sp) was strongly related to mental health but negligibly or not at all related to physical well-being. The faith factor ("religiousness") was unrelated to physical or mental well-being. 52 percent of the survivors in this survey were women. These findings support the value of the FACIT-Sp in separating people's religious involvement from their sense of spiritual well-being and that it is this sense of spiritual well-being that seems to be most related to psychological adjustment.

Another large national survey study of female family caregivers (N=252; 89% White) identified that higher levels of spirituality, as measured by the FACIT-Sp, were associated with much less psychological distress (measured by the Pearlin Stress Scale). Participants with higher levels of spirituality actually had improved well-being even as the stress caused by caregiving increased, while those with lower levels of spirituality showed the opposite pattern, suggesting a strong stress-buffering effect of spiritual well-being. This finding reinforces the need to identify low spiritual well-being when assessing the coping capacity of family caregivers as well as patients.

Ethnicity and spirituality were investigated in a qualitative study of 161 breast cancer survivors. In individual interviews, most participants (83%) spoke about some aspect of their spirituality. A higher percentage of African Americans, Latinas, and persons identified as Christians felt comforted by God than did other groups. Seven themes were identified:

1. God as a Comforting Presence

2. Questioning Faith

3. Anger at God

4. Spiritual Transformation of Self and Attitude toward Others/ Recognition of Own Mortality

5. Deepening of Faith

6. Acceptance

7. Prayer by Self

Positive religious involvement and spirituality appear to be associated with better health and a longer life expectancy, even after the researchers controlled for other variables such as health behaviors and social support, as shown in one meta-analysis.

Another study found that helper and cytotoxic T-cell counts were higher among women with metastatic breast cancer who reported greater importance of spirituality. Other investigators found that attendance at religious services was associated with better immune system functioning. Other research suggests that religious distress negatively affects health status. These associations, however, have been criticized as weak and inconsistent.

Screening and Assessment of Spiritual Concerns

Raising spiritual concerns with patients can be accomplished by the following approaches:

- Waiting for the patient to bring up spiritual concerns

- Requesting that the patient complete a paper-and-pencil assessment

- Having the physician do a spiritual inquiry or assessment by indicating her or his openness to a discussion

These approaches have different potential value and limitations. Patients may express reluctance to bring up spiritual issues, noting that they would prefer to wait for the provider to broach the subject. Standardized assessment tools vary, have generally been designed for research purposes, and need to be reviewed and utilized appropriately by the provider. Physicians, unless trained specifically to address such issues, may feel uncomfortable raising spiritual concerns with patients. However, an increasing number of models are becoming available for physician use and training.

Numerous assessment tools are pertinent to performing a religious and spiritual assessment. Several factors should be considered before choosing an assessment tool.

- Focus of the evaluation (religious practice or spiritual well-being/distress)

- Purpose of the assessment (e.g., screening for distress vs. evaluation of all patients as part of care)

- Modality of the assessment (interview or questionnaire)

- Feasibility of the assessment (staff and patient burden)

The line between assessment and intervention is blurred, and simply inquiring about an area such as religious or spiritual coping may be experienced by the patient as an opening for further exploration and validation of the importance of this experience. Evidence suggests that such an inquiry will be experienced as intrusive and distressing by only a very small proportion of patients.

Standardized Assessment Measures

One of several paper-and-pencil measures can be given to patients to assess religious and spiritual needs. These measures have the advantage of being self-administered; however, they were mostly designed as research tools, and their role for clinical assessment purposes is not as well understood. These measures may be helpful in opening up the area for exploration and for ascertaining basic levels of religious

27

engagement or spiritual well-being (or spiritual distress). Most also assume a belief in God and, therefore, may seem inappropriate for an atheist or agnostic patient, who may still be spiritually oriented. All of the measures have undergone varying degrees of psychometric development, and most are being used in investigations of the relationship between religion or spirituality, health indices, and adjustment to illness.

- **Duke Religious Index (DRI).** The DRI (or DUREL) is short (five items) and has reasonable psychometric properties examined in cancer patients. It is best used as an indicator of religious involvement rather than spirituality and has low or modest correlations with psychological well-being.

- **Systems of Belief Inventory (SBI-15R).** The SBI-15R has undergone careful psychometric development and measures two domains:

  1. Presence and importance of religious and spiritual beliefs and practices

  2. Value of support from a religious/spiritual community

The questions are worded well and may provide a good initiation for further discussion and exploration.

- **Brief Measure of Religious Coping (RCOPE).** The Brief RCOPE has two dimensions: positive religious coping and negative religious coping, with five items each. The second factor appears to uniquely identify a very important aspect of spiritual adjustment, i.e., the degree to which conflict, self-blame, or anger at God is present for an individual. A longer form of the scale, with additional dimensions, would be suitable for a more comprehensive assessment of religious/ spiritual concerns. Psychometric development is high. While high scores in negative religious coping are unusual, they are particularly powerful in predicting poor adjustment to disease.

- **Functional Assessment of Chronic Illness Therapy— Spiritual Well-Being (FACIT-Sp).** The FACIT-Sp is part of the widely used Functional Assessment of Cancer Therapy (FACT) quality-of-life battery. It was developed with an ethnically diverse cancer population and contains 12 items and 2 factors (faith, and meaning and peace), with good to excellent psychometric properties; although some evidence suggests that inner meaning and inner peace can be identified as two separate factors, such identification does not appear to substantially improve associations with other indicators of well-being. One characteristic of this scale is that the wording of items does not assume a belief in God. Therefore, it can be comfortably completed by an atheist or agnostic, yet it taps into both traditional religiousness dimensions (faith factor) and spiritual dimensions (meaning and peace factor).

The meaning and peace factor has been shown to have particularly strong associations with psychological adjustment, in that individuals who score high on this scale are much more likely to report generally enjoying life despite fatigue or pain, are less likely to desire a hastened death at the end of life, report better disease-specific and psychosocial adjustment, and report lower levels of helplessness/hopelessness. These associations have been shown to be independent of other indicators of adjustment, supporting the value of adding assessment of this dimension to standard quality-of-life evaluations. Total scores on the FACIT-Sp correlated highly over time (27 weeks) with a 10-point linear analog scale of spiritual well-being in a sample of patients with advanced cancer. The linear scale (Spiritual Well-Being Linear Analogue Self-Assessment (SWB LASA)) was worded, "How would you describe your overall spiritual well-being?" and ratings ranged from 0 (as bad as it can be) to 10 (as good as it can be).

- Spiritual Transformation Scale (STS). The STS is a 40-item measure of change in spiritual engagement after a cancer diagnosis. It has two subscales:

  1. Spiritual Growth (SG): The SG factor is highly correlated with the Positive subscale of the Religious Coping Scale (the RCOPE–Positive) (r=0.71) and the Posttraumatic Growth Inventory (r=0.68).

  2. Spiritual Decline (SD): The SD factor is correlated with the Negative subscale of the Religious Coping Scale (the RCOPE–Negative) (r=0.56) and the Center for Epidemiologic Studies Depression Scale (CES-D) (r=0.40).

Analyses show that the STS accounts for additional variance on depression, other measures of adjustment (Positive and Negative Affect Schedule (PANAS)), and the Daily Spiritual Experience Scale.

Individuals with later-stage cancer (stage III or IV) had higher SG scores, as did individuals with a recurrence rather than a new diagnosis. Individuals with higher SD scores were more likely to have not graduated from high school. A unique strength of this scale is that it is specific to change in spirituality since diagnosis; the wording of items is also generally appropriate for individuals who identify as spiritual rather than religious. Among the limitations of this scale is that development to date includes mostly observant Christians, with few minorities in the sample.

Interviewing Tools

The following are semistructured interviewing tools designed to facilitate exploration, by the physician or other healthcare provider, of religious beliefs and spiritual experiences or issues. The tools take the spiritual history approach and have the advantage of engaging the patient in dialogue, identifying possible areas of concern, and indicating the need for the provision of further resources such as referral to a chaplain or support group. These approaches, however, have not been systematically investigated as empirical measures or indices of religiousness or of spiritual well-being or distress.

- The SPIRITual History. SPIRIT is an acronym for the six domains explored by this tool:

  1. S, spiritual belief system
  2. P, personal spirituality
  3. I, integration with a spiritual community
  4. R, ritualized practices and restrictions
  5. I, implications for medical care
  6. T, terminal events planning

  The six domains cover 22 items; these may be explored in as short a time as 10 or 15 minutes, or integrated into general interviewing over several appointments. A strength of this tool is the number of questions pertinent to managing serious illness and gaining an understanding of how patient religious beliefs may affect patient care decisions.

- Faith, Importance/Influence, Community, and Address (FICA) Spiritual History. FICA is an acronym for Faith, Importance/ Influence, Community, and Address, with a set of questions to explore each area (e.g., What is your faith? How important is it? Are you part of a religious community? How would you like me as your provider to address these issues in your care?). Although developed as a spiritual history tool for use in primary care settings, it would lend itself to any patient population. The relative simplicity of the approach has led to its adoption by many medical schools.

Modes of Intervention

Various modes of intervention or assistance might be considered to address the spiritual concerns of patients. These include the following:

* Exploration by the physician or other healthcare provider within the context of usual medical care

* Encouragement for the patient to seek assistance from her or his own clergy

* Formal referral to a hospital chaplain

* Referral to a religious or faith-based therapist

* Referral to a range of support groups that are known to address spiritual issues

Two survey studies found that physicians consistently underestimate the degree to which patients want spiritual concerns addressed. An Israeli study found that patients expressed the desire that 18 percent of a hypothetical 10-minute visit be spent addressing such concerns, while their providers estimated that 12 percent of the time should be spent in this way. This study also found that while providers perceived that a patient's desire for addressing spiritual concerns related to a broader interest in complementary and alternative medicine (CAM) modalities, patients viewed CAM-related issues and spiritual/religious concerns as quite separate.

Physicians

A task force of physicians and end-of-life specialists suggested several guidelines for physicians who wish to respond to patients' spiritual concerns:

* Respect the patient's views and follow the patient's lead.

* Make a connection by listening carefully and acknowledging the patient's concerns, but avoid theological discussions or engaging in specific religious rituals.

31

- Maintain one's own integrity in relation to one's own religious beliefs and practices.

- Identify common goals for care and medical decisions.

- Mobilize other resources of support for the patient, such as referring the patient to a chaplain or encouraging contact with the patient's own clergy.

Inquiring about religious or spiritual concerns by physicians or other healthcare professionals may provide valuable and appreciated support to patients. Most cancer patients appear to welcome a dialogue about such concerns, regardless of diagnosis or prognosis. In a large survey of cancer outpatients, between 20 and 35 percent expressed the following:

- A desire for religious and spiritual resources

- Help with talking about finding meaning in life

- Help with finding hope

- Talking about death and dying

- Finding peace of mind

It is appropriate to initiate such an inquiry once initial diagnosis and treatment issues have been discussed and considered by the patient (approximately a month after diagnosis or later).

Support received from the medical team predicted the following:

- Greater quality of life

- Greater likelihood of receiving hospice care at the end of life

- Less-aggressive care for patients who have high levels of religious coping

One trial, with a sample of 115 mixed-diagnosis patients (54% under active treatment), evaluated a 5-minute semistructured inquiry into spiritual and religious concerns. The four physicians' personal religious backgrounds included two Christians, one Hindu, and one Sikh; 81 percent of patients were Christian. Unlike the history-oriented interviews noted above, this inquiry was informed by brief patient-centered counseling approaches that view the physician as an important source of empowerment to help patients identify and address personal concerns. After 3 weeks, the intervention group had larger reductions in depression, had more improvement in the quality of life, and rated their relationship with the physician more favorably. The effects for quality of life remained after statistically adjusting for change in other variables. More improvement was also seen in patients who scored lower in spiritual well-being, as measured by the Functional Assessment of Chronic Illness Therapy—Spiritual Well-Being at baseline. Acceptability was high, with physicians rating themselves as "comfortable" in providing the intervention during 85 percent of encounters. 76 percent of patients characterized the inquiry as "somewhat" to "very" useful. Physicians were twice as likely to underestimate the usefulness of the inquiry to patients rather than to overestimate it, in relation to the patient ratings.

A common concern is whether to offer to pray with patients. Although one study found that more than one-half of the patients surveyed expressed a desire to have physicians pray with them, a large proportion did not express this preference. A qualitative study of cancer patients found that patients were concerned that physicians are too busy, not interested, or even prohibited from discussing religion. At the same time, patients generally wanted their physicians to acknowledge the value of spiritual and religious issues. A suggestion was made that physicians might raise the question of prayer by asking, "Would that comfort you?"

In a study of 70 patients with advanced cancer, 206 oncology physicians, and 115 oncology nurses, all participants were interviewed about their opinions regarding the appropriateness of patient-practitioner prayer in the advanced-cancer setting. Results showed that 71 percent of advanced-cancer patients, 83 percent of oncology nurses, and 65 percent of physicians reported that it is occasionally appropriate for a practitioner to pray with a patient when the request to pray is initiated by the patient. Similarly, 64 percent of patients, 76 percent of nurses, and 59 percent of physicians reported that they consider it appropriate for a religious/spiritual healthcare practitioner to pray for a patient.

The most important guideline is to remain sensitive to the patient's preference; therefore, asking patients about their beliefs or spiritual concerns in the context of exploring how they are coping, in general, is the most viable approach in exploring these issues.

Hospital Chaplains

Traditional means of providing assistance to patients has generally been through the services of hospital chaplains. Hospital chaplains can play a key role in addressing spiritual and religious issues; chaplains are trained to work with a wide range of issues as they arise for medical patients and to be sensitive to the diverse beliefs and concerns that patients may have. Chaplains are generally available in large medical centers, but they may not be available in smaller hospitals on a reliable basis. Chaplains are rarely available in the outpatient settings where most care is now delivered.

Another traditional approach in outpatient settings is having spiritual/religious resources available in waiting rooms. This is relatively easy to do, and many such resources exist; however, a breadth of resources covering all faith backgrounds of patients is highly desirable.

Support Groups

Support groups may provide a setting in which patients may explore spiritual concerns. If spiritual concerns are important to a patient, the healthcare provider may need to identify whether a locally available group addresses these issues. The published data on the specific effects of support groups on assisting with spiritual concerns is relatively sparse, partly because this aspect of adjustment has not been systematically evaluated. A randomized trial compared the effects of a mind-body-spirit group to a standard group support program for women with breast cancer. Both groups showed improvement in spiritual well-being, although there were appreciably more differential effects for the mind-body-spirit group in the area of spiritual integration.

A study of 97 lower-income women with breast cancer who were participating in an online support group examined the relationship between a variety of psychosocial outcomes and religious expression (as indicated by the use of religious words, such as faith, God, pray, holy, or spirit). Results showed that women who communicated a deeper religiousness in their online writing to others were found to have lower levels of negative emotions, higher levels of perceived health self-efficacy, and higher functional well-being. An exploratory study of a monthly spirituality-based support group program for African American women with breast cancer suggested high levels of satisfaction in a sample that already had high levels of engagement in the religious and spiritual aspects of their lives.

One author presents a well-developed model of adjuvant psychological therapy that uses a large group format and addresses both basic coping issues and spiritual concerns and healing, using a combination of group exploration, meditation, prayer, and other spiritually-oriented exercises. In a carefully conducted longitudinal qualitative study of 22 patients enrolled in this type of intervention, researchers found that patients who were more psychologically engaged with the issues presented were more likely to survive longer. Other approaches are available but have yet to be systematically evaluated, have not explicitly addressed religious and spiritual issues, or have failed to evaluate the effects of the intervention on spiritual well-being.

Other

Other therapies may also support spiritual growth and posttraumatic benefit finding. For example, in a nonrandomized comparison of mindfulness-based stress reduction (n=60) and a healing arts program (n=44) in cancer outpatients with a variety of diagnoses, both programs significantly improved facilitation of positive growth in participants, although improvement in spirituality, stress, depression, and anger was significantly larger for the mindfulness-based stress reduction group.

Increasing Personal Awareness in Healthcare Providers

Spirituality, religion, death, and dying may be experienced by many providers as a taboo subject. The meaning of illness and the possibility of death are often difficult to address. The assessment resources noted above may be of value in introducing the topic of spiritual concerns, death, and dying to a patient in a supportive manner. In addition, reading clinical accounts by other healthcare providers can be very helpful. One such example is a qualitative study utilizing an autoethnographic approach to explore spirituality in members of an interdisciplinary palliative care team. Findings from this work yielded a collective spirituality that emerged from the common goals, values, and belonging shared by team members. Reflections of the participants offer insights into patient care for other healthcare professionals.

Issues to Consider

Although a considerable number of anecdotal accounts suggest that prayer, meditation, imagery, or other religious activity can have healing power, the empirical evidence is extremely limited and by no means consistent. On the basis of current evidence, it is questionable whether any patient with cancer should be encouraged to seek such resources as a means to healing or limiting the physical effects of the disease. However, the psychological value of support and spiritual well-being is increasingly well documented, and evidence that spiritual distress can have a negative impact on health is growing. Therefore, in exploring these issues with patients or encouraging the use of such resources, healthcare providers need to frame these resources in terms of self-understanding, clarifying questions of beliefs with an appropriate spiritual or religious leader, or seeking a sense of inner peace or awareness.

Chapter 5

Chronic Illness in Old Age

The Burden of Chronic Disease for Older Adults
Leading Causes of Death

During the twentieth century, effective public-health strategies and advances in medical treatment contributed to a dramatic increase in average life expectancy in the United States. The 30-year gain in life expectancy within the span of a century had never before been achieved. Many of the diseases that claimed our ancestors—including tuberculosis, diarrhea, and enteritis, and syphilis—are no longer the threats they once were. Although they may still present significant health challenges in the United States, these diseases are no longer the leading killers of American adults. However, other diseases have continued to be the leading causes of death every year since 1900. By 1910, heart disease became the leading cause of death every year except 1918 to 1920, when the influenza epidemic took its disastrous toll. Since 1938, cancer has held the second position every year. Heart disease and cancer pose their greatest risks as people age, as do other chronic diseases and conditions, such as stroke, chronic lower respiratory

This chapter contains text excerpted from the following sources: Text under the heading "The Burden of Chronic Disease for Older Adults" is excerpted from "The State of Aging and Health in America 2013," Centers for Disease Control and Prevention (CDC), July 9, 2013. Reviewed September 2019; Text under the heading "Supporting Older Patients with Chronic Conditions" is excerpted from "Supporting Older Patients with Chronic Conditions," National Institute on Aging (NIA), National Institutes of Health (NIH), May 17, 2017.

diseases, Alzheimer disease (AD), and diabetes (Figure 5.1). Influenza and pneumonia also continue to contribute to deaths among older adults, despite the availability of effective vaccines.

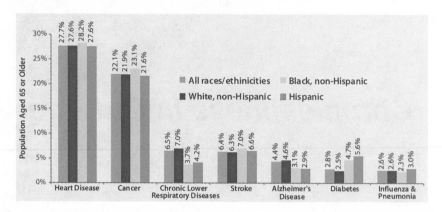

Figure 5.1. *Chronic Conditions Were the Leading Causes of Death among U.S. Adults Aged 65 or Older in 2007 to 2009.* (Source: Centers for Disease Control and Prevention (CDC), National Center for Health Statistics (NCHS). National Vital Statistics System (NVSS), 2007 to 2009.)

Diminished Quality of Life and Loss of Independence

The burden of chronic diseases encompasses a much broader spectrum of negative health consequences than death alone. People living with one or more chronic diseases often experience a diminished quality of life, generally reflected by a long period of decline and disability associated with their disease. Chronic diseases can affect a person's ability to perform important and essential activities, both inside and outside the home. Initially, they may have trouble with the instrumental activities of daily living (IADLs), such as managing money, shopping, preparing meals, and taking medications as prescribed. As functional ability—physical, mental, or both—further declines, people may lose the ability to perform more basic activities, called "activities of daily living" (ADLs), such as taking care of personal hygiene, feeding themselves, getting dressed, and toileting. The inability to perform daily activities can restrict people's engagement in life and their enjoyment of family and friends. Lack of mobility in the community or at home significantly narrows an older person's world and ability to do the things that bring enjoyment and meaning to life. Loss of the ability to care for oneself safely and appropriately means the further loss of independence and can often lead to the need for care in an institutional setting. The need for caregiving for older adults by formal, professional caregivers or by family members—and the need for long-term-care services and supports—will increase sharply during the next several decades, given the effects of chronic diseases on an aging population.

Major Contributor to Healthcare Costs

The nation's expenditures for healthcare, already the highest among developed countries, are expected to rise considerably as chronic diseases affect growing numbers of older adults. More than two-thirds of all healthcare costs are for treating chronic illnesses. Among healthcare costs for older Americans, 95 percent are for chronic diseases. The cost of providing healthcare for one person aged 65 or older is 3 to 5 times higher than the cost for someone younger than 65. By 2030, healthcare spending will increase by 25 percent, largely because the population will be older. This estimate does not take into account inflation and the higher costs of new technologies. Medicare spending is projected to increase from $555 billion in 2011 to $903 billion in 2020.

Ways to Promote and Preserve the Health of Older Adults and Reduce Costs

Death and decline associated with the leading chronic diseases are often preventable or can be delayed. Multiple opportunities exist to promote and preserve the health of older adults. The challenge is to more broadly apply what we already know about reducing the risk of chronic disease. Death is unavoidable, but the prevalence of chronic illnesses and the decline and disability commonly associated with them can be reduced.

Although the risk of developing chronic diseases increases as a person ages, the root causes of many of these diseases often begin early in life. Practicing healthy behaviors from an early age and getting recommended screenings can substantially reduce a person's risk of developing chronic diseases and associated disabilities. Research has shown that people who do not use tobacco, who get regular physical activity, and who eat a healthy diet significantly decrease their risk of developing heart disease, cancer, diabetes, and other chronic conditions.

Unfortunately, the data on health-related behaviors among people aged 55 to 64 years do not indicate a positive future for the health of older Americans. If a meaningful decline in chronic diseases among older adults is to occur, adults at younger ages, as well as our nation's children and adolescents, need to pursue health-promoting behaviors and get recommended preventive services. Communities can play a pivotal role in achieving this goal by making healthy choices easier and making changes to policies, systems, and environments that help Americans of all ages take charge of their health.

Supporting Older Patients with Chronic Conditions

Approximately 85 percent of older adults have at least one chronic health condition, and 60 percent have at least two chronic conditions, according to the Centers for Disease Control and Prevention (CDC). For many older people, coping with multiple chronic conditions is a real challenge. Learning to manage a variety of treatments while maintaining quality of life (QOL) can be problematic.

People with chronic conditions may have different needs, but they also share common challenges with other older adults, such as paying for care or navigating the complexities of the healthcare system.

Clinicians can play an important role in educating patients and families about chronic health conditions and can connect them with appropriate community resources and services.

Try to start by appreciating that people living with chronic disease are often living with loss—the loss of physical function, independence, or general well-being. Empathize with patients who feel angry, sad, lost, or bewildered. Ask, "Is it hard for you to live with these problems?" From there you can refer patients to community resources that may meet their needs or, when available, recommend a disease management program or case managers in the community.

Educating the Patient

Most older patients want to understand their medical conditions and are interested in learning how to manage them. Likewise, family members and other caregivers want this information.

Physicians typically underestimate how much patients want to know and overestimate how long they spend giving information to patients. Devoting more attention to educating patients and their caregivers may seem like a luxury, but in the long run, it can improve patients' adherence to treatment, increase patients' well-being, and save your time.

The following tips can help you inform patients and their caregivers about medical conditions and their treatment:

- Doctors' advice generally receives the greatest credence, so the doctor should introduce treatment plans. Other medical team members have an important role, including building on the original instructions.

- Let your patient know you welcome questions. Provide the name of someone on your staff whom the patient can call to have questions answered later.

- Remember, some patients would not ask questions even if they want more information. Be aware of this tendency and think about making information available even if it is not requested.

- Provide information through more than one channel. In addition to talking to the patient, you can use fact sheets, drawings, models, videos, or audio. In many cases, referrals to websites and support groups can be helpful.

- Encourage the patient or caregiver to take notes. It is helpful to offer a pad and pencil. Active involvement in recording information may promote your patient's retention and adherence.

- Repeat key points about the health problem and treatment at every office visit.

- Check that the patient and her or his caregivers understand what you say. One good approach is to ask that they repeat the main message in their own words.

- Provide encouragement. Call attention to strengths and ideas for improvement. Remember to provide continued reinforcement for a new treatment or lifestyle changes.

Explaining Diagnoses

Clear explanations of diagnoses are critical. Uncertainty about a health problem can be upsetting. When patients do not understand their medical conditions, they tend not to follow the treatment plans.

In explaining diagnoses, it is helpful to begin by finding out what the patient believes is wrong, what the patient thinks will happen, and how much more she or he wants to know. Based on the patient's responses, you can correct any misconceptions and provide appropriate types of information.

Discussing Treatment

Some older patients may refuse treatment because they do not understand what it involves or how it will improve their health. In

41

some cases, they may be frightened about side effects or have misinformation from friends and relatives with similar health problems. They may also be concerned about the cost of the treatment.

Treatment can involve lifestyle changes, such as diet and exercise, as well as medication. Make sure you develop and communicate treatment plans with the patient's input and consent. Tell the patient what to expect from the treatment, including recommended lifestyle changes, what degree of improvement is realistic, and when she or he may start to feel better.

Keep medication plans as simple and straightforward as possible. For example, minimize the number of doses per day. Tailor the plan to the patient's situation and lifestyle, and try to reduce disruption to the patient's routine. Indicate the purpose of each medication. Make it clear which medications must be taken and on what schedule. It is helpful to say which drugs the patient should take only when having particular symptoms.

After proposing a treatment plan, check with the patient about its feasibility and acceptability. Work through what the patient feels may be obstacles to maintaining the plan. They may not be medical. For instance, transportation might be an issue.

Try to resolve any misunderstandings. For example, make it clear that a referral to another doctor does not mean you are abandoning the patient. Provide oral and written instructions.

Do not assume that all of your patients are able to read. Make sure the print is large enough for the patient to read.

Encourage your patient and her or his caregivers to take an active role in discovering how to manage chronic problems. Think in terms of joint problem solving or collaborative care. Such an approach can increase the patient's satisfaction while decreasing demands on your time.

Chapter 6

Fact Sheet on End of Life

Yesterday

- In the past, death occurred at home after a short illness with help provided to the dying person through the care of family members. Treatments often focused on making the individual as comfortable as possible.

- Issues surrounding end-of-life (EOL) experiences, pain, symptom management, and advance care planning were poorly understood and little studied.

- At the time, advancements in medical health technologies were beginning to prolong life in many life-threatening situations, raising new challenges surrounding decision-making for end-of-life care.

Today

- A report from the Institute of Medicine (IOM) found widespread dissatisfaction with end-of-life care. While most individuals with serious, advanced illnesses preferred to die at home and receive a more conservative pattern of end-of-life care; the majority

This chapter includes text excerpted from "End-of-Life," Research Portfolio Online Reporting Tools (RePORT), National Institutes of Health (NIH), June 30, 2018.

died in hospitals and received more aggressive care than was desired. Many dying persons feared abandonment and untreated physical distress.

- Death is often more complicated. Many people suffer from progressive or chronic, critical illnesses that eventually reach a point when curative approaches are no longer possible. When advanced illnesses become terminal, new treatments, medications, and technologies are now available to provide greater comfort, assist in symptom and pain management, and ease the burden of illness. Patients now can choose or change the focus of their care from treatment to comfort and elect to receive palliative or hospice services in a growing number of healthcare settings.

- Research has now increased our understanding and awareness of advanced illnesses and the need to provide holistic care for those at the end of life. National Institutes of Health (NIH) studies on the management of pain and other symptoms, communication and medical decision-making, caregiving, and safe transitions between care settings for those with serious, advanced illnesses provide a foundation for current research in end-of-life care.

- End-of-life care is a major part of the national nursing research agenda. New discoveries are improving end-of-life experience. New strategies and interventions are building the biological and behavioral evidence-base that will increase health-related quality of life (QOL) and enhance excellence in the care of those with advanced illnesses.

- Hospital palliative care consultation teams are associated with significant hospital cost savings and have been shown to improve physical and psychological symptom management, caregiver well-being, and family satisfaction.

- Hospice care affirms a patient's and family's full participation in end-of-life care and serves a growing number of patients with neurologic, cardiac, or nonspecific terminal diagnoses. Various studies on the cost-effectiveness of hospice are providing evidence that hospice is a less costly approach to care for those at the end-of-life.

- Most pain can be controlled during end-of-life care, but quality management of nonpain symptoms is also needed. In one study of older nursing home hospice/palliative care patients, common nonpain symptoms (such as constipation, nausea/vomiting, fever, and diarrhea) were often undertreated in more than half of the patients.

- Approximately 25 percent of all U.S. deaths occur in the long-term-care setting, and this figure is projected to rise to 40 percent by the year 2040. Care coordination as patients transition from one form of care to another during a progressive, advanced illness can improve care and cut costs. A study showed that when elderly heart-failure patients received specialized nursing care throughout their hospital stay and at home following hospital discharge, the patients had a better quality of life and fewer hospital readmissions. Instead of costing more money for this specialized care, the study showed that the care resulted in a nearly 38 percent savings in Medicare costs (www.transitionalcare.info).

- Advance planning can help make sure that patients get the care they wish when they want it. But, many individuals and their families still struggle with a lack of continuity of care and poor communication with healthcare practitioners about their treatment wishes, especially at the end of life. A study has shown that residents with POLST (Physician Orders for Life-Sustaining Treatments) forms are less likely to receive unwanted life-sustaining treatments when compared to patients with traditional Do-Not-Resuscitate orders (www.ohsu.edu/polst). Using the POLST did not impact the degree of comfort care received for symptom management and helped individuals make more informed choices about the type and level of end-of-life care they wish to receive.

- Communication between patients, families, and providers is important across the span of end-of-life care. Up to 20 percent of all deaths in the United States occur in or shortly after an intensive care unit (ICU) stay. Many of these patients are surrounded by family members who experience stress, fear, anxiety, and depression. The desire for information and emotional support is a common theme among all ICU families. In a study, family members reported a high degree of satisfaction when opportunities were presented for inclusion in decision-making. Families benefited from providers that gave emotional support, respect, and compassion; demonstrated a willingness to answer family questions; and considered family needs. In fact, clinician–family communication was possibly the most important factor in driving family satisfaction in the ICU.

• New health technologies and information technology (IT) tools are helping to address important concerns about planning for end-of-life care. By creating outlined plans that translate individual values and goals into meaningful directives that explicitly reflect preferred healthcare wishes, new computer tools are educating users about advance care planning. These tools help to identify, clarify, and prioritize factors that influence decision-making about future medical conditions. They can help users articulate a coherent set of wishes readily interpretable by physicians, and help individuals both choose a spokesperson and prepare to engage family, friends, and healthcare providers in discussions about advance care planning.

Tomorrow

The National Institutes of Health (NIH) is poised to continue to support research that will identify new strategies to improve end-of-life care, create new interventions for pain and symptom management, identify effective, accessible treatments, and develop new health technologies to provide quality, end-of-life care to patients and families.

• Studies are exploring the different trajectories that people experience in their last years, months, and days of life. This research will help clinicians predict patient needs and design appropriate care, and will prepare loved ones for this delicate period of transition.

• New research is defining the unique end-of-life experiences and healthcare needs of each individual and family. Personalized care that incorporates cultural-ethical beliefs and practices, sensitivity to vulnerable populations and age groups, and integration of services across the course of an advanced illness will alleviate pain while maintaining awareness, address other discomforting symptoms, and help patients prepare advance directives to guide preferred plans of care.

• Studies are underway to find ways to improve communication between patients, families, and clinicians in end-of-life situations to improve the process of decision-making, help address patient concerns, and decrease stress on family caregivers.

Chapter 7

Research Findings about End-of-Life Care and Outcomes

Chapter Contents

Section 7.1 — The BEACON Study on
    End-of-Life Care 48

Section 7.2 — Telephone-Based Rehab
    Program for Cancer Patients 52

Section 7.3 — Family Involvement Improves
    End-of-Life Care 56

Section 7.1

The BEACON Study on End-of-Life Care

This section contains text excerpted from the following sources: Text under the heading "Spreading Best Practices for End-of-Life Care" is excerpted from "Spreading Best Practices for End-of-Life Care," Rehabilitation Research & Development Service (RR&D), U.S. Department of Veterans Affairs (VA), July 29, 2014. Reviewed September 2019; Text under the heading "The U.S. Department of Veterans Affairs Study Leads to Improved End-of-Life Care" is excerpted from "VA Study Leads to Improved End-of-Life Care," Rehabilitation Research & Development Service (RR&D), U.S. Department of Veterans Affairs (VA), March 26, 2014. Reviewed September 2019.

Spreading Best Practices for End-of-Life Care

At life's end, most people suffer physically, and also have significant emotional, spiritual, and social distress. This suffering can be made worse when aggressive, futile, and even harmful treatments are continued by physicians. Although palliative care treatment plans have the potential to improve the quality of end-of-life (EOL) care and reduce hospital costs, such care is not routinely available in inpatient settings in which dedicated hospice units are not available.

Most people who do not have palliative care treatment plans are likely to die in hospitals and nursing homes. Researchers led by Drs. Kathryn Burgio and Amos Bailey of the Birmingham, Alabama, U.S. Department of Veterans Affairs (VA) Medical Center created the "Best Practices for End-of-Life Care for Our Nation's Veterans" (BEACON) trial to test an intervention that could improve the quality of end-of-life care at the VA medical centers.

The four-month intervention, tested at six VA medical centers, trained hospital staff to identify actively dying patients and to implement a set of best practices traditionally used in home-based hospice care. Some of the best practices the research team encouraged staff to implement were allowing patients access to their favorite food and drinks, minimizing invasive procedures, and encouraging family members to visit their loved ones for longer periods of time.

Over the course of six years, the team found that the intervention improved the last days of veterans with respect to a number of care variables, including increasing the use of medication for pain or confusion, advance directives, and nasogastric (NG) tubes. The rates were the same for do-not-resuscitate orders, intravenous tubes, and restraints. The research team concluded that the intervention they developed has the potential to be widely distributed throughout the VA, and to improve the quality of end-of-life care in VA medical centers and other hospital settings.

The U.S. Department of Veterans Affairs Study Leads to Improved End-of-Life Care

Dr. Amos Bailey knows something about death. As an oncologist, he began referring patients to home hospice shortly after it became widely available in the late 1980s. The experience changed his outlook on care for the dying.

"I was struck that I could have two patients with the same illness, one in the hospital and another at home," says Bailey, who today is director of the Safe Harbor Palliative Care Program at the Birmingham VA Medical Center and professor of gerontology, geriatrics, and palliative care at the University of Alabama at Birmingham (UAB) School of Medicine. "When I visited the ones at home, they were so much more at peace than what I was seeing in the hospital. They had their medication at their bedside. Their families were there. There were not unnecessary dietary restrictions. Even something as simple as sitting in a recliner can make a difference. There were environmental things that made being at home much more comfortable than in the hospital."

The experience eventually led Bailey to initiate a study called "Best Practices for End-of-Life Care for our Nation's Veterans," or BEACON, which took place at six VA medical centers from 2005 to 2011. The study, which included more than 6,000 patients, was published online January 22, in the *Journal of General Internal Medicine*.

Dying at Home—Preferred, but Less Likely

Polls consistently show that most Americans would prefer to die at home. Unfortunately, according to Bailey, that is not likely. "More than half of Americans die in an institution, either a hospital or a nursing home and it appears that those numbers are rising. We need to realize people are going to die in hospitals and we need to make it a better experience."

Bailey is quick to point out that this is not necessarily a knock on hospital care. Hospitals, he says, are required to follow certain guidelines. "You cannot just leave medication out by the bedside in the hospital, and they have to worry about you falling out of that recliner," he says. "There have to be controls, but there can be a balance between home care and what is feasible in the hospital. We only die once and there is only one opportunity to provide excellent care to a patient in the last days of life."

When he came to the Birmingham VA, Dr. Bailey began to implement a comfort care order set for dying Veterans who were not able to be discharged to home or community hospice programs. This involved first identifying Veterans who were likely to die in the hospital, and then communicating with patients and families, and developing plans patterned on the best practices of home hospice care.

"It was not a perfect match," says Bailey. "It could not be. But we were able to make some significant changes. For example, we changed to sublingual medicines that dissolved under the tongue." Bailey also simplified the process for providing pain medication to dying patients, decreasing the time it took to provide relief to Veterans in pain.

He then teamed up with VA researcher Dr. Kathryn Burgio, a behavioral psychologist and also a professor at UAB. Together they studied the effects of Bailey's comfort care project. By 2003 they were able to demonstrate what Bailey describes as "remarkable" changes in the process of care. Having established the program at Birmingham, they then set out to test the effectiveness at other VA medical centers.

Changing Hospital Culture

The sites—in Florida, Georgia, Mississippi, and South Carolina— were selected as much for their proximity to Birmingham as anything else. Bailey and his team underwent routine site visits, spending several weeks at a time conducting educational visits with VA staff and then observing the results.

"The keys to excellent end-of-life care are recognizing the imminently dying patient, communicating the prognosis, identifying goals of care, and anticipating and palliating symptoms," says Burgio. To do this across multiple sites, the team developed training and education materials and leveraged the efforts of local champions to encourage culture change. The goal of the research, according to Burgio, was not just to change the practice and behavior of individual providers, but also to change the culture of the hospital.

"It is difficult to do and sometimes even harder to accept, but when a medical provider is in lifesaver mode, they are not going to be focusing on the symptoms." says Burgio. "The sooner you realize a patient is dying, the sooner you can focus on their comfort. That can mean medications for pain, delirium, or other issues." It can also mean less use of intrusive techniques like nasogastric tubes or intravenous (IV) lines.

"We talked about things that were not necessarily helpful, like feeding tubes and IVs," says Bailey. "We showed them that they did not have to stop treatment in order to model their care on what hospice does at home."

The researchers looked at 16 care variables, from the use of medication for pain or confusion to pastoral visits. They encouraged providers to allow patients access to favorite food and drinks, tried to minimize invasive procedures, and allowed families to spend more time with loved ones.

Focus on the Family

Part of the focus is on the family members, says Burgio. "We want the bereaved family members to feel like everything they want has been done and that their loved one had a comfortable death. The traumatic death of a family member can affect people for the rest of their lives and make it harder for them to deal with their grief."

From improving access to pain medications to just letting patients sit up in a chair, BEACON led to improved rates for all 16 variables. "Every one of the outcomes we measured improved after implementation of BEACON," says Burgio. Orders for pain medication went up 11 percent, while the use of feeding tubes and IVs went down. Prescriptions for death rattle went up nearly 19 percent.

The researchers hope to expand their training program and eventually disseminate the best practices they have developed not only throughout the VA, but nationwide. "Only about 15 percent of Veterans who die each year do so at a VA facility," says Bailey. "We need to be able to improve end-of-life care not just at VA facilities, but nationwide, and not just for Veterans, but for everyone."

Section 7.2

Telephone-Based Rehab Program for Cancer Patients

This section includes text excerpted from
"Telephone-Based Rehab Program Helps People with
Advanced Cancer Maintain Independence," National
Cancer Institute (NCI), April 29, 2019.

As cancer progresses, it often leads to physical disability and pain that can threaten a person's independence and devastate their quality of life (QOL).

Yet most people with advanced cancer do not receive physical therapy or engage in exercise that can help maintain function, said Andrea Cheville, M.D., a rehabilitation physician at the Mayo Clinic in Rochester, MN. For these patients, she said, small changes in physical fitness can mean the difference between being able to live independently and losing one's independence, and may also affect their ability to receive certain treatments.

A National Cancer Institute (NCI)-funded clinical trial led by Dr. Cheville found that a six-month physical rehabilitation program delivered by telephone modestly improved function and reduced pain for people with advanced cancer. The telerehabilitation program also reduced the time patients spent in hospitals and long-term-care facilities, such as nursing homes.

"Overall, the study findings add to the growing evidence that low-tech interventions can effectively improve the delivery of supportive cancer care services," wrote Manali Patel, M.D., M.P.H., of the Stanford University School of Medicine, in a commentary on the study. Embracing these low-tech approaches "may be a smart move to improve patient-reported outcomes and keep patients at home," she concluded.

The findings, published April 4, in *JAMA Oncology*, also "reiterate the importance of supportive care for patients, and particularly for patients with advanced cancer," said Karen Mustian, Ph.D., M.P.H., of the University of Rochester's Wilmot Cancer Institute, who was not involved with the study.

"We need to think of new and creative ways to be able to support patients, their care providers, and their family members in the process of managing cancer," Dr. Mustian said.

Physical Therapy for Patients with Advanced Cancer

Various factors explain why many people with advanced stages of cancer do not receive physical therapy or other rehabilitation services.

It is often hard to find physical therapists or other professionals with the specialized training needed to work with people with advanced cancer. Also, these patients may have difficulty traveling to a specialty center for care, Dr. Cheville said.

Furthermore, she said, patients may feel too overwhelmed by the disease and its treatments to seek such care.

And, Dr. Patel said, "Oncologists and other healthcare providers may also be reluctant to refer patients with cancer, especially those with advanced cancer, to physical therapy" due to concerns that the patient may be too debilitated to benefit from such a program or could even be harmed by it.

Dr. Patel, an oncologist who mainly sees patients with advanced stages of cancer, said the new findings would change her practice. That includes being more likely to refer eligible patients for physical therapy and to consider physical therapy as "a way to also provide symptom relief from pain without having to rely on pain medications alone," including opioids, she said.

Remotely Delivered Care

For the trial, dubbed COPE, Dr. Cheville and her colleagues enrolled 516 adults (257 women and 259 men) with advanced-stage cancer and moderate functional impairment. People with moderate impairment can independently get around their home and, to a more limited extent, their communities, and manage the activities of daily living such as grocery shopping, but they do so with some difficulty. The average age of study participants was approximately 66 years.

To assess the value of a telerehabilitation program that addressed function and pain, patients eligible for the trial—all of whom had been seen at one of the three Mayo Clinic medical centers (in Minnesota, Arizona, or Florida)—were randomly assigned to one of three groups.

Those in the control group (group 1) continued their usual care and activities. Those in group 2 received an individualized telerehabilitation program delivered by a physical therapist with extensive experience in cancer rehabilitation—referred to as a fitness care manager. They also received targeted rehabilitation to manage pain. Those in group 3 received the individualized telerehabilitation program plus medication-based pain management coordinated by a nurse.

At the time of enrollment, fitness care managers phoned group 2 and group 3 participants to discuss symptoms, identify goals, and discuss any physical impairments and barriers to staying active.

With supervision from a rehabilitation physician (Dr. Cheville), fitness care managers instructed patients in a simple set of strength training exercises using resistance bands and a walking program that used a pedometer to track steps. The fitness care managers monitored patients' progress and coordinated with their primary clinical team.

When needed, patients were referred to a local physical therapist to fine-tune their exercise programs or address physical impairments in consultation with the fitness care manager.

All participants were monitored for function, pain, and quality of life using short questionnaires that they could opt to answer either online or by telephone.

Modest but Meaningful Improvements with Telerehabilitation

Over the six-month study period, group 2 participants (the telerehabilitation-only group) reported improvements in function, pain, and quality of life compared with patients in the control group.

The researchers expected that group 3 participants, who received telerehabilitation plus medication-based pain management, would see the greatest improvement in pain. But, to their surprise, pain control was similar in groups 2 and 3. Also unexpectedly, telerehabilitation alone was most effective in improving function, and quality of life was not markedly better in group 3 than in the control group.

Telerehabilitation was associated with fewer and shorter hospitalizations, and hospitalized telerehabilitation participants were more likely than those in the control group to be discharged from the hospital to home, rather than to a long-term-care facility.

Although the changes in function seen with telerehabilitation alone were modest, they were clinically meaningful, Dr. Cheville said.

"Even a small change can correlate with the ability to get in and out of a chair independently, go upstairs on your own, or get in and out of a car without help. These changes can make the difference between going home from the hospital rather than going to a nursing home," she said.

Dr. Cheville's team has some ideas as to why patients in group 2 fared better overall than those in group 3 and plans to explore this question in future studies.

Cancer Therapies Alone Are Not Enough

"One of the key lessons we learned from our study is the importance of helping patients to understand that cancer care is not only about treating the cancer. We need to strategically care for the person as well" to assure their well-being, Dr. Cheville said. "Convincing patients that they need to take ownership for maintaining muscle strength and protecting their ability to function is very important."

"We should not underestimate the power of implementing telephone-based supportive care services, as was done in this study," Dr. Mustian emphasized. "We have not really adopted those models in cancer care much."

One question that remains is whether health insurance would cover such services and, if not, whether the telerehabilitation approach is cost-effective for healthcare providers, Dr. Patel noted in her commentary. Indeed, Dr. Cheville said, she and her colleagues are preparing to submit a paper that analyzes the program's cost-effectiveness.

Even without that information, the improvements in outcomes shown by the study "may be enough for cancer care providers to consider the integration of collaborative telerehabilitation into routine cancer care," Dr. Patel wrote.

Another key limitation of the study is that most of the participants were non-Hispanic Whites who had in-home caregivers. So, it is unclear whether the telerehabilitation approach can be generalized to other patient populations.

"Our next steps will involve taking what we have learned and engaging representatives from other communities to find out how we can make [this approach] better and tailor it so that it is embraced by other patient populations," Dr. Cheville said. "We see that as a critical need."

Section 7.3

Family Involvement Improves End-of-Life Care

This section includes text excerpted from "Family Involvement Improves End-of-Life-Care," Rehabilitation Research & Development Service (RR&D), U.S. Department of Veterans Affairs (VA), July 29, 2014. Reviewed September 2019.

At the end of their lives, most patients lose the ability to make decisions about their own care. When that happens, and even before, the families of many patients get involved in decision-making on their loved ones' behalf.

Researchers with the Division of Geriatrics at the San Francisco U.S. Department of Veterans Affairs (VA) Medical Center (SFVAMC) looked at the records of 34,290 Veterans who died at any of 146 VA facilities between 2010 and 2011. They divided those Veterans into two groups: those whose records showed that the Veteran's family have had documented discussions with her or his healthcare team in the last month of life, and those whose families had no involvement.

The researchers found that those Veterans whose families were involved in their care were more likely to have had a discussion about palliative care (care for patients with serious, chronic, and life-threatening illnesses that focuses on improving life and providing comfort) with their healthcare team. They were also more likely to have been visited by chaplains, and to have had a do-not-resuscitate order on file. Such orders instruct doctors, nurses, and emergency medical personnel to not attempt emergency cardiopulmonary resuscitation (CPR) should a patient's heartbeat or breathing stop.

Patients whose families were involved in their end-of-life (EOL) care were not, however, more likely to die in either a hospice or palliative care unit than those whose families had no documented discussions with the patient's healthcare team in the last month of their lives. The researchers concluded that for vulnerable patients who may lack family and friends, clinicians should support early advance care planning so that these Veterans' end-of-life wishes can be known and followed.

Part Two

Medical Management of End-of-Life Symptoms

Chapter 8

Palliative Care

Chapter Contents

Section 8.1 — What Is Palliative Care?...................................... 60

Section 8.2 — Palliative Wound Care.. 64

Section 8.3 — Palliative Care in Cancer................................... 69

Section 8.1

What Is Palliative Care?

This section includes text excerpted from "Palliative Care: The Relief You Need When You Have a Serious Illness," National Institute of Nursing Research (NINR), June 15, 2018.

Dealing with any serious illness can be difficult. However, care is available to make you more comfortable right now. It is called "palliative care." You receive palliative care at the same time that you are receiving treatments for your illness. Its primary purpose is to relieve your pain and other symptoms and improve your quality of life (QOL). Palliative care is a central part of treatment for serious or life-threatening illnesses. The information in this section will help you understand how you or someone close to you can benefit from this type of care.

Palliative care is a comprehensive treatment of the discomfort, symptoms, and stress of serious illness. It does not replace your primary treatment; palliative care works together with the primary treatment you are receiving. The goal is to prevent and ease suffering and improve your quality of life. The purpose of palliative care is to address symptoms, such as pain, breathing difficulties, or nausea, among others. Receiving palliative care does not necessarily mean you are dying.

Palliative Care Gives You a Chance to Live Your Life More Comfortably

Palliative care provides relief from symptoms including pain, shortness of breath, fatigue, constipation, nausea, loss of appetite, problems with sleep, and many other symptoms. It can also help you deal with the side effects of the medical treatments you are receiving. Perhaps most important, palliative care can help improve your quality of life and provide help to your family as well.

Palliative Care Is Different from Hospice Care

Palliative care is available to you at any time during your illness. Remember that you can receive palliative care at the same time you receive other treatments for your illness. Its availability does not depend upon whether your condition can be cured. The goal is to make you as comfortable as possible and improve your quality of life.

You do not have to be in hospice or at the end of life to receive palliative care. People in hospice always receive palliative care. Hospice focuses on a person's final months of life. To qualify for some hospice programs, patients must no longer be receiving treatments to cure their illness.

Palliative care also provides support for you and your family and can improve communication between you and your healthcare providers.

Palliative care strives to provide you with:

- Expert treatment of pain and other symptoms so you can get the best relief possible

- Open discussion about treatment choices, including treatment for your disease and management of your symptoms

- Coordination of your care with all of your healthcare providers

- Emotional support for you and your family

Palliative Care Can Be Very Effective

Researchers have studied the positive effects palliative care has on patients and their families. Few studies show that patients who receive palliative care report improvement in:

- Pain, nausea, and shortness of breath

- Communication with their healthcare providers and family members

- Emotional support

Other studies also show that starting palliative care early in the course of an illness:

- Ensures that care is more in line with patients' wishes

- Decreases stress and increases confidence in making decisions surrounding a loved one's care

- Meets the emotional and spiritual needs of patients and their families

Palliative Care Can Improve Your Quality of Life in a Variety of Ways

Together with your primary healthcare provider, your palliative care team provides pain and symptom control with every part of your treatment. Team members spend as much time as it takes with you and your family to help you fully understand your condition, care options, and other needs. They also help you make smooth transitions between all the settings where you may receive care (the hospital, nursing facilities, or home care).

This results in well-planned, complete treatment for all of your symptoms throughout your illness—treatment that takes care of you in your present condition and anticipates your future needs.

Palliative Care Is a Team Approach to Patient-Centered Care

Every palliative care team is different. Your palliative care team may include:

• Doctors

• Nurses

• Social workers

• Religious or spiritual advisors

• Pharmacists

• Nutritionists

• Counselors and others

Palliative care supports you and those who love you by making you comfortable. It also helps you set goals for the future that lead to a meaningful, enjoyable life while you get treatment for your illness.

How Do You Know If You Need Palliative Care?

Many adults and children living with serious illnesses, such as cancer, heart disease, lung disease, kidney failure, multiple sclerosis, acquired immune deficiency syndrome (AIDS), and cystic fibrosis, among others, experience physical symptoms and emotional distress related to their diseases. Sometimes these symptoms are due to the medical treatments they are receiving.

You may want to consider palliative care if you or your loved one:

• Suffers from pain or other symptoms due to ANY serious illness

• Has physical or emotional pain that is NOT under control

• Needs help understanding their illness and discussing treatment

Start Palliative Care as Soon as You Find Out That You Have a Serious Illness

It is never too early to start palliative care. In fact, palliative care occurs at the same time as all other treatments for your illness and does not depend upon the course of your disease.

There is no reason to wait. Palliative care teams understand that pain and other symptoms affect your quality of life and can leave you lacking the energy or motivation to pursue the things you enjoy. They also know that the stress of what you are going through can have a big impact on your family. And they can assist you and your loved ones as you cope with the experience of living with a serious illness.

Palliative Care Involves Working Together as a Team

Patients who may want palliative care often wonder how it will affect their relationships with their current healthcare providers. Some of their questions include:

- Will I have to give up my primary healthcare provider?
- Who do I ask for palliative care?
- Will I offend my healthcare provider if I ask questions?

Most important, you do NOT give up your own healthcare provider to get palliative care. The palliative care team and your healthcare provider work together.

Most clinicians appreciate the extra time and information the palliative care team provides to their patients. You may have to ask your healthcare provider for a referral to get palliative care services. Tell your healthcare provider you are thinking about palliative care and ask how to access palliative care in your area.

Where Is Palliative Care Provided?

Palliative care can be provided in the hospital, at outpatient clinics, or at home. The process begins when either your healthcare provider refers you to the palliative care team or you ask your healthcare provider for a referral. Palliative care is provided by a team of professionals, including medical and nursing specialists, social workers, pharmacists, nutritionists, religious or spiritual advisors, and others.

Who Pays for Palliative Care

Most insurance plans cover at least part of the palliative care services, just as they would other medical services. Medicare and Medicaid also typically cover palliative care. If you have concerns about the cost of palliative care, then a social worker, care manager, or financial advisor at your hospital or clinic can help you.

How Does Palliative Care Address Pain?

If you have an illness causing you pain that is not relieved by drugs such as acetaminophen or ibuprofen, the palliative care team may recommend trying stronger medicines.

As always, if you have concerns about taking medications, talk to your palliative care team. They can tell you about how various medications work, what their side effects are, and how to get the most effective pain relief.

Do Not Wait to Get the Help You Deserve. Ask for Palliative Care and Start Feeling Better Now.

If you think you need palliative care, ask for it now. Tell your healthcare provider that you would like to add palliative care to your treatment and ask to meet with the palliative care team or ask for a referral for palliative care.

Section 8.2

Palliative Wound Care

"Palliative Wound Care," © 2017 Omnigraphics.
Reviewed September 2019.

Whereas typical medical treatment focuses on healing, the aim of palliative care is to treat symptoms and improve the quality of life (QOL) for terminally ill patients and their families. More than one-third of hospice patients and other individuals with serious illnesses suffer from such issues as pressure ulcers (bedsores), surgical wounds, and other skin problems as a result of the deterioration of the body and multi-organ systems failure. Palliative wound care is an effective method for relieving pain, treating infection, preventing new wounds from developing, and helping the patient and her or his family make the most of the remaining time they have together.

Management of Palliative Wound Care

Palliative care takes a coordinated approach to treating wounds and lessening symptoms, with the ultimate goal of ensuring patient comfort and sense of well-being. Generally, this means local wound care (treatment of the wound itself) and pain management.

Local Wound Care

Although healing is not always possible in palliative care, proper treatment of wounds can help prevent infection and improve the patient's state of mind. Wound care addresses such issues as:

- **Bleeding.** The repeated dressing and re-dressing of wounds often results in the tearing of tissue, which can lead to bleeding, increased discomfort, and infection. Topical vasoconstrictors are often used to stem blood flow, and a variety of sealants or barriers may be applied to the surface. Dressings with silicone adhesives may be used, since they are less likely to cause trauma to the wound with repeated applications.

- **Exudates.** These are clear or pus-like liquids that ooze out of cuts or areas of inflammation. Normally exudates are beneficial and central to the healing process, but in the case of chronic wounds they can cause problems such as infection of the wound or inflammation of the surrounding skin. The most common ways to manage exudates are through the use of the proper dressings and the application of topical steroids.

- **Infection.** Open wounds can easily become contaminated with bacteria, often leading to infection, which can spread and cause additional problems. And in the case of chronically ill patients, who frequently have compromised immune systems, this can be particularly dangerous. The best practice is to prevent infection in the first place. This is accomplished by using wound dressings with antimicrobial agents, applying topical antibiotics, and cleansing and debriding (removing dead tissue) the area when changing dressings.

- **Odor.** Unpleasant odor is a common problem with wounds, particularly those in which infection has set in, and in additional to being a sign of physical issues this has a tendency to negatively affect the patient's mental state. The first step in addressing or preventing odor is the proper cleansing of the wound, along with the application of topical antibiotics to treat infection and the use of specialized dressings.

Pain Management

Pressure ulcers and other skin problems can be especially painful, and unfortunately they are extremely common among terminally ill patients and others requiring palliative care. Therefore, controlling pain is one of the most important components in palliative wound care and is perhaps the one with the most impact on the patient's well-being and quality of life. Pain management may include:

- **Prevention.** The best way to manage pain is to prevent it as much as possible in the first place. This often means using special dressings that do not stick to wounds and training caregivers in the proper way to change dressings. Bedridden patients are usually turned frequently to prevent pressure ulcers, but in some cases, as when certain wounds are present, this procedure can increase pain, so less frequent turning may be called for. Debridement, although necessary, can be extremely painful, so in some cases medical professionals may need to administer a local anesthetic prior to the procedure.

- **Assessment.** Since pain is a subjective experience, assessing the degree to which it affects any given individual can be difficult. But since palliative care includes involving the patient in decision-making, her or his own description of pain must be taken into account by caregivers. In addition, a variety of tools—numerical scales, charts, and drawings—are often used, as are physiological and behavior observations by medical professionals.

- **Topical anesthetics.** The application of pain-relief medication directly to the wound has the advantage of bypassing the circulatory system, thus avoiding many side effects and often allowing for lower doses. Common topical anesthetics include lidocaine, benzydamine, sucralfate, and morphine gel, sometimes with antibiotics added to help prevent infection. Dressings that contain slow-release pain-relief pain medication, such as ibuprofen, have also proven effective.

- **Systemic analgesics.** These medications can be administered orally, by injection, or through an IV, and work by being absorbed into the bloodstream where they affect the body's pain receptors. Generally, the treatment of moderate pain will begin with such medications as acetaminophen and nonsteroidal anti-inflammatory drugs. More severe pain often requires the use of opioid (narcotic) analgesics, such as morphine, meperidine, nalbuphine, butorphanol, and fentanyl. Although these medications relieve pain, they tend to reduce the patient's mental status or, in large doses, make her or him sleep most of the time, so doctors need to balance their benefits against quality of life.

- **Alternative methods.** A number of methods for controlling pain without medication—or with lower doses of medication— have proven effective in some cases. These include gentle massage, physical therapy, acupuncture, and relaxation techniques, such as biofeedback and hypnosis. Transcutaneous electrical nerve stimulation, or TENS, which employs low-voltage electrical current for pain relief, has also been used with good results. And many patients respond well to pet therapy, as the presence of an animal and stoking its fur can have a very soothing effect.

Locations for Palliative Wound Care

Palliative wound care can take place in a hospital, an outpatient clinic (if the patient is ambulatory), at home, or in a hospice. In all cases, the palliative care team will typically consist of doctors, nurses, and social workers, as well as the patient and family members, who are integral part of the management process. In some cases, other specialists, including massage therapists, pharmacists, and nutrition- ists, may be part of the team. Each location has its advantages and disadvantages, which depend on the illness, the severity of symptoms, the patient's preferences, and access to qualified caregivers.

- **Hospital care.** During the early stages of an illness, patients are generally treated in a hospital. And even when treatment is completed or discontinued, many hospitals now have specialists on staff to provide palliative care, although unless the hospital has a hospice or other dedicated facility, this is usually only available for a limited time.

- **Outpatient palliative care.** If a patient is ambulatory, specialized wound care may be provided at a clinic that is outfitted and staffed for palliative care. The advantage of this type of care is that the patient and family are able to maintain close to their normal routines, while the illness is managed as required by a team of professionals.

- **Palliative care at home.** Most patients prefer to live at home, rather than in a care facility. And with the many types of professional support available through a variety of hospital programs, government agencies, and private sources, many individuals with serious illnesses are able to do so. Generally, this means working with a team of visiting nurses, social workers, and other professionals—as well as the cooperation of family members—to ensure that adequate care is available as needed.

- **Hospice care.** When illnesses have progressed too far for home or outpatient care, palliative care in a hospice may be recommended. In most instances, hospices are for terminally ill patients who may have only months to live. Here, although the level of care is not as intense as in a hospital, the patient can be observed more closely and professional help is generally more readily available. But, as with all palliative care, the emphasis is on patient comfort and quality of life.

References

1. Graves, Marilyn L., MSN, RN, CHPN, CWOCN, and Virginia Sun, Ph.D., RN. "Providing Quality Wound Care at the End of Life," Medscape.com, n.d.

2. Hughes, Ronda G. Ph.D., MHS, RN, et al. "Palliative Wound Care at the End of Life," Home Health Care Management & Practice (HHCMP), April 2005.

3. "Managing Pain Beyond Drugs," Web MD, August 14, 2015.

4. Tippett, Aletha W., MD. "Palliative Wound Treatment Promotes Healing," Wounds, January 2015.

5. Woo, Kevin Y., Ph.D., RN, ACNP, GNC(C), FAPWCA, et al. "Palliative Wound Care Management Strategies for Palliative Patients and Their Circles of Care," Clinical Management, March 2015.

Section 8.3

Palliative Care in Cancer

This section includes text excerpted from "Palliative Care in Cancer," National Cancer Institute (NCI), October 20, 2017.

What Is Palliative Care?

Palliative care is care given to improve the quality of life (QOL) of patients who have a serious or life-threatening disease, such as cancer. Palliative care is an approach to care that addresses the person as a whole, not just their disease. The goal is to prevent or treat, as early as possible, the symptoms and side effects of the disease and its treatment, in addition to any related psychological, social, and spiritual problems. Palliative care is also called "comfort care," "supportive care," and "symptom management." Patients may receive palliative care in the hospital, an outpatient clinic, a long-term care facility, or at home under the direction of a physician.

Who Gives Palliative Care?

Palliative care is usually provided by palliative care specialists, healthcare practitioners who have received special training and/ or certification in palliative care. They provide holistic care to the patient and family or caregiver focusing on the physical, emotional, social, and spiritual issues cancer patients may face during the cancer experience. Often, palliative care specialists work as part of a multidisciplinary team that may include doctors, nurses, registered dieticians, pharmacists, chaplains, psychologists, and social workers. The palliative care team works in conjunction with your oncology care team to manage your care and maintain the best possible quality of life for you. Palliative care specialists also provide caregiver support, facilitate communication among members of the healthcare team, and help with discussions focusing on goals of care for the patient.

What Issues Are Addressed in Palliative Care?

The physical and emotional effects of cancer and its treatment may be very different from person to person. Palliative care can address a broad range of issues, integrating an individual's specific needs into care. A palliative care specialist will take the following issues into account for each patient:

- **Physical.** Common physical symptoms include pain, fatigue, loss of appetite, nausea, vomiting, shortness of breath, and insomnia.

- **Emotional and coping.** Palliative care specialists can provide resources to help patients and families deal with the emotions that come with a cancer diagnosis and cancer treatment. Depression, anxiety, and fear are only a few of the concerns that can be addressed through palliative care.

- **Spiritual.** With a cancer diagnosis, patients and families often look more deeply for meaning in their lives. Some find the disease brings them closer to their faith or spiritual beliefs, whereas others struggle to understand why cancer happened to them. An expert in palliative care can help people explore their beliefs and values so that they can find a sense of peace or reach a point of acceptance that is appropriate for their situation.

- **Caregiver needs.** Family members are an important part of cancer care. Like the patient, they have changing needs. It is common for family members to become overwhelmed by the extra responsibilities placed upon them. Many find it hard to care for a sick relative while trying to handle other obligations, such as work, household duties, and caring for other family members. Uncertainty about how to help their loved one with medical situations, inadequate social support, and emotions such as worry and fear can also add to caregiver stress. These challenges can compromise caregivers' own health. Palliative care specialists can help families and friends cope and give them the support they need.

- **Practical needs.** Palliative care specialists can also assist with financial and legal worries, insurance questions, and employment concerns. Discussing the goals of care is also an important component of palliative care. This includes talking about advance directives and facilitating communication among family member, caregivers, and members of the oncology care team.

When Is Palliative Care Used in Cancer Care?

Palliative care may be provided at any point along the cancer care continuum, from diagnosis to the end of life. When a person receives palliative care, she or he may continue to receive cancer treatment.

How Does a Person Access Palliative Care?

Your oncologist (or someone on your oncology care team) is the first person you should ask about palliative care. She or he may refer you to a palliative care specialist, depending on your physical and emotional needs. Some national organizations have databases for referrals.

What Is the Difference between Palliative Care and Hospice?

Palliative care can begin at any point along the cancer care continuum, but hospice care begins when curative treatment is no longer the goal of care and the sole focus is quality of life. Palliative care can help patients and their loved ones make the transition from treatment meant to cure or control the disease to hospice care by:

- Preparing them for physical changes that may occur near the end of life

- Helping them cope with the different thoughts and emotional issues that arise

- Providing support for family members

Who Pays for Palliative Care

Private health insurance usually covers palliative care services. Medicare and Medicaid also pay for some kinds of palliative care. For example, Medicare Part B pays for some medical services that address symptom management. Medicaid coverage of some palliative care services varies by state. If patients do not have health insurance or are unsure about their coverage, they should check with a social worker or their hospital's financial counselor.

Chapter 9

Chronic Illnesses and End-of-Life Care

In the early 20th-century public-health advances that addressed infectious diseases and poor nutrition greatly improved life expectancy. Now, as scientific understanding and technological advances have made acute and episodic illness (such as heart attack and stroke) survivable, chronic disease has become one of the most important challenges facing the U.S. healthcare system. More and more people are living with not just one chronic illness, such as diabetes, heart disease or depression, but with two or more conditions. In fact, 31.5 percent of all Americans, almost a third of the population, are now living with multiple chronic conditions (MCC). The healthcare needs of people with MCC are often complex. About 71 percent of all healthcare spending in the United States goes towards treating people with MCC. Although MCC affects a large percentage of working-age Americans (49% of those aged 45–64), prevalence increases with age — 80 percent of people 65 and older live with MCC. And as the U.S. population ages, and people live longer, the number of people with MCC is expected

---

This chapter contains text excerpted from the following sources: Text in this chapter begins with excerpts from "Multiple Chronic Conditions Chartbook," Agency for Healthcare Research and Quality (AHRQ), U.S. Department of Health and Human Services (HHS), April 2014. Reviewed September 2019; Text under the heading "Caregiving for Chronic Illness" is excerpted from "Caregiving for Family and Friends—A Public Health Issue," Centers for Disease Control and Prevention (CDC), July 30, 2019.

to continue to grow. It will be important to monitor the prevalence of multiple chronic conditions over time, to understand patterns of disease, the costs to the healthcare system and individuals, and the effect on quality of life (QOL).

Caregiving for Chronic Illness

Caregiving is an important public-health issue that affects the quality of life for millions of individuals. Caregivers provide assistance with another person's social or health needs. Caregiving may include help with one or more activities important for daily living, such as bathing and dressing, paying bills, shopping, and providing transportation. It also may involve emotional support and help with managing a chronic disease or disability. Caregiving responsibilities can increase and change as the recipient's needs increase, which may result in additional strain on the caregiver.

Caregivers can be unpaid family members or friends or paid caregivers. Informal or unpaid caregivers are the backbone of long-term care provided in people's homes. In particular, middle-aged and older adults provide a substantial portion of this care in the United States, as they care for children, parents, or spouses. These informal caregivers are the focus of this brief.

Caregiving can affect the caregiver's life in a myriad of ways including her or his ability to work, engage in social interactions and relationships, and maintain good physical and mental health. Caregiving can also bring great satisfaction and strengthen relationships, thus enhancing the caregivers' quality of life. As the population ages and disability worsens, it is critical to understand the physical and mental-health burden on caregivers, the range of tasks caregivers may perform, and the societal and economic impacts of long-term chronic diseases or disability.

Chapter 10

Pain Management and Assessment

Chapter Contents

Section 10.1—Pain: An Overview 76

Section 10.2—Cancer Pain Control... 80

Section 10.3—Pain Assessment in Patients with
Dementia 93

Section 10.1

Pain: An Overview

This section includes text excerpted from "Pain: You Can Get Help," National Institute on Aging (NIA), National Institutes of Health (NIH), February 28, 2018.

Acute Pain and Chronic Pain

There are two kinds of pain. Acute pain begins suddenly, lasts for a short time, and goes away as your body heals. You might feel acute pain after surgery or if you have a broken bone, infected tooth, or kidney stones.

Pain that lasts for three months or longer is called "chronic pain." This pain often affects older people. For some people, chronic pain is caused by a health condition such as arthritis. It may also follow acute pain from an injury, surgery, or other health issue that has been treated, like postherpetic neuralgia after shingles.

Living with any type of pain can be hard. It can cause many other problems. For instance, pain can:

• Get in the way of your daily activities

• Disturb your sleep and eating habits

• Make it difficult to continue working

• Be related to depression or anxiety

• Keep you from spending time with friends and family

Describing Pain

Many people have a hard time describing pain. Think about these questions when you explain how the pain feels:

• Where does it hurt?

• When did the pain start? Does it come and go?

• What does it feel like? Is the pain sharp, dull, or burning? Would you use some other words to describe it?

• Do you have other symptoms?

• When do you feel the pain? In the morning? In the evening? After eating?

- Is there anything you do that makes the pain feel better or worse? For example, does using a heating pad or ice pack help? Does changing your position from lying down to sitting up make it better?

- What medicines, including over-the-counter (OTC) medications and nonmedicine therapies have you tried, and what was their effect?

Your doctor or nurse may ask you to rate your pain on a scale of 0 to 10, with 0 being no pain and 10 being the worst pain you can imagine. Or, your doctor may ask if the pain is mild, moderate, or severe. Some doctors or nurses have pictures of faces that show different expressions of pain and ask you to point to the face that shows how you feel. Your doctor may ask you to keep a diary of when and what kind of pain you feel every day.

Attitudes about Pain

Everyone reacts to pain differently. Some people feel they should be brave and not complain when they hurt. Other people are quick to report pain and ask for help.

Worrying about pain is common. This worry can make you afraid to stay active, and it can separate you from your friends and family. Working with your doctor, you can find ways to continue to take part in physical and social activities despite having pain.

Some people put off going to the doctor because they think pain is part of aging and nothing can help. This is not true!

It is important to see a doctor if you have a new pain. Finding a way to manage pain is often easier if it is addressed early.

Treating Pain

Treating, or managing chronic pain is important. Some treatments involve medications, and some do not. Your treatment plan should be specific to your needs.

Most treatment plans focus on both reducing pain and increasing ways to support daily function while living with pain.

Talk with your doctor about how long it may take before you feel better. Often, you have to stick with a treatment plan before you get relief. It is important to stay on a schedule. Sometimes this is called "staying ahead" or "keeping on top" of your pain. Be sure to tell your doctor about any side effects. You might have to try different treatments until you find a plan that works for you. As your pain lessens, you can likely become more active and will see your mood lift and sleep improve.

Medicines to Treat Pain

Your doctor may prescribe one or more of the following pain medications. Talk with your doctor about their safety and the right dose to take.

- **Acetaminophen** may help all types of pain, especially mild-to-moderate pain. Acetaminophen is found in OTC and prescription medicines. People who have more than three drinks per day or who have liver disease should not take acetaminophen.

- **Nonsteroidal anti-inflammatory drugs (NSAIDs)** include aspirin, naproxen, and ibuprofen. Long-term use of some NSAIDs can cause side effects, like internal bleeding or kidney problems, which make them unsafe for many older adults. You may not be able to take ibuprofen if you have high blood pressure.

- **Narcotics** (also called "opioids") are used for moderate to severe pain and require a doctor's prescription. They may be habit-forming. They can also be dangerous when taken with alcohol or certain other drugs. Examples of narcotics are codeine, morphine, and oxycodone.

- **Other medications** are sometimes used to treat pain. These include antidepressants, anticonvulsive medicines, local painkillers like nerve blocks or patches, and ointments and creams.

As people age, they are at risk for developing more side effects from medications. It is important to take exactly the amount of pain medicine your doctor prescribes. Do not chew or crush your pills if they are supposed to be swallowed whole. Talk with your doctor or pharmacist if you are having trouble swallowing your pills.

Mixing any pain medication with alcohol or other drugs can be dangerous. Make sure your doctor knows all the medicines you take, including OTC drugs and dietary supplements, as well as the amount of alcohol you drink.

What Other Treatments Help with Pain

In addition to drugs, there are a variety of complementary and alternative approaches that may provide relief. Talk to your doctor

78

about these treatments. It may take both medicine and other treatments to feel better.

- Acupuncture uses hair-thin needles to stimulate specific points on the body to relieve pain.

- Biofeedback helps you learn to control your heart rate, blood pressure, muscle tension, and other body functions. This may help reduce your pain and stress level.

- Cognitive-behavioral therapy is a form of short-term counseling that may help reduce your reaction to pain.

- Distraction can help you cope with acute pain, taking your mind off your discomfort.

- Electrical nerve stimulation uses electrical impulses to relieve pain.

- Guided imagery uses directed thoughts to create mental pictures that may help you relax, manage anxiety, sleep better, and have less pain.

- Hypnosis uses focused attention to help manage pain.

- Massage therapy can release tension in tight muscles.

- Mind–body stress reduction combines mindfulness meditation, body awareness, and yoga to increase relaxation and reduce pain.

- Physical therapy uses a variety of techniques to help manage everyday activities with less pain and teaches you ways to improve flexibility and strength.

Help Yourself Feel Better

There are things you can do yourself that might help you feel better. Try to:

- Keep a healthy weight. Putting on extra pounds can slow healing and make pain worse. A healthy weight might help with pain in the knees, back, hips, or feet.

- Be physically active. Pain might make you inactive, which can lead to more pain and loss of function. Activity can help.

- Get enough sleep. It can reduce pain sensitivity, help healing, and improve your mood.

- Avoid tobacco, caffeine, and alcohol. They can get in the way of treatment and increase pain.

- Join a pain support group. Sometimes, it can help to talk to other people about how they deal with pain. You can share your thoughts while learning from others.

Pain at the End of Life

Not everyone who is dying is in pain. But, if a person has pain at the end of life, there are ways to help. Experts believe it is best to focus on making the person comfortable, without worrying about possible addiction or drug dependence.

Section 10.2

Cancer Pain Control

This section includes text excerpted from "Support for People with Cancer—Cancer Pain Control," National Cancer Institute (NCI), January 2019.

Cancer pain can range from mild to very severe. Some days it can be worse than others. It can be caused by the cancer itself, the treatment, or both.

You may also have pain that has nothing to do with your cancer. Some people have other health issues or headaches and muscle strains. Always check with your doctor before taking any over-the-counter (OTC) medicine to relieve everyday aches and pains. This will help ensure that there will be no interactions with other drugs or safety concerns to know about.

Different Types of Pain

Here are the common terms used to describe different types of pain:

- **Acute pain** ranges from mild to severe. It comes on quickly and lasts a short time.

- **Chronic pain** ranges from mild to severe and persists or progresses over a long period of time.

- **Breakthrough pain** is an intense rise in pain that occurs suddenly or is felt for a short time. It can occur by itself or in relation to a certain activity. It may happen several times a day, even when you are taking the right dose of medicine. For example, it may happen as the current dose of your medicine is wearing off.

What Causes Cancer Pain

Cancer and its treatment cause most cancer pain. Major causes of pain include:

- **Pain from medical tests.** Some methods used to diagnose cancer or see how well treatment is working can be painful. Examples may be a biopsy, spinal tap, or bone marrow test. Do not let concerns about pain stop you from having tests done. Talk with your doctor ahead of time about the steps that will be taken to lessen any potential pain.

- **Pain from a tumor.** If the cancer grows bigger or spreads, it can cause pain by pressing on the tissues around it. For example, a tumor can cause pain if it presses on bones, nerves, the spinal cord, or body organs.

- **Pain from treatment.** Chemotherapy, radiation therapy, surgery, and other treatments may cause pain for some people. Some examples of pain from treatment are:

  - **Neuropathic pain.** This is pain that may occur if treatment damages the nerves. The pain is often burning, sharp, or shooting. The cancer itself can also cause this kind of pain.

  - **Phantom pain.** You may still feel pain or other discomfort coming from a body part that has been removed by surgery. Doctors are not sure why this happens, but it is real.

  - **Joint pain** (called "arthralgia"). This kind of pain is associated with the use of aromatase inhibitors, a type of hormonal therapy.

How much pain you feel depends on different things. These include the cause of the pain and how you experience it in your body. Everyone is different.

Talking about Your Pain

Pain control is part of treatment. Talking openly is key. The most important member of the team is you. You are the only one who knows what your pain feels like. Talking about pain is important. It gives your healthcare team the feedback they need to help you feel better.

Some people with cancer do not want to talk about their pain because they:

• Think that they will distract their doctors from working on ways to help treat their cancer

• Worry that they would not be seen as "good" patients

• Worry that they would not be able to afford pain medicine

As a result, people sometimes get so used to living with their pain that they forget what it is like to live without it.

• Tell your healthcare team if you are:

  • Taking any medicine to treat other health problems

  • Taking more or less of the pain medicine than prescribed

  • Allergic to certain drugs

  • Using any OTC medicines, home remedies, or herbal or alternative therapies

This information could affect the pain control plan your doctor suggests for you. If you feel uneasy talking about your pain, bring a family member or friend to speak for you. Or let your loved one take notes and ask questions. Remember, open communication between you, your loved ones, and your healthcare team will lead to better pain control.

Know How to Describe Your Pain
Assess Pain Threshold

The first step in getting your pain under control is talking honestly about it. Try to talk with your healthcare team and your loved ones about what you are feeling.

You will be asked to describe and rate your pain. This provides a way for your doctor to assess your pain threshold, which is the point at which a person becomes aware of pain. Knowing this will help measure how well your pain control plan is working.

Your doctor may ask you to describe your pain in a number of ways. A pain scale is the most common way. The scale uses the numbers 0 to 10, where 0 is no pain, and 10 is the worst. Some doctors show their patients a series of faces and ask them to point to the face that best describes how they feel. You will also need to talk about any new pain you feel.

This also means telling them:

- Where you have pain

- What it feels like (sharp, dull, throbbing, constant, burning, or shooting)

- How strong your pain is

- How long it lasts

- What lessens your pain or makes it worse

- When it happens (what time of day, what you are doing, and what is going on)

- If it gets in the way of daily activities

Use a Pain Diary

Many patients have found it helpful to keep a record of their pain. Some people use a pain diary or journal. Others create a list or a computer spreadsheet. Choose the way that works best for you.

Your record could list:

- When you take pain medicine

- Name and dose of the medicine you are taking

- Any side effects you have

- How much the medicine lowers the pain level

- How long the pain medicine works

- Other pain relief methods you use to control your pain

- Any activity that is affected by pain, or makes it better or worse

- Things that you cannot do at all because of the pain

Share your record with your healthcare team. It can help them figure out how helpful your pain medicines are, or if they need to change your pain control plan.

Share Your Beliefs about Medicines

Some people do not want to take medicine, even when it is prescribed by the doctor. Taking it may be against religious or cultural beliefs. Or there may be other personal reasons why someone would not take medicine.

If you feel any of these ways about pain medicine, it is important to share your views with your healthcare team. If you prefer, ask a friend or family member to share them for you. Talking openly about your beliefs will help your healthcare team find a plan that works best for you.

Pain-Control Plan

Make your pain-control plan work for you. Your pain-control plan will be designed for you and your body. Everyone has a different pain-control plan. Even if you have the same type of cancer as someone else, your plan may be different.

Take your pain medicine on schedule to keep the pain from starting or getting worse. This is one of the best ways to stay on top of your pain. Do not skip doses. Once you feel pain, it is harder to control and may take longer to get better.

Here are some other things you can do:

- Bring your list of medicines to each visit.

- Bring your pain record or diary.

- If you are seeing more than one doctor, make sure each one sees your list of medicines, especially if she or he is going to change or prescribe medicine.

- Do not wait for the pain to get worse.

- Never take someone else's medicine or share medicine. What helped a friend or relative may not help you.

- Do not get medicine from other countries or the Internet without telling your doctor.

- Ask your doctor to change your pain-control plan if it is not working.

Follow the Dose

The best way to control pain is to stop it before it starts or prevent it from getting worse. Do not wait until the pain gets bad or unbearable before taking your medicine. Pain is easier to control when it is mild. And you need to take pain medicine often enough to stay ahead of your pain. Follow the dose schedule your doctor gives you. Do not try to "hold off" between doses. If you wait:

- Your pain could get worse.

- It may take longer for the pain to get better or go away.

- You may need larger doses to bring the pain under control.

Keep a List of All Your Medicines

Make a list of all the medicines you are taking. If you need to, ask a member of your family or healthcare team to help you.

Your healthcare team needs to know what you take and when. Tell them each drug you are taking, no matter how harmless you think it might be. Even OTC, herbs, and supplements can interfere with cancer treatment. Or they could cause serious side effects or reactions.

How to Tell When You Need a New Pain-Control Plan

Here are a few things to watch out for and tell your healthcare team about:

- Your pain is not getting better or going away.

- Your pain medicine does not work as long as your doctor said it would.

- You have breakthrough pain.

- You have side effects that do not go away.

- Pain interferes with things like eating, sleeping, or working.

- The schedule or the way you take the medicine does not work for you.

Do not give up hope. Your pain can be managed. If you are still having pain that is hard to control, you may want to talk with your healthcare team about seeing a pain or palliative care specialist. Whatever you do, do not give up. If one medicine does not work, there is almost always another one to try. And unlike other medicines, there is no "right" dose for many pain medicines. Your dose may be more or less than someone else's. The right dose is the one that relieves your pain and makes you feel better.

Medicines to Treat Cancer Pain

There is more than one way to treat pain. Your doctor prescribes medicine based on the kind of pain you have and how severe it is. In studies, these medicines have been shown to help control cancer pain. Doctors use three main groups of drugs for pain: OTC, prescription and nonopioid medicines, and opioids. You may also hear the term "analgesics" used for these pain relievers. Some are stronger than others. It helps to know the different kinds of medicines, why and how they are used, how you take them, and what side effects you might expect.

Over-the-Counter for Mild-to-Moderate Pain

Over-the-counter (OTC) drugs can be used to treat mild-to-moderate pain. On a scale of 0 to 10, an OTC may be used if you rate your pain from 1 to 4. These medicines are stronger than most people realize. In many cases, they are all you will need to relieve your pain. You just need to be sure to take them regularly.

You can buy most OTC drugs without a prescription. But you still need to talk with your doctor before taking them. Some of them may have things added to them that you need to know about. And they do have side effects. Common ones, such as nausea, itching, or drowsiness, usually go away after a few days. Do not take more than the label says unless your doctor tells you to do so.

Over-the-counter drugs include:

Acetaminophen, which you may know as "Tylenol®"

- Acetaminophen reduces pain. It is not helpful with inflammation. Most of the time, people do not have side effects from a normal dose of acetaminophen. However, it is important to know: Regularly taking large doses can damage the liver.

- Drinking alcohol with this drug may cause liver damage.

Always tell the doctor if you are taking acetaminophen because:

- Sometimes it is used in other medicines, so you may be taking more than you should Acetaminophen can lower a fever. If you are on chemotherapy, your doctor may not want you to take the medicine too often. It could cover up a fever, which would hide the fact you might have an infection.

- Nonsteroidal anti-inflammatory drugs (NSAIDs), such as ibuprofen (which you may know as "Advil®" or "Motrin®") and aspirin help control pain and inflammation. With NSAIDs, the most common side effect is stomach upset or indigestion, especially in older people. Eating food or drinking milk when you take these drugs may stop this from happening.

Other side effects NSAIDs may cause:

- Bleeding of the stomach lining (especially if you drink alcohol)
- Kidney problems, especially in the elderly or those with existing kidney problems
- Heart problems, especially in those who already have heart disease (however, aspirin does not cause heart problems)
- Blood clotting problems, which means it is harder to stop bleeding after you have cut or hurt yourself.

When taking NSAIDs, tell your doctor if:
- Your stools become darker than normal
- You notice bleeding from your rectum
- You have an upset stomach
- You have heartburn symptoms
- You cough up blood

Important to Remember When Taking Nonsteroidal Anti-Inflammatory Drugs

Some people have conditions that NSAIDs can make worse. In general, you should avoid these drugs if you:
- Are allergic to aspirin
- Are on steroid medicines
- Have stomach ulcers or a history of ulcers, gout, or bleeding disorders

- Are taking prescription medicines for arthritis
- Have kidney problems
- Have heart problems
- Are planning surgery within a week
- Are taking blood-thinning medicine (such as heparin or Coumadin®)

Talk to your healthcare team before taking NSAIDs. As with acetaminophen, NSAIDs can lower fever. If you are on chemotherapy, your doctor may not want you to take them too often. The medicines can cover up a fever, hiding the fact that you might have an infection.

Other Prescription Medicines for Pain

Doctors also prescribe other types of medicine to relieve cancer pain. They can be used along with nonopioids and opioids. Some include:

- **Antidepressants.** Some drugs can be used for more than one purpose. For example, antidepressants are used to treat depression, but they may also help relieve tingling and burning pain. Nerve damage from radiation, surgery, or chemotherapy can cause this type of pain.

- **Antiseizure medicines (anticonvulsants).** Like antidepressants, anticonvulsants or antiseizure drugs can also be used to help control tingling or burning from nerve injury.

- **Steroids.** Steroids are mainly used to treat pain caused by swelling.

Opioids for Moderate-to-Severe Pain

If you are having moderate to severe pain, your doctor may recommend that you take stronger drugs called "opioids." Opioids are sometimes called "narcotics." You must have a doctor's prescription to take them.

Opioids may be long-acting or short-acting. Short-acting means that the drug begins working quickly and is prescribed as needed depending on your pain levels. Long-acting drugs are absorbed in the body more slowly, but they last longer and are taken regularly as prescribed. Short-acting is often prescribed in addition with long-acting to treat breakthrough pain.

Common short-acting opioids include:

- Buprenorphine
- Codeine
- Diamorphine
- Fentanyl®
- Hydrocodone
- Hydromorphone (e.g., Dilaudid®)
- Methadone
- Morphine®
- Oxycodone®
- Oxymorphone
- Tapentadol
- Tramadol

Long-acting opioids include:

- MS Contin®
- Oxycontin®
- Duragesic®

Getting Relief with Opioids

Over time, people who take opioids for pain sometimes find that they need to take larger doses to get relief. This is caused by more pain, the cancer getting worse, or medicine tolerance. When a medicine does not give you enough pain relief, your doctor may increase the dose and how often you take it. She or he can also prescribe a stronger drug. Both methods are safe and effective under your doctor's care. Do not increase the dose of medicine on your own.

Tolerance, Physical Dependence, and Addiction

People with cancer often need opioids for pain. When your health-care team discusses your options for taking opioids, you may hear the terms "tolerance," "physical dependence," and "addiction." It may be helpful to understand the difference between the three.

Some patients with cancer pain stop getting pain relief from opioids if they take them for a long time. This is called "tolerance." The development of tolerance is not addiction. Larger amounts or a different opioid may be needed if your body stops responding to the original dose. Your healthcare team will work with you to either increase your dose or change your medicine.

Physical dependence occurs when the body gets used to a certain level of the opioid and has withdrawal symptoms if the drug is suddenly stopped or taken in much smaller doses. Withdrawal consists of unpleasant physical or psychological symptoms, such as anxiety, sweating, nausea, and vomiting, to name a few. This is not the same as addiction, though people with addiction will experience physical dependence. Physical dependence can happen with the chronic use of many drugs—including many prescription drugs, even if taken as instructed.

Addiction is a chronic disease characterized by:

• Compulsive drug seeking

• The inability to stop use despite harmful consequences

• Failure to meet work, social, or family obligations

• Sometimes tolerance and withdrawal

Although many patients who are prescribed opioids for cancer pain use them safely, some patients are at greater risk for addiction than others. It is very important for you to share any personal or family history of drug or alcohol abuse with your healthcare team. Other factors in your life may also increase your risk of addiction. It is common for cancer patients to worry that they will become addicted to pain medicines. Your doctor will carefully prescribe and monitor your opioid doses so that you are treated for pain safely. Do not be afraid to take these medicines. Controlling your pain is one of the goals for your care.

Managing and Preventing Side Effects

Side effects vary with each person. It is important to talk to your doctor often about any side effects you are having. If needed, she or he can change your medicines or the doses you are taking. They can also add other medicines to your pain-control plan to help your side effects.

Do not let any side effects stop you from getting your pain managed. Your healthcare team can talk with you about other ways to relieve them. There are solutions to getting your pain under control. Less common side effects include:

- Dizziness

- Confusion

- Breathing problems (Call your doctor right away if this occurs)

- Itching

- Trouble urinating

- Altered sleep patterns (nightmares)

Constipation

Almost everyone taking opioids has some constipation. This happens because opioids cause the stool to move more slowly through your system, so your body takes more time to absorb water from the stool. The stool then becomes hard. Keep in mind that constipation will only go away if it is treated.

You can control or prevent constipation by taking these steps:

- Ask your doctor about giving you laxatives and stool softeners (drugs to help you pass stool from your body) when you first start taking opioids. Taking these right when you start taking pain medicine may prevent the problem.

- Drink plenty of liquids. Drinking 8 to 10 glasses of liquid each day will help keep stools soft.

- Eat foods high in fiber, including raw fruits with the skin left on, vegetables, and whole-grain breads and cereals.

- Exercise as much as you are able. Any movement, such as light walking, will help.

- Call your doctor if you have not had a bowel movement in 2 days or more.

Drowsiness

Some opioids cause drowsiness. Or, if your pain has kept you from sleeping, you may sleep more at first when you begin taking opioids.

The drowsiness could go away after a few days. If you are tired or drowsy:

- Do not walk up and down stairs alone.

- Do not drive or use machines, equipment, or anything else that requires focus.

Call your doctor if the drowsiness does not go away after a few days. She or he may adjust the dose you are taking or change drugs.

Nausea and Vomiting

Nausea and vomiting may go away after a few days of taking opioids. However, if your nausea or vomiting prevents you from taking your medicine, or affects your ability to eat and drink, call your doctor right away. These tips may help:

- Stay in bed for an hour or so after taking your medicine if you feel sick when walking around. This kind of nausea is like feeling seasick. Some OTC drugs may help, too. But be sure to check with your doctor before taking any other medicines.

- Your doctor may want to change or add medicines, or prescribe antinausea drugs.

- Ask your doctor if something else could be making you feel sick. It might be related to your cancer or another medicine you are taking. Constipation can also add to nausea.

Starting a new pain medicine Some pain medicines can make you feel sleepy when you first take them. This usually goes away within a few days. Also, some people get dizzy or feel confused. Tell your doctor if any of these symptoms persist. Changing your dose or the type of medicine can usually solve the problem.

Section 10.3

Pain Assessment in Patients with Dementia

This section includes text excerpted from "Prevalence and Management of Pain, by Race and Dementia among Nursing Home Residents: United States, 2004," Centers for Disease Control and Prevention (CDC), November 6, 2015. Reviewed September 2019.

Pain is common among nursing home residents, and effective pain management has an impact on improving quality of life. Previous research has shown race differences in pain reporting and management in various settings, with racial and ethnic minority groups less likely than White residents to report pain and receive adequate treatment. Other studies have documented cognitive impairment as a barrier in the detection and self-report of pain, with the underreporting likely resulting in undertreatment. However, the relationships among race, dementia, and pain reporting and management remain understudied. This section explores the combined impact of race and a diagnosis of dementia on reporting or showing signs of pain and pain management among nursing home residents.

Does Pain Vary by Race? Does Pain Vary by a Diagnosis of Dementia?

Overall among nursing home residents, 23 percent reported or showed signs of pain in the 7 days prior to the interview.

Non-White residents were less likely to report or show signs of pain than White residents. Nursing home residents with dementia were also less likely to report or show signs of pain compared with residents who did not have dementia.

Among all residents, 17 percent of non-White residents compared with 24 percent of White residents reported or showed signs of pain. Seventeen percent of those with dementia reported or showed signs of pain in the 7 days prior to the interview compared with 29 percent of those without dementia (Figure 10.1).

A similar association between dementia status and reporting of pain existed among both White and non-White residents, with a significantly greater proportion of residents without dementia reporting or showing signs of pain compared with residents with dementia. Non-White residents with dementia (12%) were least likely to report or show signs of pain, and White residents without dementia (31%) were most likely to report or show signs of pain (Figure 10.2).

93

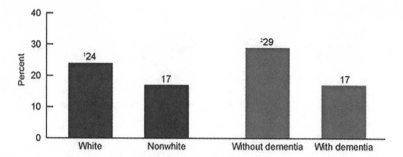

Figure 10.1. *Adjusted Percentages of Nursing Home Residents with Pain, by Race and Dementia Diagnosis: United States, 2004.* (Source: Centers for Disease Control and Prevention (CDC)/National Center for Health Statistics (NCHS), National Nursing Home Survey (NNHS), 2004.)

[1]*Significantly different from non-White residents (p<0.05).*
[2]*Significantly different from residents with dementia (p<0.05).*
Notes: Dementia included the following International Classification of Diseases, Ninth Revision codes: 290.0, 294.1, 294.0, 294.11, 294.8, 310, 331.0, 331, and 797. Data were adjusted for any current diagnosis of arthritis, cancer, pressure ulcers at stage II or higher, age, and sex.

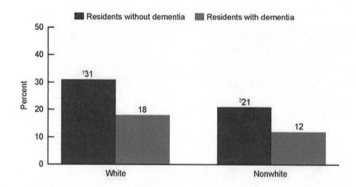

Figure 10.2. *Adjusted Percentages of Nursing Home Residents with Pain among White and Non-White Residents, by Dementia Diagnosis: United States, 2004.* (Source: Centers for Disease Control and Prevention (CDC)/ National Center for Health Statistics (NCHS), National Nursing Home Survey (NNHS), 2004.)

[1]*Significantly different from White residents with dementia (p<0.05).*
[2]*Significantly different from non-White residents with dementia (p<0.05).*
Notes: Dementia included the following International Classification of Diseases, Ninth Revision codes: 290.0, 294.1, 294.0, 294.11, 294.8, 310, 331.0, 331, and 797. Data were adjusted for any current diagnosis of arthritis, cancer, pressure ulcers at stage II or higher, age, and sex.

Did Residents with Pain Receive Appropriate Pain Management?

Although the use of medications for pain management may vary by age, sex, and clinical condition, appropriate care for pain is either standing orders for pain medication or receipt of services from a special program for pain management, particularly among nursing home residents with moderate to severe pain. Figure 10.3 gives the overall distribution of pain management strategies used for nursing home residents with pain, without adjusting for age, sex, or clinical diagnosis. Among nursing home residents with pain, 44 percent neither had standing orders nor received special services for pain management, 46 percent either had standing orders or received special services, and another 10 percent had both standing orders and received special services for pain management (Figure 10.3).

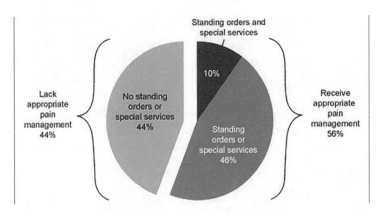

Figure 10.3. *Percentage of Nursing Home Residents with Pain, by Pain Management Strategy, 2004.* (Source: Centers for Disease Control and Prevention (CDC)/National Center for Health Statistics (NCHS), National Nursing Home Survey (NNHS), 2004.)

Notes: Special services refer to special programs for pain management. Appropriate pain management is receiving standing orders for pain medication or special services from a special program for pain management.

Among Residents with Pain, Does Appropriate Pain Management Vary by Race or Diagnosis of Dementia?

There were no statistically significant differences in lack of appropriate pain management by dementia diagnosis (44% of those with dementia and 45% of those without dementia) or race (45% of White residents and 48% of non-White residents) (not shown).

If one considers race and dementia diagnosis simultaneously, a similar percentage of White residents with or without dementia and non-White residents without dementia lacked appropriate pain management (43%, 46%, and 44%, respectively) (Figure 10.4). However, lack of appropriate pain management differed between non-White residents with dementia and White residents with dementia; 56 percent of non-White residents with dementia lacked appropriate pain management compared with 43 percent of White residents with dementia ($p<.05$).

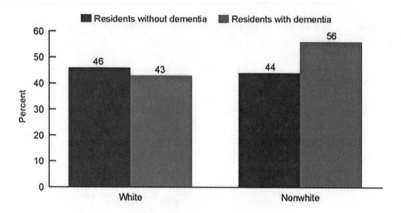

Figure 10.4. *Adjusted Percentages of Nursing Home Residents with Pain Who Lack Appropriate Pain Management among the White and Non-White Residents, by Dementia Diagnosis, 2004.* (Source: Centers for Disease Control and Prevention (CDC)/National Center for Health Statistics (NCHS), National Nursing Home Survey (NNHS), 2004.)

Notes: Dementia included the following International Classification of Diseases, Ninth Revision codes: 290.0, 294.1, 294.0, 294.11, 294.8, 310, 331.0, 331, and 797. Data were adjusted for any current diagnosis of arthritis, cancer, pressure ulcers at stage II or higher, age, and sex.

Chapter 11

Managing and Treating Fatigue

Chapter Contents

Section 11.1—Fatigue: More Than Being Tired 98

Section 11.2—Cancer and Fatigue 101

Section 11.3—Coping with Fatigue after Cancer
Treatment 114

Section 11.1

Fatigue: More Than Being Tired

This section includes text excerpted from "Fatigue in Older Adults," National Institute on Aging (NIA), National Institutes of Health (NIH), July 22, 2019.

Everyone feels tired now and then. But, after a good night's sleep, most people feel refreshed and ready to face a new day. If you continue to feel tired for weeks, it is time to see your doctor. She or he may be able to help you find out what is causing your fatigue. In fact, your doctor may even suggest you become more active, as exercise may reduce fatigue and improve your quality of life (QOL).

Some Illnesses Cause Fatigue

Sometimes, fatigue can be the first sign that something is wrong in your body. For example, people with rheumatoid arthritis (RA), a painful condition that affects the joints, often complain of fatigue. People with cancer may feel fatigued from the disease, treatments, or both.

Many medical problems and treatments can add to fatigue. These include:

- Taking certain medications, such as antidepressants, antihistamines, and medicines for nausea and pain

- Having medical treatments, such as chemotherapy and radiation, or recovering from major surgery

- Infections

- Chronic diseases, such as diabetes, heart disease, kidney disease, liver disease, thyroid disease, and chronic obstructive pulmonary disease (COPD)

- Untreated pain and diseases such as fibromyalgia

- Anemia

- Sleep apnea and other sleep disorders

Managing a health problem may make the fatigue go away. Your doctor can help.

Can Emotions Cause Fatigue?

Are you fearful about the future? Do you worry about your health and who will take care of you? Are you afraid you are no longer needed? Emotional stresses like these can take a toll on your energy. Fatigue can be linked to many conditions, including:

- Anxiety

- Depression

- Grief from the loss of family or friends

- Stress from financial or personal problems

- Feeling that you no longer have control over your life

Not getting enough sleep can also contribute to fatigue. Regular physical activity can improve your sleep. It may also help reduce feelings of depression and stress while improving your mood and overall well-being. Yoga, meditation, or cognitive-behavioral therapy (CBT) could also help you get more rest. Talk with your doctor if your mental well-being is affecting your sleep or making you tired.

What Else Causes Fatigue

Some lifestyle habits can make you feel tired. Here are some things that may be draining your energy:

- **Staying up too late.** A good night's sleep is important to feeling refreshed and energetic. Try going to bed and waking up at the same time every day.

- **Having too much caffeine.** Drinking caffeinated drinks such as soda, tea, or coffee late in the day can keep you from getting a good night's sleep. Limit the amount of caffeine you have during the day and avoid it in the evening.

- **Drinking too much alcohol.** Alcohol changes the way you think and act. It may also interact with your medicines.

- **Eating junk food.** Say "no thanks" to food with empty calories, such as fried foods and sweets, which have few nutrients and are high in fat and sugars. Choose nutritious foods to get the energy you need to do the things you enjoy.

- **Getting too little or too much exercise.** Regular exercise can boost your energy levels, but do not overdo it.

Can Boredom Cause Fatigue?

Being bored can make you feel tired. That may sound strange, but it is true. If you were very busy during your working years, you may feel lost about how to spend your time when you retire. When you wake up in the morning, you may see long days stretching before you with nothing planned. It does not have to be that way.

Engaging in social and productive activities that you enjoy, like volunteering in your community, may help maintain your well-being. Think about what interests you and what skills or knowledge you have to offer and look for places to volunteer.

How Can I Feel Less Tired?

Some changes to your lifestyle can make you feel less tired. Here are some suggestions:

- **Keep a fatigue diary** to help you find patterns throughout the day when you feel more or less tired.

- **Exercise regularly.** Almost anyone, at any age, can do some type of physical activity. If you have concerns about starting an exercise program, ask your doctor if there are any activities you should avoid. Moderate exercise may improve your appetite, energy, and outlook. Some people find that exercises combining balance and breathing (for example, tai chi or yoga) improve their energy.

- **Try to avoid long naps** (over 30 minutes) late in the day. Long naps can leave you feeling groggy and may make it harder to fall asleep at night.

- **Stop smoking.** Smoking is linked to many diseases and disorders, such as cancer, heart disease, and breathing problems, which can drain your energy.

- **Ask for help if you feel swamped.** Some people have so much to do that just thinking about their schedules can make them feel tired. Working with others may help a job go faster and be more fun.

When Should I See a Doctor for Fatigue?

If you have been tired for several weeks with no relief, it may be time to call your healthcare provider. She or he will ask questions about your sleep, daily activities, appetite, and exercise and will likely give you a physical exam and order lab tests.

Your treatment will be based on your history and the results of your exam and lab tests. Your doctor may prescribe medications to target underlying health problems, such as anemia or irregular thyroid activity. She or he may suggest that you eat a well-balanced diet and begin an exercise program.

Chronic Fatigue Syndrome

Chronic fatigue syndrome (CFS), also known as "myalgic encephalomyelitis" (ME), is a condition in which fatigue lasts 6 months or longer and is not related to other diseases or conditions. People with CFS experience symptoms that make it hard to do daily tasks such as dressing or bathing. Along with severe fatigue that does not get better with rest, CFS symptoms can include problems with sleep, memory and concentrating, pain, dizziness, sore throat, and tender lymph nodes.

Section 11.2

Cancer and Fatigue

This section includes text excerpted from "Fatigue (PDQ®)—Patient Version," National Cancer Institute (NCI), May 15, 2019.

Cancer-Related Fatigue and Quality of Life

Cancer treatments such as chemotherapy, radiation therapy (RT), and biologic therapy can cause fatigue in cancer patients. Fatigue is also a common symptom of some types of cancer. Patients describe fatigue as feeling tired, weak, worn out, heavy, slow, or that they have no energy to get up and go. Fatigue in cancer patients may be called "cancer fatigue," "cancer-related fatigue," and "cancer treatment-related fatigue."

Fatigue related to cancer is different from fatigue that healthy people feel. When a healthy person is tired by day-to-day activities, their fatigue can be relieved by sleep and rest. Cancer-related fatigue is different. Cancer patients get tired after less activity than people who do not have cancer. Also, cancer-related fatigue is not completely relieved by sleep and rest and may last for a long time. Fatigue usually decreases after cancer treatment ends, but patients may still feel some fatigue for months or years.

Fatigue can affect all areas of life by making the patient too tired to take part in daily activities, relationships, social events, and community activities. Patients may miss work or school, spend less time with friends and family, or spend more time sleeping. In some cases, physical fatigue leads to mental fatigue and mood changes. This can make it hard for the patient to pay attention, remember things, and think clearly. Money may become a problem if the patient needs to take leave from a job or stop working completely. Job loss can lead to the loss of health insurance. All these things can lessen the patient's quality of life (QOL) and self-esteem. Getting help with fatigue may prevent some of these problems and improve the quality of life.

Causes of Cancer-Related Fatigue

Doctors do not know all the reasons cancer patients have fatigue. Many conditions may cause fatigue at the same time, such as:

- Cancer treatment with chemotherapy, radiation therapy, and some biologic therapies

- Anemia (a lower than normal number of red blood cells (RBCs))

- Hormone levels that are too low or too high

- Trouble breathing or getting enough oxygen

- Heart trouble

- Infection

- Pain

- Stress

- Loss of appetite or not getting enough calories and nutrients

- Dehydration (loss of too much water from the body, such as from severe diarrhea or vomiting)

- Changes in how well the body uses food for energy

- Loss of weight, muscle, and/or strength

- Medicines that cause drowsiness
- Problems getting enough sleep
- Being less active
- Other medical conditions

Fatigue is common in people with advanced cancer who are not receiving cancer treatment.

Fatigue Caused by Cancer Treatment

Doctors are trying to better understand how cancer treatments, such as surgery, chemotherapy, and radiation therapy cause fatigue. Some studies show that fatigue is caused by:

- The need for extra energy to repair and heal body tissue damaged by treatment.
- The buildup of toxic substances that are left in the body after cells are killed by cancer treatment.
- The effect of biologic therapy on the immune system.
- Changes in the body's sleep–wake cycle.

When they begin cancer treatment, many patients are already tired from medical tests, surgery, and the emotional stress of coping with the cancer diagnosis. After treatment begins, fatigue may get worse. Patients who are older, have advanced cancer, or receive more than one type of treatment (for example, both chemotherapy and radiation therapy) are more likely to have long-term fatigue.

Fatigue and Chemotherapy

Patients treated with chemotherapy usually feel the most fatigue in the days right after each treatment. Then the fatigue decreases until the next treatment. Fatigue usually increases with each cycle. Some studies have shown that patients have the most severe fatigue about midway through all the cycles of chemotherapy. Fatigue decreases after chemotherapy is finished, but patients may not feel back to normal until a month or more after the last treatment. Many patients feel fatigued for months or years after the treatment ends.

Fatigue during chemotherapy may be increased by the following:

- Pain
- Depression

- Anxiety

- Anemia. Some types of chemotherapy stop the bone marrow from making enough new RBCs, causing anemia (too few RBCs to carry oxygen to the body)

- Lack of sleep caused by some anticancer drugs

Fatigue and Radiation Therapy

Many patients receiving radiation therapy have fatigue that keeps them from being as active as they want to be. After radiation therapy begins, fatigue usually increases until midway through the course of treatments and then stays about the same until treatment ends. For many patients, fatigue improves after radiation therapy stops. However, in some patients, fatigue will last months or years after the treatment ends. Some patients never have the same amount of energy they had before treatment.

Cancer-related fatigue has been studied in patients with breast cancer and prostate cancer. The amount of fatigue they felt and the time of day the fatigue was worst was different in different patients.

In men with prostate cancer, fatigue was increased by having the following symptoms before radiation therapy started:

- Poor sleep

- Depression

In women with breast cancer, fatigue was increased by the following:
- Working while receiving radiation therapy
- Having children at home
- Depression
- Anxiety
- Trouble sleeping
- Younger age
- Being underweight
- Having advanced cancer or other medical conditions

Fatigue and Biologic Therapy

Biologic therapy often causes flu-like symptoms. These symptoms include being tired physically and mentally, fever, chills, muscle pain, headache, and not feeling well in general. Some patients may also have problems thinking clearly. Fatigue symptoms depend on the type of biologic therapy used.

Fatigue and Surgery

Fatigue is often a side effect of surgery, but patients usually feel better with time. However, fatigue caused by surgery can be worse when the surgery is combined with other cancer treatments.

Fatigue Caused by Anemia

Anemia is a common cause of fatigue. Anemia affects the patient's energy level and quality of life. Anemia may be caused by the following:

- The cancer
- Cancer treatments
- A medical condition not related to the cancer

The effects of anemia on a patient depend on the following:

- How quickly the anemia occurs
- The patient's age
- The amount of plasma (the fluid part of the blood) in the patient's blood
- Other medical conditions the patient has

Fatigue Caused by Anxiety and Depression

Anxiety and depression are the most common psychological causes of fatigue in cancer patients.

The emotional stress of cancer can cause physical problems, including fatigue. It is common for cancer patients to have changes in moods and attitudes. Patients may feel anxiety and fear before and after a cancer diagnosis. These feelings may cause fatigue. The effect of the disease on the patient's physical, mental, social, and financial well-being can increase emotional distress.

About 15 to 25 percent of patients who have cancer get depressed, which may increase fatigue caused by physical factors. The following are signs of depression:

- Feeling tired mentally and physically

- Loss of interest in life

- Problems thinking

- Loss of sleep

- Feeling a loss of hope

Some patients have more fatigue after cancer treatments than others do.

Fatigue Caused by Poor Sleep

Not sleeping well may cause fatigue. Some people with cancer are not able to get enough sleep. The following problems related to sleep may cause fatigue:

- Waking up during the night

- Not going to sleep at the same time every night

- Sleeping during the day and less at night

- Not being active during the day

Poor sleep affects people in different ways. For example, the time of day that fatigue is worse may be different. Some patients who have trouble sleeping may feel more fatigue in the morning. Others may have severe fatigue in both the morning and the evening.

Even in patients who have poor sleep, fixing sleep problems does not always improve fatigue. A lack of sleep may not be the cause of the fatigue.

Attention Fatigue

Fatigue may be increased when it is hard for patients to learn and remember. During and after cancer treatment, patients may find they cannot pay attention for very long and have a hard time thinking, remembering, and understanding. This is called "attention fatigue." Sleep helps to relieve attention fatigue, but sleep may not be enough when the fatigue is related to cancer. Taking part in restful activities and spending time outdoors may help relieve attention fatigue.

Nutritional Side Effects Cause Fatigue

Side effects related to nutrition may cause or increase fatigue. The body's energy comes from food. Fatigue may occur if the body does not take in enough food to give the body the energy it needs. For many patients, the effects of cancer and cancer treatments make it hard to eat well. In people with cancer, three major factors may affect nutrition:

- A change in the way the body is able to use food. A patient may eat the same amount as before having cancer, but the body may not be able to absorb and use all the nutrients from the food. This is caused by cancer or its treatment.

- A decrease in the amount of food eaten because of low appetite, nausea, vomiting, diarrhea, or a blocked bowel

- An increase in the amount of energy needed by the body because of a growing tumor, infection, fever, or shortness of breath

Other Medications Cause Fatigue

Medicines other than chemotherapy may add to fatigue. Patients may take medicines for cancer symptoms, such as pain, or conditions other than the cancer. These medicines may cause the patient to feel sleepy. Opioids, antidepressants, and antihistamines have this side effect. If many of these medicines are taken at the same time, fatigue may be worse.

Taking opioids over time may lower the amount of sex hormones made in the testicles and ovaries. This can lead to fatigue as well as sexual problems and depression.

Assessment of Fatigue

An assessment is done to find out the level of fatigue and how it affects the patient's daily life. There is no test to diagnose fatigue, so it is important for the patient to tell family members and the healthcare team if fatigue is a problem. To assess fatigue, the patient is asked to describe how bad the fatigue is, how it affects daily activities, and what makes the fatigue better or worse. The doctor will look for causes of fatigue that can be treated. An assessment of fatigue includes a physical exam and blood tests.

Physical Exam

This is an exam of the body to check general signs of health or anything that seems unusual. The doctor will check for problems, such as trouble breathing or loss of muscle strength. The patient's walking, posture, and joint movements will be checked.

Rating the Level of Fatigue

The patient is asked to rate the level of fatigue (how bad the fatigue is). There is no standard way to rate fatigue. The doctor may ask the patient to rate the fatigue on a scale from 0 to 10. Other ways to rate fatigue check for how much fatigue affects the patient's quality of life.

A Series of Questions

- When the fatigue started, how long it lasts, and what makes it better or worse

- Symptoms or side effects, such as pain, the patient is having from the cancer or the treatments

- Medicines being taken

- Sleeping and resting habits

- Eating habits and changes in appetite or weight

- How fatigue affects daily activities and lifestyle

- How the fatigue affects being able to work

- Whether the patient has depression, anxiety, or pain

- Health habits and past illnesses and treatments

Blood Tests to Check for Anemia

The most common blood tests to check if the number of red blood cells is normal are:

- **Complete blood count (CBC) with differential:** A procedure in which a sample of blood is taken and checked for the following:

  - The number of red blood cells and platelets

  - The number and type of white blood cells (WBCs)

  - The amount of hemoglobin (the protein that carries oxygen) in the red blood cells

  - The portion of the blood sample made up of red blood cells

- **Peripheral blood smear:** A procedure in which a sample of blood is checked for the number and kinds of white blood cells, the number of platelets, and changes in the shape of blood cells.

- **Other blood tests** may be done to check for other conditions that affect red blood cells. These include a bone marrow aspiration and biopsy or a Coombs' test. Blood tests to check the levels of vitamin B_{12}, iron, and erythropoietin may also be done.

A fatigue assessment is repeated to see if there is a pattern for when fatigue starts or becomes worse. Fatigue may be worse right after a chemotherapy treatment, for example. The same method of measuring fatigue is used at each assessment. This helps show changes in fatigue over time.

Treatment of Fatigue
Relieving Related Conditions

Fatigue in cancer patients is often treated by relieving related conditions, such as anemia and depression. Treatment of fatigue depends on the symptoms and whether the cause of fatigue is known. When the cause of fatigue is not known, treatment is usually given to relieve symptoms and teach the patient ways to cope with fatigue.

Treatment of Anemia

Treating anemia may help decrease fatigue. When known, the cause of the anemia is treated. When the cause is not known, treatment of anemia is supportive care and may include the following:

- **Change in diet**

  Eating more foods rich in iron and vitamins may be combined with other treatments for anemia.

- **Transfusions of red blood cells**

  Transfusions work well to treat anemia. Possible side effects of transfusions include an allergic reaction, infection, graft-versus-host disease (GvHD), immune system changes, and too much iron in the blood.

- **Medicine**

  Drugs that cause the bone marrow to make more red blood cells may be used to treat anemia-related fatigue in patients receiving chemotherapy. Epoetin alfa and darbepoetin alfa are two of these drugs. This type of drug may shorten survival time, increase the risk of serious heart problems, and cause some tumors to grow faster or recur. The U.S. Food and Drug Administration (FDA) has not approved these drugs for the treatment of fatigue. Discuss the risks and benefits of these drugs with your doctor.

Treatment of Pain

If pain is making fatigue worse, the patient's pain medicine may be changed or the dose may be increased. If too much pain medicine is making fatigue worse, the patient's pain medicine may be changed or the dose may be decreased.

Treatment of Depression

Fatigue in patients who have depression may be treated with anti-depressant drugs. Psychostimulant drugs may help some patients have more energy and a better mood, and help them think and concentrate. The use of psychostimulants for treating fatigue is still being studied. The FDA has not approved psychostimulants for the treatment of fatigue.

Psychostimulants have side effects, especially with long-term use. Different psychostimulants have different side effects. Patients who have heart problems or who take anticancer drugs that affect the heart may have serious side effects from psychostimulants. These drugs have warnings on the label about their risks. Talk to your doctor about the effects these drugs may have and use them only under a doctor's care. Some of the possible side effects include the following:

- Trouble sleeping

- Euphoria (feelings of extreme happiness)

- Headache

- Nausea

- Anxiety

- Mood changes

- Loss of appetite

- Nightmares

- Paranoia (feelings of fear and distrust of other people)

- Serious heart problems

The doctor may prescribe low doses of a psychostimulant to be used for a short time in patients with advanced cancer who have severe fatigue. Talk to your doctor about the risks and benefits of these drugs.

Treatment of Fatigue Using Drugs

Certain drugs are being studied for fatigue related to cancer such as:

- **Bupropion** is an antidepressant that is being studied to treat fatigue in patients with or without depression.

- **Dexamethasone** is an anti-inflammatory drug being studied in patients with advanced cancer. In one clinical trial, patients who received dexamethasone reported less fatigue than the group that received a placebo. More trials are needed to study the link between inflammation and fatigue.

Treatment of Fatigue Using Dietary Supplements

Certain dietary supplements are being studied for fatigue related to cancer such as:

- L-carnitine is a supplement that helps the body make energy and lowers inflammation that may be linked to fatigue.

- Ginseng is an herb used to treat fatigue which may be taken in capsules of ground ginseng root. In a clinical trial, cancer patients who were either in treatment or had finished treatment, received either ginseng or placebo. The group receiving ginseng had less fatigue than the placebo group.

Other Treatments

Treatment of fatigue may include teaching the patient ways to increase energy and cope with fatigue in daily life.

Exercise

Exercise (including walking) may help people with cancer feel better and have more energy. The effect of exercise on fatigue in cancer patients is being studied. One study reported that breast cancer survivors who took part in enjoyable physical activity had less fatigue and pain and were better able to take part in daily activities. In clinical trials, some patients reported the following benefits from exercise:

- More physical energy

- Better appetite

- More able to do the normal activities of daily living

- Better quality of life

- More satisfaction with life

- A greater sense of well-being

- More able to meet the demands of cancer and cancer treatment

Moderate activity for three to five hours a week may help cancer-related fatigue. You are more likely to follow an exercise plan if you choose a type of exercise that you enjoy. The healthcare team can help you plan the best time and place for exercise and how often to exercise. Patients may need to start with light activity for short periods of time and build up to more exercise little by little. Studies have shown that exercise can be safely done during and after cancer treatment.

Mind and body exercises, such as qigong, tai chi, and yoga may help relieve fatigue. These exercises combine activities, such as movement, stretching, balance, and controlled breathing with spiritual activity such as meditation.

A Schedule of Activity and Rest

Changes in daily routine make the body use more energy. A regular routine can improve sleep and help the patient have more energy to be active during the day. A program of regular times for activity and rest help to make the most of a patient's energy. A healthcare professional can help patients plan an exercise program and decide which activities are the most important to them.

The following sleep habits may help decrease fatigue:

- Lie in bed for sleep only

- Take naps for no longer than one hour

- Avoid noise (like television and radio) during sleep

Cancer patients should not try to do too much. Health professionals have information about support services to help with daily activities and responsibilities.

Talk Therapy

Therapists use talk therapy (counseling) to treat certain emotional or behavioral disorders. This kind of therapy helps patients change how they think and feel about certain things. Talk therapy may help decrease a cancer patient's fatigue by working on problems related to cancer that make fatigue worse, such as:

• Stress from coping with cancer

• Fear that the cancer may come back

• Feeling hopeless about fatigue

• Not enough social support

• A pattern of sleep and activity that changes from day to day

Self-Care for Fatigue

Learning about the risk of cancer-related fatigue and how to reduce fatigue may help you cope with it better and improve the quality of life. For example, some patients in treatment worry that having fatigue means the treatment is not working. Anxiety over this can make fatigue even worse. Some patients may feel that reporting fatigue is complaining. Knowing that fatigue is a normal side effect that should be reported and treated may make it easier to manage.

Working with the healthcare team to learn about the following may help patients cope with fatigue:

• How to cope with fatigue as a normal side effect of treatment

• The possible medical causes of fatigue, such as not enough fluids, electrolyte imbalance, breathing problems, or anemia

• How patterns of rest and activity affect fatigue

• How to schedule important daily activities during times of less fatigue, and give up less important activities

• The kinds of activities that may help you feel more alert (walking, gardening, bird-watching)

• The difference between fatigue and depression

• How to avoid or change situations that cause stress

• How to avoid or change activities that cause fatigue

- How to change your surroundings to help decrease fatigue

- Exercise programs that are right for you and decrease fatigue

- The importance of eating enough food and drinking enough fluids

- Physical therapy for patients who have nerve problems or muscle weakness

- Respiratory therapy for patients who have trouble breathing

- How to tell if treatments for fatigue are working

Fatigue after Cancer Treatment Ends

Fatigue continues to be a problem for many cancer survivors long after treatment ends and the cancer is gone. Studies show that some patients continue to have moderate-to-severe fatigue years after treatment. Long-term therapies, such as tamoxifen can also cause fatigue. In children who were treated for brain tumors and cured, fatigue may continue after treatment. The causes of fatigue after treatment ends are different than the causes of fatigue during treatment. Treating fatigue after treatment ends also may be different from treating it during cancer therapy. Since fatigue may greatly affect the quality of life for cancer survivors, long-term follow-up care is important.

Section 11.3

Coping with Fatigue after Cancer Treatment

This section includes text excerpted from "Facing Forward—Life after Cancer Treatment," National Cancer Institute (NCI), March 2018.

Fatigue

Some cancer survivors report that they still feel tired or worn out. In fact, fatigue is one of the most common complaints during the first year of recovery.

Rest or sleep does not cure the type of fatigue that you may have. Doctors do not know its exact causes. The causes of fatigue are different for people who are receiving treatment than they are for those who have finished.

- Fatigue during treatment can be caused by cancer therapy. Other problems can also play a part in fatigue, like anemia (having too few red blood cells (RBCs)) or having a weak immune system. Poor nutrition, not drinking enough liquids, and depression can also be causes. Pain can make fatigue worse.

- Researchers are still learning about what may cause fatigue after treatment.

How long will fatigue last? There is no normal pattern. For some, fatigue gets better over time. Some people, especially those who have had bone marrow transplants, may still feel energy loss years later.

Some people feel very frustrated when fatigue lasts longer than they think it should and when it gets in the way of their normal routine. They may also worry that their friends, family, and coworkers will get upset with them if they continue to show signs of fatigue.

Getting Help

Talk with your doctor or nurse about what may be causing your fatigue and what can be done about it. Ask about:

- How any medicines you are taking or other medical problems you have might affect your energy level

- How you can control your pain, if pain is a problem for you

- Exercise programs that might help, such as walking

- Relaxation exercises

- Changing your diet or drinking more fluids

- Medicines or nutritional supplements that can help

- Specialists who might help you, such as physical therapists, occupational therapists, nutritionists, or mental-healthcare providers

Coping with Fatigue

Here are some ideas:

- Plan your day

- Be active at the time of day when you feel most alert and energetic

- Save your energy by changing how you do things. For example, sit on a stool while you cook or wash dishes

- Take short naps or rest breaks between activities

- Try to go to sleep and wake up at the same time every day

- Do what you enjoy, but do less of it. Focus on old or new interests that do not tire you out. For example, try to read something brief or listen to music.

- Let others help you. They might cook meals, run errands, or do the laundry. If no one offers, ask for what you need. Friends and family might be willing to help but may not know what to do. Choose how to spend your energy. Try to let go of things that do not matter as much now.

- Think about joining a support group. Talking about your fatigue with others who have had the same problem may help you find new ways to cope.

Chapter 12

Acute Respiratory Distress Syndrome

What Is Acute Respiratory Distress Syndrome?

Acute respiratory distress syndrome (ARDS) is a lung condition that leads to low oxygen levels in the blood. ARDS can be life-threatening because your body's organs need oxygen-rich blood to work well. People who develop ARDS often are very ill with another disease or have major injuries. They might already be in the hospital when they develop ARDS.

To understand ARDS, it helps to understand how the lungs work. When you breathe, air passes through your nose and mouth into your windpipe. The air then travels to your lungs' air sacs. These sacs are called "alveoli." Small blood vessels called "capillaries" run through the walls of the air sacs. Oxygen passes from the air sacs into the capillaries and then into the bloodstream. Blood carries the oxygen to all parts of the body, including the body's organs.

In ARDS, infections, injuries, or other conditions cause fluid to buildup in the air sacs. This prevents the lungs from filling with air and moving enough oxygen into the bloodstream. As a result, the body's organs (such as the kidneys and brain) do not get the oxygen they need. Without oxygen, the organs may not work well or at all.

This chapter includes text excerpted from "ARDS," National Heart, Lung, and Blood Institute (NHLBI), May 18, 2014. Reviewed September 2019.

People who develop ARDS often are in the hospital for other serious health problems. Rarely, people who are not hospitalized have health problems that lead to ARDS, such as severe pneumonia. If you have trouble breathing, call your doctor right away. If you have severe shortness of breath, call 911.

More people are surviving ARDS now than in the past. One likely reason for this is that treatment and care for the condition have improved. Survival rates for ARDS vary depending on age, the underlying cause of ARDS, associated illnesses, and other factors.

Some people who survive recover completely. Others may have lasting damage to their lungs and other health problems. Acute respiratory distress syndrome is also called "acute lung injury," "adult respiratory distress syndrome," "increased-permeability pulmonary edema," and "noncardiac pulmonary edema." In the past, ARDS was called "stiff lung," "shock lung," and "wet lung."

Causes of Acute Respiratory Distress Syndrome

Many conditions or factors can directly or indirectly injure the lungs and lead to ARDS. Some common ones are:

- **Sepsis.** This is a condition in which bacteria infect the bloodstream.

- **Pneumonia.** This is an infection in the lungs.

- Severe bleeding caused by an injury to the body.

- An injury to the chest or head, like a severe blow.

- Breathing in harmful fumes or smoke.

- Inhaling vomit or stomach contents from the mouth.

It is not clear why some very sick or seriously injured people develop ARDS and others do not. Researchers are trying to find out why ARDS develops and how to prevent it.

Risk Factors of Acute Respiratory Distress Syndrome

People at risk for ARDS have a condition or illness that can directly or indirectly injure their lungs.

Direct Lung Injury

Conditions that can directly injure the lungs include:

- **Pneumonia.** This is an infection in the lungs.

- Breathing in harmful fumes or smoke

- Inhaling vomit or stomach contents from the mouth

- **Using a ventilator.** This is a machine that helps people breathe; rarely, it can injure the lungs.

- **Nearly drowning**

Indirect Lung Injury

Conditions that can indirectly injure the lungs include:

- **Sepsis.** This is a condition in which bacteria infect the bloodstream

- **Severe bleeding** caused by an injury to the body or having many blood transfusions

- An injury to the chest or head, such as a severe blow

- **Pancreatitis.** This is a condition in which the pancreas becomes irritated or infected. The pancreas is a gland that releases enzymes and hormones.

- **Fat embolism.** This is a condition in which fat blocks an artery. A physical injury, such as a broken bone, can lead to a fat embolism

- **Drug reaction**

Signs, Symptoms, and Complications of Acute Respiratory Distress Syndrome

The first signs and symptoms of ARDS are feeling like you cannot get enough air into your lungs, rapid breathing, and a low blood oxygen level.

Other signs and symptoms depend on the cause of ARDS. They may occur before ARDS develops. For example, if pneumonia is causing ARDS, you may have a cough and fever before you feel short of breath.

Sometimes people who have ARDS develop signs and symptoms, such as low blood pressure, confusion, and extreme tiredness. This may mean that the body's organs, such as the kidneys and heart, are not getting enough oxygen-rich blood.

People who develop ARDS often are in the hospital for other serious health problems. Rarely, people who are not hospitalized have health problems that lead to ARDS, such as severe pneumonia. If you have trouble breathing, call your doctor right away. If you have severe shortness of breath, call 911.

Complications from Acute Respiratory Distress Syndrome

If you have ARDS, you can develop other medical problems while in the hospital. The most common problems are:

- **Infections.** Being in the hospital and lying down for a long time can put you at risk for infections, such as pneumonia. Being on a ventilator also puts you at a higher risk for infections.

- **A pneumothorax (collapsed lung).** This is a condition in which air or gas collects in the space around the lungs. This can cause one or both lungs to collapse. The air pressure from a ventilator can cause this condition.

- **Lung scarring.** ARDS causes the lungs to become stiff (scarred). It also makes it hard for the lungs to expand and fill with air. Being on a ventilator also can cause lung scarring.

- **Blood clots.** Lying down for long periods can cause blood clots to form in your body. A blood clot that forms in a vein deep in your body is called a "deep vein thrombosis." This type of blood clot can break off, travel through the bloodstream to the lungs, and block blood flow. This condition is called "pulmonary embolism."

Diagnosis of Acute Respiratory Distress Syndrome

Your doctor will diagnose ARDS-based on your medical history, a physical exam, and test results.

Medical History

Your doctor will ask whether you have or have recently had conditions that could lead to ARDS. Your doctor also will ask whether you have heart problems, such as heart failure. Heart failure can cause fluid to build up in your lungs.

Physical Exam

Acute respiratory distress syndrome may cause abnormal breathing sounds, such as crackling. Your doctor will listen to your lungs

120

with a stethoscope to hear these sounds. She or he also will listen to your heart and look for signs of extra fluid in other parts of your body. Extra fluid may mean you have heart or kidney problems. Your doctor will look for a bluish color on your skin and lips. A bluish color means your blood has a low level of oxygen. This is a possible sign of ARDS.

Diagnostic Tests

You may have ARDS or another condition that causes similar symptoms. To find out, your doctor may recommend one or more of the following tests.

Initial Tests

The first tests done are:

- **An arterial blood gas test.** This blood test measures the oxygen level in your blood using a sample of blood taken from an artery. A low blood oxygen level might be a sign of ARDS.

- **Chest x-ray.** This test creates pictures of the structures in your chest, such as your heart, lungs, and blood vessels. A chest x-ray can show whether you have extra fluid in your lungs.

- **Blood tests,** such as a complete blood count, blood chemistries, and blood cultures. These tests help find the cause of ARDS, such as an infection.

- **A sputum culture.** This test is used to study the spit you have coughed up from your lungs. A sputum culture can help find the cause of an infection.

Other Tests

Other tests used to diagnose ARDS include:

- **Chest computed tomography scan, or chest CT scan.** This test uses a computer to create detailed pictures of your lungs. A chest CT scan may show lung problems, such as fluid in the lungs, signs of pneumonia, or a tumor.

- **Heart tests that look for signs of heart failure.** Heart failure is a condition in which the heart cannot pump enough blood to meet the body's needs. This condition can cause fluid to buildup in your lungs.

Treatment of Acute Respiratory Distress Syndrome

Acute respiratory distress syndrome is treated in a hospital's intensive care unit (ICU). Current treatment approaches focus on improving blood oxygen levels and providing supportive care. Doctors also will try to pinpoint and treat the underlying cause of the condition.

Oxygen Therapy

One of the main goals of treating ARDS is to provide oxygen to your lungs and other organs (such as your brain and kidneys). Your organs need oxygen to work properly.

Oxygen usually is given through nasal prongs or a mask that fits over your mouth and nose. However, if your oxygen level does not rise or it is still hard for you to breathe, your doctor will give you oxygen through a breathing tube. She or he will insert the flexible tube through your mouth or nose and into your windpipe.

Before inserting the tube, your doctor will squirt or spray a liquid medicine into your throat (and possibly your nose) to make it numb. Your doctor also will give you medicine through an intravenous (IV) line in your bloodstream to make you sleepy and relaxed. The breathing tube will be connected to a machine that supports breathing (a ventilator). The ventilator will fill your lungs with oxygen-rich air.

Your doctor will adjust the ventilator as needed to help your lungs get the right amount of oxygen. This also will help prevent injury to your lungs from the pressure of the ventilator. You will use the breathing tube and ventilator until you can breathe on your own. If you need a ventilator for more than a few days, your doctor may do a tracheotomy.

This procedure involves making a small cut in your neck to create an opening to the windpipe. The opening is called a "tracheostomy." Your doctor will place the breathing tube directly into the windpipe. The tube is then connected to the ventilator.

Supportive Care

Supportive care refers to treatments that help relieve symptoms, prevent complications, or improve the quality of life (QOL). Supportive approaches used to treat ARDS include:

- Medicines to help you relax, relieve discomfort, and treat pain

- Ongoing monitoring of heart and lung function (including blood pressure and gas exchange)

- **Nutritional support.** People who have ARDS often suffer from malnutrition. Thus, extra nutrition may be given through a feeding tube.

- **Treatment for infections.** People who have ARDS are at a higher risk for infections, such as pneumonia. Being on a ventilator also increases the risk of infections. Doctors use antibiotics to treat pneumonia and other infections.

- **Prevention of blood clots.** Lying down for long periods can cause blood clots to form in the deep veins of your body. These clots can travel to your lungs and block blood flow (a condition called "pulmonary embolism"). Blood-thinning medicines and other treatments, such as compression stockings (stockings that create gentle pressure up the leg) are used to prevent blood clots.

- **Prevention of intestinal bleeding.** People who receive long-term support from a ventilator are at increased risk of bleeding in the intestines. Medicines can reduce this risk.

- **Fluids.** You may be given fluids to improve blood flow through your body and to provide nutrition. Your doctor will make sure you get the right amount of fluids. Fluids are usually given through an IV line inserted into one of your blood vessels.

Living with Acute Respiratory Distress Syndrome

Some people fully recover from ARDS. Others continue to have health problems. After you go home from the hospital, you may have one or more of the following problems:

- **Shortness of breath.** After treatment, many people who have ARDS recover close-to-normal lung function within six months. For others, it may take longer. Some people have breathing problems for the rest of their lives.

- **Tiredness and muscle weakness.** Being in the hospital and on a ventilator (a machine that supports breathing) can cause your muscles to weaken. You also may feel very tired following treatment.

- **Depression.** Many people who have had ARDS feel depressed for a while after treatment.

- **Problems with memory and thinking clearly.** Certain medicines and a low blood oxygen level can cause these problems.

123

These health problems may go away within a few weeks, or they may last longer. Talk with your doctor about how to deal with these issues.

Getting Help

You can take steps to recover from ARDS and improve your quality of life. For example, ask your family and friends to help with everyday activities. If you smoke, quit. Smoking can worsen lung problems. Talk to your doctor about programs and products that can help you quit. Also, try to avoid secondhand smoke and other lung irritants, such as harmful fumes. If you have trouble quitting smoking on your own, consider joining a support group. Many hospitals, workplaces, and community groups offer classes to help people quit smoking.

Go to pulmonary rehabilitation (rehab) if your doctor recommends it. Rehab might include exercise training, education, and counseling. Rehab can teach you how to return to normal activities and stay active. Your rehab team might include doctors, nurses, and other specialists. They will work with you to create a program that meets your needs.

Emotional Issues and Support

Living with ARDS may cause fear, anxiety, depression, and stress. Talk about how you feel with your healthcare team. Talking with a professional counselor also can help. If you are very depressed, your doctor may recommend medicines or other treatments that can improve your quality of life.

Joining a patient support group may help you adjust to living with ARDS. You can see how other people who have the same symptoms have coped with them. Talk to your doctor about local support groups or check with an area medical center.

Support from family and friends also can help relieve stress and anxiety. Let your loved ones know how you feel and what they can do to help you.

Chapter 13

Artificial Hydration and Nutrition

Patients suffering from life-threatening illness may, at some point, lose interest in food and fluids or may not be able to take them by mouth. Artificial hydration and nutrition is a treatment methodology that allows patients to receive food and fluids when they are no longer able to chew or swallow. This technique works not only for people at the end of their life but also for those who are recovering from surgery or suffering from temporary illness, such as diarrhea, nausea, and vomiting.

Types of Artificial Hydration and Nutrition

There are different ways to provide artificial hydration and nutrition.

Intravenous Hydration

In intravenous (IV) hydration, fluids are injected directly into the patient's vein through a small needle that is hooked up to a plastic tube. This method involves only a few risks, such as:

- Infection or bleeding at the site of insertion of the needle

- Swelling and breathing problems due to overload of fluid

"Artificial Hydration and Nutrition," © 2020 Omnigraphics. Reviewed September 2019.

Hypodermoclysis is a method similar to IV hydration by which the fluid is administered under the skin instead of in a vein.

Total Parenteral Nutrition

Total parenteral nutrition (TPN) involves the delivery of nutrition through a central line inserted in the armpit or neck and threaded through a vein. This method poses an increased risk of infection in the central line, which is highly dangerous to the patient.

Nasogastric Tubes

In this method, a tube is inserted into the nostril of the patient and made to pass to the stomach. A liquid formula delivered through the nasogastric (NG) tube then provides artificial hydration and nutrition. The tube can be left in only for a short period of one to four weeks. This method has a higher risk of causing pneumonia and thereby reducing the survival rate of patients.

Gastrostomy Tubes

In this method, a gastrostomy (G) tube is placed into the wall of the stomach through surgery. Percutaneous endoscopic gastrostomy (PEG) is a similar method in which the tube is placed endoscopically. Both methods are considered to be less risky than the other methods. However, there is a chance of developing pneumonia via these methods, too.

Frequently Asked Questions about Artificial Hydration and Nutrition

Is Artificial Hydration and Nutrition Different from Normal Intake of Food and Fluids?

Yes, the artificial hydration and nutrition medical treatment is completely different than eating and drinking. In artificial hydration and nutrition, the patient cannot feel the taste or texture of food and fluid. Moreover, it can be administered only by medical professionals, who ultimately decide what type and how much nutrition to be given and who monitor the side effects as well.

Can Artificial Hydration and Nutrition Save Lives?

Artificial hydration and nutrition can be effective for patients suffering from temporary illness, such as dehydration, nausea, vomiting, diarrhea, etc. It can also help patients recover faster after surgery. However, it may not be beneficial to someone who is at the end of her or his life. In some cases, artificial hydration and nutrition may add to the discomfort of a dying person by causing bloating, irritation, swelling, diarrhea, and breathing problems.

Can a Patient Refuse to Take Artificial Hydration and Nutrition?

Legally, every patient has the right to decide to accept, refuse, or discontinue artificial hydration and nutrition. If the patient is able to communicate, she or he can directly convey this decision to the physician. When the patient is no longer able to talk, her or his advanced directives will be followed. However, when there is an uncertainty about the decision of the patient, the treatment will usually be continued.

References

1. Morrow, Angela. "Artificial Nutrition and Hydration," Verywell Health, May 12, 2019.

2. "Artificial Hydration and Nutrition," American Academy of Family Physicians (AAFP), January 15, 2018.

3. "Artificial Nutrition (Food) and Hydration (Fluids) at the End of Life," National Hospice and Palliative Care Organization (NHPCO), 2015.

Chapter 14

Nutrition in Cancer Care

Overview of Nutrition in Cancer Care
Good Nutrition Is Vital

Nutrition is a process in which food is taken in and used by the body for growth, to keep the body healthy, and to replace tissue. Good nutrition is important for the good health of cancer patients. Eating the right kinds of foods before, during, and after cancer treatment can help the patient feel better and stay stronger. A healthy diet includes eating and drinking enough of the foods and liquids that have important nutrients (vitamins, minerals, protein, carbohydrates, fat, and water) the body needs.

Healthy Eating Habits Are Important

Healthy eating habits are important during and after cancer treatment. Nutrition therapy is used to help cancer patients keep a healthy bodyweight, maintain strength, keep body tissue healthy, and decrease side effects both during and after treatment.

Healthcare Team: Dietitian or Nutritionist Is a Must

A registered dietitian is an important part of the healthcare team. A registered nutritionist as a healthcare professional helps with cancer

---

This chapter includes text excerpted from "Nutrition in Cancer Care (PDQ®)— Patient Version," National Cancer Institute (NCI), March 16, 2018.

treatment and recovery. A dietitian will work with patients, their families, and the rest of the medical team to manage the patient's diet during and after cancer treatment.

Cancer Affects Nutrition

Cancer and cancer treatments may cause side effects that affect nutrition. For many patients, the effects of cancer and cancer treatments make it hard to eat well. Cancer treatments that affect nutrition include:

- Chemotherapy
- Hormone therapy
- Radiation therapy
- Surgery
- Immunotherapy
- Stem cell transplant

When the head, neck, esophagus, stomach, intestines, pancreas, or liver are affected by the cancer treatment, it is hard to take in enough nutrients to stay healthy.

Cancer Causes Malnutrition

Cancer and cancer treatments may cause malnutrition. Cancer and cancer treatments may affect taste, smell, appetite, and the ability to eat enough food or absorb the nutrients from food. This can cause malnutrition, which is a condition caused by a lack of key nutrients. Alcohol abuse and obesity may increase the risk of malnutrition.

Malnutrition can cause the patient to be weak, tired, and unable to fight infection or finish cancer treatment. Malnutrition may be made worse if the cancer grows or spreads.

Eating the right amount of protein and calories is important for healing, fighting infection, and having enough energy.

Anorexia and Cachexia Cause Malnutrition

Anorexia and cachexia are common causes of malnutrition in cancer patients. Anorexia is the loss of appetite or desire to eat. It is a common symptom in patients with cancer. Anorexia may occur early in the disease or later, if the cancer grows or spreads. Some patients already have anorexia when they are diagnosed with cancer. Most patients who have advanced cancer will have anorexia. Anorexia is the most common cause of malnutrition in cancer patients.

Cachexia is a condition marked by weakness, weight loss, and fat and muscle loss. It is common in patients with tumors that affect eating and digestion. It can occur in cancer patients who are eating well, but are not storing fat and muscle because of tumor growth.

Some tumors change the way the body uses certain nutrients. The body's use of protein, carbohydrates, and fat may be affected, especially by tumors of the stomach, intestines, or head and neck. A patient may seem to be eating enough, but the body may not be able to absorb all the nutrients from the food. Cancer patients may have anorexia and cachexia at the same time.

Effects of Cancer Treatment on Nutrition
Chemotherapy and Hormone Therapy

Chemotherapy affects cells all through the body. Chemotherapy uses drugs to stop the growth of cancer cells, either by killing the cells or by stopping them from dividing. Healthy cells that normally grow and divide quickly may also be killed. These include cells in the mouth and digestive tract. Hormone therapy adds, blocks, or removes hormones. It may be used to slow or stop the growth of certain cancers. Some types of hormone therapy may cause weight gain. Chemotherapy and hormone therapy cause different nutrition problems. Side effects from chemotherapy may cause problems with eating and digestion. When more than one chemotherapy drug is given, each drug may cause different side effects or when drugs cause the same side effects, the side effects may be more severe.

The following side effects are common:

- Loss of appetite

- Nausea

- Vomiting

- Dry mouth

- Sores in the mouth or throat

- Changes in the way food tastes

- Trouble swallowing

- Feeling full after eating a small amount of food

131

- Constipation

- Diarrhea

Patients receiving hormone therapy may need changes in their diet to prevent weight gain

Radiation Therapy
Radiation Therapy Kills Cells

Radiation therapy kills cancer cells and healthy cells in the treatment area. How severe the side effects are depends on the following:

- The part of the body that is treated

- The total dose of radiation and how it is given

Radiation Therapy Harms Nutrition

Radiation therapy may affect nutrition. Radiation therapy to any part of the digestive system has side effects that cause nutrition problems. Most of the side effects begin two to three weeks after radiation therapy begins and go away a few weeks after it is finished. Some side effects can continue for months or years after treatment ends.

The following are some of the more common side effects:

- **For radiation therapy to the brain or head and neck**
  - Loss of appetite
  - Nausea
  - Vomiting
  - Dry mouth or thick saliva. Medication may be given to treat a dry mouth.
  - Sore mouth and gums
  - Changes in the way food tastes
  - Trouble swallowing
  - Pain when swallowing
  - Being unable to fully open the mouth
- **For radiation therapy to the chest**
  - Loss of appetite
  - Nausea

- Vomiting
- Trouble swallowing
- Pain when swallowing
- Choking or breathing problems caused by changes in the upper esophagus
- **For radiation therapy to the abdomen, pelvis, or rectum**
  - Nausea
  - Vomiting
  - Bowel obstruction
  - Colitis
  - Diarrhea

Radiation therapy may also cause tiredness, which can lead to a decrease in appetite

Surgery
Surgery Causes Nutrition Problems

Surgery increases the body's need for nutrients and energy. The body needs extra energy and nutrients to heal wounds, fight infection, and recover from surgery. If the patient is malnourished before surgery, it may cause problems during recovery, such as poor healing or infection. For these patients, nutrition care may begin before surgery. Surgery to the head, neck, esophagus, stomach, or intestines may affect nutrition. Most cancer patients are treated with surgery. Surgery that removes all or part of certain organs can affect a patient's ability to eat and digest food.

The following are nutrition problems caused by surgery:

- Loss of appetite
- Trouble chewing
- Trouble swallowing
- Feeling full after eating a small amount of food

Immunotherapy
Immunotherapy May Affect Nutrition

The side effects of immunotherapy are different for each patient and the type of immunotherapy drug given. The following nutrition problems are common:

- Tiredness

- Fever

- Nausea

- Vomiting

- Diarrhea

Stem Cell Transplant
Stem Cell Transplant Increases Nutrition Needs

Patients who receive a stem cell transplant have special nutrition needs. Chemotherapy, radiation therapy, and other medicines used before or during a stem cell transplant may cause side effects that keep a patient from eating and digesting food as usual. Common side effects include the following:

- Mouth and throat sores

- Diarrhea

Patients who receive a stem cell transplant have a high risk of infection. Chemotherapy or radiation therapy given before the transplant decreases the number of white blood cells, which fight infection. It is important that these patients learn about safe food handling and avoid foods that may cause infection.

After a stem cell transplant, patients are at risk for acute or chronic graft-versus-host disease (GVHD). GVHD may affect the gastrointestinal tract or liver and change the patient's ability to eat or absorb nutrients from food.

Nutrition Assessment in Cancer Care
Healthcare Team Questions Diet and Weight History

Screening is used to look for health problems that affect the risk of poor nutrition. This can help find out if the patient is likely to become malnourished, and if nutrition therapy is needed.

The healthcare team may ask questions about the following:

- Weight changes over the past year

- Changes in the amount and type of food eaten

- Problems that have affected eating, such as loss of appetite, nausea, vomiting, diarrhea, constipation, mouth sores, dry mouth, changes in taste and smell, or pain

- Ability to walk and do other activities of daily living (dressing, getting into or out of a bed or chair, taking a bath or shower, and using the toilet)

A physical exam is done to check the body for general health and signs of disease. The patient is checked for signs of loss of weight, fat, and muscle, and for fluid buildup in the body.

Counseling and Diet Changes Improve Nutrition

A registered dietitian can work with patients and their families to counsel them on ways to improve the patient's nutrition. The registered dietitian gives care based on the patient's nutrition and diet needs. Changes to the diet are made to help decrease symptoms from cancer or cancer treatment. These changes may be in the types and amount of food, how often a patient eats, and how food is eaten (for example, at a certain temperature or taken with a straw).

A registered dietitian works with other members of the healthcare team to check the patient's nutritional health during cancer treatment and recovery. In addition to the dietitian, the healthcare team may include the following:

- Physician
- Nurse
- Social worker
- Psychologist

Nutrition Therapy Depends on Care Plan

The goal of nutrition therapy in patients with advanced cancer is to give patients the best possible quality of life and control symptoms that cause distress. Patients with advanced cancer may be treated with anticancer therapy and palliative care, palliative care alone, or may be in hospice care. Nutrition goals will be different for each patient. Some types of treatment may be stopped if they are not helping the patient. As the focus of care goes from cancer treatment to hospice or end-of-life care, nutrition goals may become less aggressive, and a change to care meant to keep the patient as comfortable as possible.

Treatment of Symptoms

When side effects of cancer or cancer treatment affect normal eating, changes can be made to help the patient get the nutrients they need. Eating foods that are high in calories, protein, vitamins, and minerals is important. Meals should be planned to meet the patient's nutrition needs and tastes in food. The following are some of the more common symptoms caused by cancer and cancer treatment and ways to treat or control them.

Anorexia

The following may help cancer patients who have anorexia (loss of appetite or desire to eat):

- Eat foods that are high in protein and calories. The following are high-protein food choices:

  - Beans

  - Chicken

  - Fish

  - Meat

  - Yogurt

  - Eggs

- Add extra protein and calories to food, such as using protein-fortified milk.

- Eat high-protein foods first in your meal when your appetite is strongest.

- Sip only small amounts of liquids during meals.

- Drink milkshakes, smoothies, juices, or soups if you do not feel like eating solid foods.

- Eat foods that smell good.

- Try new foods and new recipes.

- Try blenderized drinks that are high in nutrients (check with your doctor or registered dietitian first).

- Eat small meals and healthy snacks often throughout the day.

- Eat larger meals when you feel well and are rested.

- Eat your largest meal when you feel hungriest, whether at breakfast, lunch, or dinner.

- Make and store small amounts of favorite foods so they are ready to eat when you are hungry.

- Be as active as possible so that you will have a good appetite.

- Brush your teeth and rinse your mouth to relieve symptoms and aftertastes.

- Talk to your doctor or registered dietitian if you are having eating problems, such as nausea, vomiting, or changes in how foods taste and smell.

If these diet changes do not help with anorexia, tube feedings may be needed so that you will get enough nutrients each day. Medicines may be given to increase appetite.

Nausea

The following may help cancer patients control nausea:

- Choose foods that appeal to you. Do not force yourself to eat food that makes you feel sick. Do not eat your favorite foods, to avoid linking them to being sick.

- Eat foods that are bland, soft, and easy-to-digest, rather than heavy meals.

- Eat dry foods, such as crackers, bread sticks, or toast throughout the day.

- Eat foods that are easy on your stomach, such as white toast, plain yogurt, and clear broth.

- Eat dry toast or crackers before getting out of bed if you have nausea in the morning.

- Eat foods and drink liquids at room temperature (not too hot or too cold).

- Slowly sip liquids throughout the day.

- Suck on hard candies such as peppermints or lemon drops if your mouth has a bad taste.

- Stay away from food and drink with strong smells.

- Eat five or six small meals every day instead of three large meals.

- Sip on only small amounts of liquid during meals to avoid feeling full or bloated.

- Do not skip meals and snacks. An empty stomach may make your nausea worse.

- Rinse your mouth before and after eating.

- Do not eat in a room that has cooking odors or that is very warm. Keep the living space at a comfortable temperature and well-ventilated.

- Sit up or lie with your head raised for one hour after eating.

- Plan the best times for you to eat and drink.

- Relax before each cancer treatment.

- Wear clothes that are loose and comfortable.

- Keep a record of when you feel nausea and why.

- Talk with your doctor about using antinausea medicine.

Vomiting

The following may help cancer patients control vomiting:

- Do not eat or drink anything until the vomiting stops.

- Drink small amounts of clear liquids after vomiting stops.

- After you are able to drink clear liquids without vomiting, drink liquids, such as strained soups, or milkshakes, that are easy on your stomach.

- Eat five or six small meals every day instead of three large meals.

- Sit upright and bend forward after vomiting.

- Ask your doctor to order medicine to prevent or control vomiting.

Dry Mouth

The following may help cancer patients with a dry mouth:

- Eat foods that are easy to swallow.

- Moisten food with sauce, gravy, or salad dressing.

- Eat foods and drinks that are very sweet or tart, such as lemonade, to help make more saliva.

- Chew gum or suck on hard candy, ice pops, or ice chips.

- Sip water throughout the day.
- Do not drink any type of alcohol, beer, or wine.
- Do not eat foods that can hurt your mouth (such as spicy, sour, salty, hard, or crunchy foods).
- Keep your lips moist with lip balm.
- Rinse your mouth every one to two hours. Do not use mouthwash that contains alcohol.
- Do not use tobacco products and avoid secondhand smoke.
- Ask your doctor or dentist about using artificial saliva or similar products to coat, protect, and moisten your mouth and throat.

Mouth Sores

The following can help patients who have mouth sores:

- Eat soft foods that are easy to chew, such as milkshakes, scrambled eggs, and custards.
- Cook foods until soft and tender.
- Cut food into small pieces. Use a blender or food processor to make food smooth.
- Suck on ice chips to numb and soothe your mouth.
- Eat foods cold or at room temperature. Hot foods can hurt your mouth.
- Drink with a straw to move liquid past the painful parts of your mouth.
- Use a small spoon to help you take smaller bites, which are easier to chew.
- Stay away from the following:
  - Citrus foods, such as oranges, lemons, and limes
  - Spicy foods
  - Tomatoes and ketchup
  - Salty foods
  - Raw vegetables
  - Sharp and crunchy foods
  - Drinks with alcohol

- Do not use tobacco products.

- Visit a dentist at least two weeks before starting immunotherapy, chemotherapy, or radiation therapy to the head and neck.

- Check your mouth each day for sores, white patches, or puffy and red areas.

- Rinse your mouth three to four times a day. Mix ¼ teaspoon baking soda, teaspoon salt, and one cup warm water for a mouth rinse. Do not use mouthwash that contains alcohol.

- Do not use toothpicks or other sharp objects.

Taste Changes

The following may help cancer patients who have taste changes:

- Eat poultry, fish, eggs, and cheese instead of red meat.

- Add spices and sauces to foods (marinate foods).

- Eat meat with something sweet, such as cranberry sauce, jelly, or applesauce.

- Try tart foods and drinks.

- Use sugar-free lemon drops, gum, or mints if there is a metallic or bitter taste in your mouth.

- Use plastic utensils and do not drink directly from metal containers if foods have a metal taste.

- Try to eat your favorite foods, if you are not nauseated. Try new foods when feeling your best.

- Find nonmeat, high-protein recipes in a vegetarian or Chinese cookbook.

- Chew food longer to allow more contact with taste buds, if food tastes dull but not unpleasant.

- Keep food and drinks covered, drink through a straw, turn a kitchen fan on when cooking, or cook outdoors if smells bother you.

- Brush your teeth and take care of your mouth. Visit your dentist for checkups.

Sore Throat and Trouble Swallowing

The following may help cancer patients who have a sore throat or trouble swallowing:

- Eat soft foods that are easy to chew and swallow, such as milkshakes, scrambled eggs, oatmeal, or other cooked cereals.

- Eat foods and drinks that are high in protein and calories.

- Moisten food with gravy, sauces, broth, or yogurt.

- Stay away from the following foods and drinks that can burn or scratch your throat:

  - Hot foods and drinks

  - Spicy foods

  - Foods and juices that are high in acid

  - Sharp or crunchy foods

  - Drinks with alcohol

- Cook foods until soft and tender.

- Cut food into small pieces. Use a blender or food processor to make food smooth.

- Drink with a straw.

- Eat 5 or 6 small meals every day instead of 3 large meals.

- Sit upright and bend your head slightly forward when eating or drinking, and stay upright for at least 30 minutes after eating.

- Do not use tobacco.

- Talk to your doctor about tube feedings if you cannot eat enough to stay strong.

Lactose Intolerance

The following may help patients who have symptoms of lactose intolerance:

- Use lactose-free or low-lactose milk products. Most grocery stores carry food (such as milk and ice cream) labeled "lactose free" or "low lactose."

- Choose milk products that are low in lactose, such as hard cheeses (e.g., cheddar) and yogurt.

- Try products made with soy or rice (such as soy and rice milk and frozen desserts). These products do not contain lactose.

- Avoid dairy products that give you problems. Eat small portions of dairy products, such as milk, yogurt, or cheese, if you can.

- Try nondairy drinks and foods with calcium added.

- Eat calcium-rich vegetables, such as broccoli and greens.

- Take lactase tablets when eating or drinking dairy products. Lactase breaks down lactose so it is easier to digest.

- Prepare your own low-lactose or lactose-free foods.

Weight Gain

The following may help cancer patients prevent weight gain:

- Eat a lot of fruits and vegetables.

- Eat foods that are high in fiber, such as whole-grain breads, cereals, and pasta.

- Choose lean meats, such as lean beef, pork trimmed of fat, and poultry (such as chicken or turkey) without skin.

- Choose low-fat milk products.

- Eat less fat (eat only small amounts of butter, mayonnaise, desserts, and fried foods).

- Cook with low-fat methods, such as broiling, steaming, grilling, or roasting.

- Eat less salt.

- Eat foods that you enjoy so you feel satisfied.

- Eat only when hungry. Consider counseling or medicine if you eat because of stress, fear, or depression. If you eat because you are bored, find activities you enjoy.

- Eat smaller amounts of food at meals.

- Exercise daily.

- Talk with your doctor before going on a diet to lose weight.

Types of Nutrition Support

Nutrition support helps patients who cannot eat or digest food normally. It is best to take in food by mouth whenever possible. Some patients may not be able to take in enough food by mouth because of problems from cancer or cancer treatment. Nutrition support can be given in different ways. In addition to counseling by a dietitian, and changes to the diet, nutrition therapy includes nutritional supplement drinks, and enteral and parenteral nutrition support. Nutritional supplement drinks help cancer patients get the nutrients they need. They provide energy, protein, fat, carbohydrates, fiber, vitamins, and minerals. They are not meant to be the patient's only source of nutrition.

A patient who is not able to take in the right amount of calories and nutrients by mouth may be fed using the following:

- **Enteral nutrition:** Nutrients are given through a tube inserted into the stomach or intestines.

- **Parenteral nutrition:** Nutrients are infused into the bloodstream.

The nutrients are given in liquid formulas that have water, protein, fats, carbohydrates, vitamins, and/or minerals. Nutrition support can improve a patient's quality of life during cancer treatment, but may cause problems that should be considered before making the decision to use it. The patient and healthcare team should discuss the harms and benefits of each type of nutrition support.

Enteral Nutrition

Enteral nutrition is also called "tube feeding."

Enteral nutrition is giving the patient nutrients in liquid form (formula) through a tube that is placed into the stomach or small intestine. The following types of feeding tubes may be used:

- A nasogastric tube is inserted through the nose and down the throat into the stomach or small intestine. This is used when enteral nutrition is only needed for a few weeks.

- A gastrostomy tube is inserted into the stomach or a jejunostomy tube is inserted into the small intestine through an opening made on the outside of the abdomen. This is usually used for long-term enteral feeding or for patients who cannot use a tube in the nose and throat.

The type of formula used is based on the specific needs of the patient. There are formulas for patients who have special health conditions, such as diabetes, or other needs, such as religious or cultural diets.

Parenteral Nutrition

Parenteral nutrition carries nutrients directly into the bloodstream. Parenteral nutrition is used when the patient cannot take food by mouth or by enteral feeding. Parenteral feeding does not use the stomach or intestines to digest food. Nutrients are given to the patient directly into the blood, through a catheter inserted into a vein. These nutrients include proteins, fats, vitamins, and minerals.

The catheter may be placed into a vein in the chest or in the arm. A central venous access catheter is placed beneath the skin and into a large vein in the upper chest. The catheter is put in place by a surgeon. This type of catheter is used for long-term parenteral feeding.

The patient is checked often for infection or bleeding at the place where the catheter enters the body.

Medicines to Treat Loss of Appetite and Weight Loss
Nutrition Therapy

Medicine may be given with nutrition therapy to treat loss of appetite and weight loss. It is important that cancer symptoms and side effects that affect eating and cause weight loss are treated early. Both nutrition therapy and medicine can help lessen the effects that cancer and its treatment have on weight loss.

Medication

Different types of medicine may be used to treat loss of appetite and weight loss. Medicines that improve appetite and cause weight gain, such as prednisone and megestrol, may be used to treat loss of appetite and weight loss. Studies have shown that the effect of these medicines may not last long or there may be no effect. Treatment with a combination of medicines may work better than treatment with one medicine. Patients who are treated with a combination of medicines may have more side effects.

Nutrition Needs at End of Life
Nutrition Needs Change

For patients at the end of life, the goals of nutrition therapy are focused on relieving symptoms rather than getting enough nutrients.

Common symptoms that can occur at the end of life include the following:

- Anorexia (loss of appetite)

- Dry mouth

- Swallowing problems

- Nausea

- Vomiting

Patients who have problems swallowing may find it easier to swallow thick liquids than thin liquids.

Patients often do not feel much hunger at all and may need very little food. Sips of water, ice chips, and mouth care can decrease thirst in the last few days of life. Good communication with the healthcare team is important to understand the patient's changes in nutrition needs.

Patients and Families Decide Regarding Nutrition

Patients and families decide how much nutrition and fluids will be given at the end of life. Cancer patients and their caregivers have the right to make informed decisions. The patient's religious and cultural preferences may affect their decisions. The healthcare team may work with the patient's religious and cultural leaders when making decisions. The healthcare team and a registered dietitian can explain the benefits and risks of using nutrition support for patients at the end of life. In most cases, there are more harms than benefits.

The risks of nutrition support at the end of life include the following:

- Sepsis (bacteria or their toxins in the blood or tissues) with the use of parenteral nutrition

- Aspiration (the accidental breathing in of food or fluid into the lungs) with the use of enteral nutrition

- Sores and breakdown of the skin where the enteral feeding tube is inserted

- Diarrhea with the use of enteral and parenteral nutrition

- Complications caused by fluid overload (a condition where there is too much fluid in the blood) with the use of enteral and parenteral nutrition

Nutrition Trends in Cancer
Some Cancer Patients Try Special Diets to Improve Their Prognosis

Cancer patients may try special diets to make their treatment work better, prevent side effects from treatment, or to treat the cancer itself. However, for most of these special diets, there is no evidence that shows they work.

Vegetarian or Vegan Diet

It is not known if following a vegetarian or vegan diet can help side effects from cancer treatment or the patient's prognosis. If the patient already follows a vegetarian or vegan diet, there is no evidence that shows they should switch to a different diet.

Macrobiotic Diet

A macrobiotic diet is a high-carbohydrate, low-fat, plant-based diet. No studies have shown that this diet will help cancer patients.

Ketogenic Diet

A ketogenic diet limits carbohydrates and increases fat intake. The purpose of the diet is to decrease the amount of glucose (sugar) the tumor cells can use to grow and reproduce. It is a hard diet to follow because exact amounts of fats, carbohydrates and proteins are needed. However, the diet is safe.

Several clinical trials are recruiting glioblastoma patients to study whether a ketogenic diet affects glioblastoma tumor activity. Patients with glioblastoma who want to start a ketogenic diet should talk to their doctor and work with a registered dietitian. However, it is not yet known how the diet will affect the tumor or its symptoms.

Some Cancer Patients May Take Dietary Supplements

A dietary supplement is a product that is added to the diet. It is usually taken by mouth, and usually has one or more dietary ingredients. Cancer patients may take dietary supplements to improve their symptoms or treat their cancer.

Vitamin C

Vitamin C is a nutrient that the body needs in small amounts to function and stay healthy. It helps fight infection, heal wounds, and keep tissues healthy. Vitamin C is found in fruits and vegetables. It can also be taken as a dietary supplement.

Probiotics

Probiotics are live microorganisms used as dietary supplements to help with digestion and normal bowel function. They may also help keep the gastrointestinal tract healthy.

Studies have shown that taking probiotics during radiation therapy and chemotherapy can help prevent diarrhea caused by those treatments. This is especially true for patients receiving radiation therapy to the abdomen. Cancer patients who are receiving radiation therapy to the abdomen or chemotherapy that is known to cause diarrhea may be helped by probiotics.

Melatonin

Melatonin is a hormone made by the pineal gland (tiny organ near the center of the brain). Melatonin helps control the body's sleep cycle. It can also be made in a laboratory and taken as a dietary supplement.

Several small studies have shown that taking a melatonin supplement with chemotherapy and/or radiation therapy for treatment of solid tumors may be helpful. It may help reduce side effects of treatment. Melatonin does not appear to have side effects.

Oral Glutamine

Oral glutamine is an amino acid that is being studied for the treatment of diarrhea and mucositis (inflammation of the lining of the digestive system, often seen as mouth sores) caused by chemotherapy or radiation therapy. Oral glutamine may help prevent mucositis or make it less severe.

Cancer patients who are receiving radiation therapy to the abdomen may benefit from oral glutamine. Oral glutamine may reduce the severity of diarrhea. This can help the patients continue with their treatment plan.

Chapter 15

Delirium

Chapter Contents

Section 15.1—What Is Delirium?.. 150
Section 15.2—Delirium among Cancer Patients...................... 155

Section 15.1

What Is Delirium?

This section contains text excerpted from the following sources: Text beginning with the heading "Delirium—Sudden Confusion or Change in Behavior" is excerpted from "Delirium or Sudden Confusion in Elderly Adults," U.S. Department of Veterans Affairs (VA), June 13, 2018; Text under the heading "Delirium in Older Patients" is excerpted from "The Dilemma of Delirium in Older Patients," National Institute on Aging (NIA), National Institutes of Health (NIH), August 26, 2013. Reviewed September 2019.

Delirium—Sudden Confusion or Change in Behavior

For elderly adults who have dementia, feeling confused may be expected. But when the confusion comes on suddenly, or the older adult becomes difficult to arouse, this could be a condition called "delirium." This type of sudden confusion may be the first sign that the person has another illness and needs medical help right away.

One myth we often hear about aging is that it is not unusual to be confused when you are old. It is true that we can expect many changes as part of normal aging. But a sudden change in cognitive function—or the way we think and process information—is not one of them.

Even if there has simply been a change in the elder's thinking or behavior, most caregivers and family members will know that something is not right. It is important to contact a doctor as soon as possible so that she or he can find the cause of the delirium and treat the underlying problem. This section will help you learn more about how to recognize when sudden confusion is an emergency and what you can do about it.

When Is Delirium an Emergency?

If you notice that an elderly adult has become suddenly confused or is not acting like her/himself, you may need to get help. Signs to watch for include:

• They cannot focus on attention or make eye contact

• You cannot fully wake them up

• They are mumbling or their speech does not make sense

• They are seeing or hearing things that are not there

• They have become agitated without any obvious cause

Behavior like this may be the first sign of a medical emergency called "sudden confusion" or "delirium."

- Elderly adults who have any of these symptoms should see their primary care doctor right away

- If you notice any of these symptoms in the hospital, tell a staff member immediately

It is important to remember that sudden confusion is different than other common changes in thinking that can happen as we age, such as dementia. With dementia, confusion happens slowly over time. With sudden confusion that needs medical treatment, the older adult's thinking abilities change quickly, often with no warning.

What Should I Do When Faced with Delirium?

Sudden confusion in seniors can be very scary—both for the person who experiences it and the loved ones who witness it. Get medical help as soon as possible, then focus on keeping the older adult safe while they are confused.

People with sudden confusion may focus inward, showing a lack of interest in or attention to the things around them. Or they may become restless and agitated, reacting strongly to things they see, hear, or feel. It is important to remember that feeling confused can be frightening. Do your best to remain calm as you try to figure out the cause of their distress.

Some people with sudden confusion may punch, yell, kick, or act aggressively. That is why it is important to focus on keeping the confused person safe until you find out what is causing their distress. If possible, try to help them walk or change positions since this may help ease discomfort. You may try to gently reorient the person to reality, but remember that their confusion may cause them to see reality in a different way. It will help comfort them to meet them in their world until the confusion is resolved.

Can Delirium Be Prevented?

You can take a few simple steps to avoid—or help your loved ones avoid—sudden confusion.

Knowing the risk factors for sudden confusion is the first step. These include:

- Older age

- Dementia
- Sudden confusion in the past
- Multiple medications
- Problems seeing or hearing
- Not getting enough to eat or drink
- Chronic physical illness
- Alcohol or drug use
- Depression
- Problems in the brain or nervous system
- Functional disability

Steps to Counter Risk Factors of Delirium

- Making sure the elderly adult gets enough calories and fluids
- Correcting vision or hearing problems with glasses, hearing aids, or other devices
- Helping ensure the elderly adult has good sleep habits and does not become overly tired or nap excessively during the day
- Trying to involve the elderly adult in activities that challenge the brain, like puzzles, reading, talking about current events, or sharing memories of the past
- Reviewing medications and dosages carefully at each doctor visit and asking questions to help make sure they are not given any longer than necessary

Having one or more risk factors makes an elderly adult more likely to develop sudden confusion. But a sudden event, such as a severe illness, infection, or fracture is often what disrupts the brain and causes sudden confusion. This type of confusion is a medical emergency. It is important to identify the cause quickly and to start treatment as soon as possible.

Delirium in Older Patients

Ill and hospitalized older people sometimes experience episodes of delirium, a state of confusion and disorientation. For centuries considered a transient and reversible condition, delirium in older people is still viewed by many to be a normal consequence of surgery, chronic disease, or infections.

There is mounting evidence, however, that delirium may be associated with increased risk for dementia and may contribute to morbidity and death. A study found that in a group of 553 people age 85 and older, those with a history of delirium had an eight-fold increase in risk for developing dementia. The researchers also found that among the participants with dementia, delirium was associated with an acceleration of dementia severity, loss of independent functioning, and higher mortality. These findings showed that delirium is a strong risk factor for dementia and cognitive decline in the oldest old.

Growing Momentum and Awareness of Delirium

At the National Institute on Aging (NIA) and throughout the geriatric research community, momentum is building to better understand the mechanisms involved in delirium and to improve ways to recognize and treat the condition.

National Institute on Aging supports several clinical trials focused on finding effective drugs and protocols to prevent or reduce the impact of delirium in hospitalized older people. The goal is to identify a variety of interventions that reduce delirium for patients in intensive care, including the testing of supplements, pain medications, and sedatives that may alleviate delirium in pre and postoperative patients.

"The research and medical communities are becoming more aware and interested in the impact delirium may have on the long-term cognitive health of older patients," said Dr. Molly Wagster, chief of NIA's Behavioral and Systems Neuroscience Branch."

"At this stage, unfortunately, there are more questions than answers. In order to treat or prevent delirium, it will be important to determine why some older people are more susceptible to developing it during hospital stays or as a result of trauma or illness."

In addition to supporting the clinical trials, NIA, in collaboration with the American Geriatrics Society (AGS), sponsored a conference on delirium in early 2014 through a cooperative grant mechanism. As part of the AGS Bedside-to-Bench conference series, the meeting covered a wide array of delirium-related research topics, including biomarkers, genetic risk factors, neuroimaging, inflammation, brain injuries, drug and nondrug interventions, and animal models. Recommendations from the meeting will inform research on this topic for years to come.

These activities join efforts already underway of the American Delirium Society (ADS), a group formed by researchers and clinicians seeking better understanding of the science of delirium and its prevention, treatment, and long-term consequences. The group hosts an annual conference that draws a mix of clinicians and scientists from many different disciplines and specialties.

Attitudes about Delirium Evolving

Dr. Joseph Flaherty of the Division of Geriatrics at Saint Louis University, a leading member of ADS, says that attitudes about delirium are slowly evolving among medical practitioners.

"As a medical student 20 years ago, I was taught delirium was completely reversible. That is simply not the case for many older patients," he said. "Over the past 15 years, interest has grown in identifying ways not only to reverse the condition, but to prevent it from occurring in the first place."

He applauds NIA funding of delirium drug trials, but also suggests that changes in nursing and hospital protocols today could help prevent the onset or reduce the severity of delirium.

"Changing the hospital environment and culture to match what the older patient with delirium or at risk for delirium needs is critical," Dr. Flaherty said."

Examples of such changes include allowing hospitalized older people to sleep undisturbed between 10 p.m. and 6 a.m. so that their normal sleep cycle is less disrupted, not using physical restraints, and giving staff concrete nonpharmacologic methods to deal with agitation that may occur with delirium.

"There are very promising, nonpharmacological methods being tested that may enable hospitals and nursing facilities to prevent, treat, and manage delirium," he said. "For example, the new standard in intensive care units (ICUs) is to get patients up and out of their beds within 1 to 2 days, even if they are connected to a ventilator. This reduces the number of days with delirium and time spent in intensive care."

Dr. Flaherty said these new methods may also improve the odds of regaining normal cognitive as well as physical function.

Section 15.2

Delirium among Cancer Patients

This section includes text excerpted from "Delirium and Cancer Treatment," National Cancer Institute (NCI), September 14, 2018.

Delirium is a confused mental state that includes changes in awareness, thinking, judgment, sleeping patterns, as well as behavior. Although delirium can happen at the end of life, many episodes of delirium are caused by medicine or dehydration and are reversible.

The symptoms of delirium usually occur suddenly (within hours or days) over a short period of time and may come and go. Although delirium may be mistaken for depression or dementia, these conditions are different and have different treatments.

Types of Delirium

The three main types of delirium include:

- Hypoactive delirium: The patient seems sleepy, tired, or depressed

- Hyperactive delirium: The patient is restless, anxious, or suddenly agitated and uncooperative

- Mixed delirium: The patient changes back and forth between hypoactive delirium and hyperactive delirium

Causes of Delirium

Your healthcare team will work to find out what is causing delirium, so that it can be treated. Causes of delirium may include:

- Advanced cancer

- Older age

- Brain tumors

- Dehydration

- Infection

- Taking certain medicines, such as high doses of opioids

- Withdrawal from or stopping certain medicines

155

Early monitoring of someone with these risk factors for delirium may prevent it or allow it to be treated more quickly.

Changes caused by delirium can be upsetting for family members and dangerous to the person with cancer, especially if judgment is affected. People with delirium may be more likely to fall, unable to control their bladder and/or bowels, and more likely to become dehydrated. Their confused state may make it difficult to talk with others about their needs and make decisions about care. Family members may need to be more involved in decision-making.

Ways to Treat Delirium in People with Cancer

Steps that can be taken to treat symptoms related to delirium include:

- **Treat the causes of delirium:** If medicines are causing delirium, then reducing the dose or stopping them may treat delirium. If conditions such as dehydration, poor nutrition, and infections are causing the delirium, then treating these may help.

- **Control surroundings:** If the symptoms of delirium are mild, it may help to keep the room quiet and well lit, with a clock or calendar and familiar possessions. Having family members around and keeping the same caregivers, as much as possible, may also help.

- **Consider medicines:** Medicines are sometimes given to treat the symptoms of delirium. However, these medicines have serious side effects and patients receiving them require careful observation by a doctor.

- **Sometimes sedation may help:** After discussion with family members, sedation is sometimes used for delirium at the end of life, if it does not get better with other treatments. The doctor will discuss the decisions involved in using sedation to treat delirium with the family.

Part Three

Medical Decisions Surrounding the End of Life

Chapter 16

Preferences for Care at the End of Life

Patients with Chronic Illness Need Advance Planning

The majority of people who die in the United States (80 to 85 percent) are Medicare beneficiaries age 65 and over, and most die from chronic conditions, such as heart disease, cerebrovascular disease, chronic obstructive pulmonary disease (COPD), diabetes, Alzheimer disease (AD), and renal failure. Only about 22 percent of deaths in people aged 65 and over are from cancer.

People with terminal cancer generally follow an expected course, or "trajectory," of dying. Many maintain their activities of daily living until about two months prior to death, after which most functional disability occurs.

In contrast, people with chronic diseases such as heart disease or COPD go through periods of slowly declining health marked by sudden severe episodes of illness requiring hospitalization, from which the patient recovers. This pattern may repeat itself over and over, with the patient's overall health steadily declining, until the patient dies. For these individuals, there is considerable uncertainty about when death is likely to occur.

This chapter includes text excerpted from "Advance Care Planning, Preferences for Care at the End of Life," Agency for Healthcare Research and Quality (AHRQ), U.S. Department of Health and Human Services (HHS), March 12, 2003. Reviewed September 2019.

Patients who suffer from chronic conditions, such as stroke, dementia, or the frailty of old age go through a third trajectory of dying, marked by a steady decline in mental and physical ability that finally results in death. Patients are not often told that their chronic disease is terminal, and estimating a time of death for people suffering from chronic conditions is much more difficult than it is for those dying of cancer.

When patients are hospitalized for health crises resulting from their chronic incurable disease, medical treatment cannot cure the underlying illness, but it is still effective in resolving the immediate emergency and thus possibly extending the patient's life. At any one of these crises the patient may be close to death, yet there often is no clearly recognizable threshold between being very ill and actually dying. Patients may become too incapacitated to speak for themselves, and decisions about which treatments to provide or withhold are usually made jointly between the patient's physician and family or surrogate.

Patients Value Advance Care Planning Discussions

According to patients who are dying and their families who survive them, lack of communication with physicians and other healthcare providers causes confusion about medical treatments, conditions and prognoses, and the choices that patients and their families need to make. One Agency for Healthcare Research and Quality (AHRQ) study indicated that about one-third of patients would discuss advance care planning if the physician brought up the subject and about one-fourth of patients had been under the impression that advance care planning was only for people who were very ill or very old. Only five percent of patients stated that they found discussions about advance care planning too difficult.

Many AHRQ-funded studies have shown that discussing advance care planning and directives with their doctor increased patient satisfaction among patients age 65 years and over. Patients who talked with their families or physicians about their preferences for end-of-life care:

- Experienced less fear and anxiety

- Felt they had more ability to influence and direct their medical care

- Believed that their physicians had a better understanding of their wishes

- Indicated a greater understanding and comfort level than they had before the discussion

Compared to surrogates of patients who did not have an advance directive, surrogates of patients with an advance directive who had discussed its content with the patient, reported greater understanding, better confidence in their ability to predict the patient's preferences, and a stronger belief in the importance of having an advance directive.

Finally, patients who had advance planning discussions with their physicians continued to discuss and talk about these concerns with their families. Such discussions enabled patients and families to reconcile their differences in end-of-life care and could help the family and physician come to an agreement if they should need to make decisions for the patient.

Opportunities Exist for Advance Planning Discussions

Many AHRQ studies indicate that physicians can conduct advance care planning discussions with some patients during routine outpatient office visits. Hospitalization for a serious and progressive illness offers another opportunity. The Patient Self-Determination Act (PSDA) requires facilities such as hospitals that accept Medicare and Medicaid money to provide written information to all patients concerning their rights under State law to refuse or accept treatment and to complete advance directives.

Patients often send cues to their physicians that they are ready to discuss end-of-life care by talking about wanting to die or asking about hospice. Certain situations, such as approaching death or discussions about prognoses or treatment options that have poor outcomes, also lend themselves to advance care planning discussions. Predicting when patients are near death is difficult, but providers can ask themselves the question: are the patients "sick enough today that it would not be surprising to find that they had died within the next year (or few months, or 6 months)?"

A Structured Process for Discussions Is Helpful

Researchers sponsored by AHRQ have suggested a five-part process that physicians can use to structure discussions on end-of-life care:

1. **Initiate a guided discussion.** During this discussion, the physicians should share their medical knowledge of hypothetical scenarios and treatments applicable to a patient's particular situation and find out the patient's preferences for

providing or withholding treatments under certain situations. The hypothetical scenarios should cover a range of possible prognoses and any disability that could result from treatment. By presenting various hypothetical scenarios and probable treatments and noting when the patient's preferences change from "treat" to "do not treat," the physician can begin to identify the patient's personal preferences and values.

The physician can also determine if the patient has an adequate understanding of the scenario, the treatment, and possible outcomes. One AHRQ-funded study indicated that elderly patients have enough knowledge about advance directives, cardiopulmonary resuscitation (CPR), and artificial nutrition/hydration on which to base decisions for treatment at the end of life, but they do not always understand their realistic chances for a positive outcome. Other research indicates that patients significantly overestimate their probability of survival after receiving CPR and have little or no understanding of mechanical ventilation. In one study, after patients were told their probability of survival, over half changed their treatment preference from wanting CPR to refusing CPR. Patients also may not know of the risks associated with the use of mechanical ventilation that a physician is aware of, such as neurological impairment or cardiac arrest.

2. **Introduce the subject of advance care planning and offer information.** Patients should be encouraged to complete both an advance directive and durable power of attorney. The patient should understand that when no advance directive or durable power of attorney exists, patients essentially leave treatment decisions to their physicians and family members. Physicians can provide this information themselves; refer the patient to other educational sources, including brochures or videos; and recommend that the patient talk with the clergy or a social worker to answer questions or address concerns.

3. **Prepare and complete advance care planning documents.** Advance care planning documents should contain specific instructions. AHRQ studies indicate that the standard language contained in advance directives often is not specific enough to be effective in directing care. Many times, instructions do not state the cutoff point of the patient's illness

that should be used to discontinue treatment and allow the person to die. Terms such as "no advanced life support" are too vague to offer guidance on specific treatments. If a patient does not want to be on a ventilator, the physician should ask the patient if this is true under all circumstances or only specific circumstances. One AHRQ-funded study found that because patient preferences were not clear in advance directives, life-sustaining treatment was discontinued only when it was clearly medically futile.

4. **Review the patient's preferences on a regular basis and update documentation.** Patients should be reminded that advance directives can be revised at any time. Although AHRQ studies show that patients' preferences were stable over time when considering hypothetical situations, other research indicates that patients often changed their minds when confronted with the actual situation or as their health status changed. Some patients who stated that they would rather die than endure a certain condition did not choose death once that condition occurred.

    Other research shows that patients who had an advance directive maintained stable treatment preferences 86 percent of the time over a two year period, while patients who did not have an advance directive changed their preferences 59 percent of the time. Both patients with and patients without a living will be more likely to change their preferences and desire increased treatment once they became hospitalized, suffered an accident, became depressed, or lost the functional ability or social activity. Another study linked changes in depression to changes in preferences for CPR. Increased depression was associated with patients' changing their initial preference for CPR to a refusal of CPR, while less depression was associated with patients' changing their preference from refusal of CPR to acceptance of CPR. It is difficult for people to fully imagine what a prospective health state might be like. Once they experience that health state, they may find it more or less tolerable than they imagined.

    During reviews of advance directives, physicians should note which preferences stay the same and which change. Preferences that change indicate that the physician needs to investigate the basis for the change.

5. **Apply the patient's desires to actual circumstances.**
   Conflicts sometimes arise during discussions about end-of-life decision-making. AHRQ-sponsored research indicates that if patients desired nonbeneficial treatments or refused beneficial treatments, most physicians stated that they would negotiate with them, trying to educate and convince them to either forgo a nonbeneficial treatment or to accept a beneficial treatment. If the treatment was not harmful, expensive, or complicated, about one-third of physicians would allow the patient to receive a nonbeneficial treatment. Physicians stated that they would also enlist the family's help or seek a second opinion from another physician.

Many patients do not lose their decision-making capacity at the end of life. Physicians and family members can continue discussing treatment preferences with these patients as their condition changes. However, physicians and families may encounter the difficulty of knowing when an advance directive should become applicable for patients who are extremely sick and have lost their decision-making capacity but are not necessarily dying. There is no easy answer to this dilemma. One AHRQ study found that advance directives were invoked only once patients had crossed a threshold to be "absolutely, hopelessly ill." The patients' physicians and surrogates determined that boundary on an individual basis. AHRQ studies have shown that patients' treatment was generally consistent with their preferences if those preferences were clearly stated in an advance directive and the physician was aware that they had an advance directive.

Even if patients require a decision for a situation that was not anticipated and addressed in their advance directive, physicians and surrogates still can make an educated determination based on the knowledge they have about the patients' values, goals, and thresholds for treatment. AHRQ research indicates that patients choose a treatment based on the quality of the prospective health state, the invasiveness and length of treatment, and possible outcomes.

Patients Have Preference Patterns for Hypothetical Situations

Many AHRQ-funded studies indicate that patients are more likely to accept treatment for conditions they consider better than death and to refuse treatment for conditions they consider worse than death. Results from the study conducted on health states considered worse than death. Patients also were more likely to accept treatments that were less invasive, such as CPR, than invasive treatments, such as mechanical ventilation. Patients were more likely to accept short-term or simple treatments, such as antibiotics, than long-term invasive treatments, such as permanent tube feeding.

Patient Preference Patterns Can Predict Other Choices

Acceptance or refusal of invasive and noninvasive treatments under certain circumstances can predict what other choices the patient would make under the same or different circumstances. According to AHRQ research, patients' refusal of noninvasive treatments was predictive of their refusal of invasive treatments, and accepting invasive treatments predicted their acceptance of noninvasive treatments. Refusal of noninvasive treatments, such as antibiotics strongly predicted that invasive treatments, such as major surgery would also be refused. Decisions with the strongest predictive ability were refusing antibiotics or simple tests and accepting major surgery or dialysis.

An AHRQ research also reveals that patients were more likely to refuse treatment under hypothetical conditions as their prognosis became worse. For example, more adults would refuse both invasive and noninvasive treatments for a scenario of dementia with a terminal illness than for dementia only. Adults were also more likely to refuse treatment for a scenario of a persistent vegetative state than for a coma with a chance of recovery. More patients preferred treatment if there was even a slight chance for recovery from a coma or a stroke. Fewer patients would want complicated and invasive treatments if they had a terminal illness. Finally, patients were more likely to want treatment if they would remain cognitively intact rather than impaired.

Chapter 17

End-of-Life Care for Dementia

As they reach the end of life, people suffering from dementia can present special challenges for caregivers. People can live with diseases such as Alzheimer disease (AD) or Parkinson disease-related dementia for years, so it can be hard to think of these as terminal diseases. But, they do cause death.

Making Difficult End-of-Life Decisions for a Person with Dementia

Dementia causes a gradual loss of thinking, remembering, and reasoning abilities, making it difficult for those who want to provide supportive care at the end of life to know what is needed. Because people with advanced dementia can no longer communicate clearly, they cannot share their concerns. Is Uncle Bert refusing food because he is not hungry or because he is confused? Why does Grandma Sakura seem agitated? Is she in pain and needs medication to relieve it, but cannot tell you?

As these conditions progress, caregivers may find it hard to provide emotional or spiritual comfort. How can you let Grandpa know how

This chapter includes text excerpted from "End-of-Life Care for People with Dementia," National Institute on Aging (NIA), National Institutes of Health (NIH), May 17, 2017.

much his life has meant to you? How do you make peace with your mother if she no longer knows who you are? Someone who has severe memory loss might not take spiritual comfort from sharing family memories or understand when others express what an important part of their life this person has been. Palliative care or hospice can be helpful in many ways to families of people with dementia.

Sensory connections—targeting someone's senses, such as hearing, touch, or sight—can bring comfort. Being touched or massaged can be soothing. Listening to music, white noise, or sounds from nature seem to relax some people and lessen their agitation.

When dementia-like AD is first diagnosed, if everyone understands that there is no cure, then plans for the end of life can be made before thinking and speaking abilities fail and the person with AD can no longer legally complete documents, such as advance directives.

End-of-life care decisions are more complicated for caregivers if the dying person has not expressed the kind of care she or he would prefer. Someone newly diagnosed with AD might not be able to imagine the later stages of the disease.

Quality of life (QOL) is an important issue when making healthcare decisions for people with dementia. For example, medicines are available that may delay or keep symptoms from becoming worse for a little while. Medicines also may help control some behavioral symptoms in people with mild-to-moderate AD.

However, some caregivers might not want drugs prescribed for people in the later stages of AD. They may believe that the person's QOL is already so poor that medicine is unlikely to make a difference. If the drug has serious side effects, it may be even more likely to decide against it.

When making care decisions for someone else near the end of life, consider the goals of care and weigh the benefits, risks, and side effects of the treatment. You may have to make a treatment decision based on the person's comfort at one end of the spectrum and extending life or maintaining abilities for a little longer at the other.

With dementia, a person's body may continue to be physically healthy while her or his thinking and memory are deteriorating. This means that caregivers and family members may be faced with very difficult decisions about how treatments that maintain physical health, such as installing a pacemaker, fit within the care goals.

Dementia's Unpredictable Progression

Dementia often progresses slowly and unpredictably. Experts suggest that signs of the final stage of AD include some of the following:

- Being unable to move around on one's own

- Being unable to speak or make oneself understood

- Needing help with most, if not all, daily activities, such as eating and self-care

- Eating problems such as difficulty swallowing

Because of their unique experience with what happens at the end of life, hospice and palliative care experts might be able to help identify when someone in the final stage of AD is in the last days or weeks of life.

Support for Dementia Caregivers at the End of Life

Caring for people with AD or other dementias at home can be demanding and stressful for the family caregiver. Depression is a problem for some family caregivers, as is fatigue because many feel they are always on call. Family caregivers may have to cut back on work hours or leave work altogether because of their caregiving responsibilities.

Many family members taking care of a person with advanced dementia at home feel relief when death happens—for themselves and for the person who died. It is important to realize such feelings are normal. Hospice—whether used at home or in a facility (such as a nursing home)—gives family caregivers needed support near the end of life, as well as help with their grief, both before and after their family member dies.

Chapter 18

End-of-Life Care for Advanced Cancer

Quality Care at the End of Life
What Does Care before Dying Mean?

Your care continues even after all treatments have stopped. End-of-life care is more than what happens moments before dying. Care is needed in the days, weeks, and sometimes even months before death. During this time, many patients feel it is important to:

- Have their pain and symptoms controlled

- Avoid a long process of dying

- Feel a sense of control over what is happening to them

- Cause less emotional and financial burden on the family

- Become closer with loved ones

Your doctors and family need to know the kind of end-of-life care you want.

This chapter includes text excerpted from "Planning the Transition to End-of-Life Care in Advanced Cancer (PDQ®)—Patient Version," National Cancer Institute (NCI), November 24, 2015. Reviewed September 2019.

Making End-of-Life Care Decisions Early

You may be able to think about your options more clearly if you talk about them before the decisions need to be made. It is a good idea to let your doctors, family, and caregivers know your wishes before there is an emergency.

End-of-Life Care Decisions to Be Made
Care Decisions for Advanced Stages of Cancer

Care decisions for the last stages of cancer can be about treatments and procedures, pain control, place of care, and spiritual issues.

Chemotherapy

Some patients choose to begin new chemotherapy treatment in the end stages of cancer. Others wish to let the disease take its course when a cure is not expected. In the end stages of cancer, chemotherapy usually does not help you live longer and it may lower the quality of the time that remains. Each person and each cancer is different. Talking with your doctor about the effects of treatment and your quality of life (QOL) can help you make a decision. You can ask if the treatment will make you comfortable or if it will help you live longer.

Pain and Symptom Control

Controlling pain and other symptoms can help you have a better QOL in the end stages of cancer. Pain and symptom control can be part of your care in any place of care, such as the hospital, home, and hospice.

Cardiopulmonary Resuscitation

It is important to decide if you will want to have cardiopulmonary resuscitation (CPR). CPR is a procedure used to try to restart the heart and breathing when it stops. In advanced cancer, the heart, lungs, and other organs begin to fail and it is harder to restart them with CPR. Your doctor can help you understand how CPR works and talk with you about whether CPR is likely to work for you.

People who are near the end of life may choose not to have CPR done. Your decision about having CPR is personal. Your own spiritual or religious views about death and dying may help you decide. If you decide you do not want CPR, you can ask your doctor to write a do-not-resuscitate (DNR) order. This tells other healthcare professionals not to perform CPR if your heart or breathing stops. You can remove the DNR order at any time.

Talk with your doctors and other caregivers about CPR as early as possible (for example, when being admitted to the hospital), in case you are not able to make the decision later. If you do choose to have your doctor write a DNR, it is important to tell all your family members and caregivers about it.

In the United States, if there is no DNR order, you will be given CPR to keep you alive.

Ventilator Use

A ventilator is a machine used to help you breathe and keep you alive after normal breathing stops. It does not treat a disease or condition. It is used only for life support. You can tell doctors whether you would want to be put on a ventilator if your lungs stop working or if you cannot breathe on your own after CPR. If your goal of care is to live longer, you may choose to have a ventilator used. Or you may choose to have a ventilator for only a certain length of time. It is important to tell your family and healthcare providers what you want before you have trouble breathing.

Religious and Spiritual Support

Your religious or spiritual beliefs may help you with end of life decisions. Clergy and chaplains can give counseling. You can also talk with a member of your church, a social worker, or even other people who have cancer.

Talking with Your Doctor about End-of-Life Care
Starting the Conversation

Some doctors do not ask patients about end-of-life issues. If you want to make choices about these issues, talk with your doctors so that your wishes can be carried out. Open communication can help you and your doctors make decisions together and create a plan of care that meets your goals and wishes. If your doctor is not comfortable talking about end-of-life plans, you can talk to other specialists for help.

Deciding End-of-Life Issues

Prognosis, treatment goals, and making decisions are some of the end-of-life issues to discuss with your doctor.

173

Understanding Prognosis

Having a good understanding of your prognosis is important when making decisions about your care and treatment during advanced cancer. You will probably want to know how long you have to live. That is a hard question for doctors to answer. It can be different for each person and depends on the type of cancer, where it has spread, and whether you have other illnesses. Treatments can work differently for each person. Your doctor can talk about the treatment options with you and your family and explain the effects they may have on your cancer and your quality of life (QOL). Knowing the benefits and risks of available treatments can help you decide on your goals of care for the last stages of cancer.

Deciding on Your Care Goals

Your care goals for advanced cancer depend in part on whether the QOL or length of life is more important to you. Your goals of care may change as your condition changes or if new treatments become available. Tell your doctor what your goals of care are, even if you are not asked. It is important that you and your doctor are working toward the same goals.

Taking Part in Decision-Making

Do you want to take part in making the decisions about your care? Or would you rather have your family and your doctors make those decisions? This is a personal choice and your family and doctors need to know what you want.

Preparing for End-of-Life Issues

Early communication with your doctors can help you feel more prepared for end-of-life issues. Many patients who start talking with their doctors early about end-of-life issues report feeling better prepared. Better communication with your doctors may make it easier to deal with concerns about being older, living alone, relieving symptoms, spiritual well-being, and how your family will cope in the future.

Ways to Improve Communication with Your Doctors

Tell your doctor how you and your family wish to receive information and the type of information you want. Also, ask how you can get information at times when you cannot meet face-to-face.

Remembering what your doctor said and even remembering what you want to ask can be hard to do. Some of the following may help communication and help you remember what was said:

- Have a family member go with you when you meet with your doctor.

- Make a list of the questions you want to ask the doctor during your visit.

- Get the information in writing.

- Record the discussion with tape recorders, smartphones, or on video.

- Ask if your doctor or clinic offers any of the following:

  - A cancer consultation preparation package, which includes aids such as a question idea sheet, booklets on decision making and patient rights, and information about the clinic.

  - A talk with a psychologist about advance planning and end-of-life issues.

  - An end of life preference interview, which includes a list of questions that can help you explain your wishes about the end of life.

Supportive Care, Palliative Care, and Hospice
Care Is Vital Despite No Cure

Even when treatments can no longer cure the cancer, medical care is still needed, such as supportive and palliative care or hospice.

Supportive Care

Supportive care is given to prevent or treat, as early as possible, the symptoms of cancer, side effects caused by treatments, and psychological, social, and spiritual problems related to the cancer or its treatment. During active treatment to cure cancer, supportive care helps you stay healthy and comfortable enough to continue receiving the cancer treatments. In the last stages of cancer, when a cure is no longer the goal, supportive care is used for side effects that continue.

Palliative Care

Palliative care is specialized medical care for people with serious or life-threatening illnesses. The focus of palliative care is relief from pain and other symptoms, both during active treatment and when treatment has been stopped. Palliative care is offered in some hospitals, outpatient centers, and in the home.

Palliative care helps to improve your QOL by preventing and relieving suffering. When you are more comfortable, your family's QOL may also be better. Palliative care includes treating physical symptoms such as pain and helping you and your family with emotional, social, and spiritual concerns. When palliative treatment is given at the end of life, the focus is on relieving symptoms and distress caused by the process of dying and to make sure your goals of care are followed.

Hospice Care

When treatment is no longer helping, you may choose hospice. Hospice is a program that gives care to people who are near the end of life and have stopped treatment to cure or control their cancer. Hospice care focuses on QOL rather than the length of life. The hospice team offers physical, emotional, and spiritual support for patients who are expected to live no longer than six months. The goal of hospice is to help patients live each day to the fullest by making them comfortable and relieving their symptoms. This may include supportive and palliative care to control pain and other symptoms so you can be as alert and comfortable as possible. Services to help with the emotional, social, and spiritual needs of you and your family are also an important part of hospice care.

Hospice programs are designed to keep the patient at home with family and friends, but hospice care may also be given in hospice centers and in some hospitals and nursing homes. The hospice team includes doctors, nurses, spiritual advisors, social workers, nutritionists, and volunteers. Team members are specially trained on issues that occur at the end of life. The hospice program continues to give help, including grief counseling, to the family after their loved one dies. Ask your doctor for information if you wish to receive hospice care.

Advance Planning
Early Decisions Decrease Stress

Making end-of-life care decisions early can ease your mind and decrease stress on your family. There may come a time when you cannot tell the healthcare team what you want. When that happens, would you prefer to have your doctor and family make decisions? Or would you rather make decisions early, so your wishes will be known and can be followed when the time comes? If not planned far ahead of time, the end-of-life decisions must be made by someone other than you.

Planning ahead for end-of-life care helps with the following:

- Makes sure your doctors and family know what your wishes are

- Allows you to refuse the use of treatments

- Decreases the emotional stress on your family, who would have to make decisions if you are not able to

- Reduces the cost of care, if you choose not to receive life-saving procedures

- Eases your mind to have these decisions already made

You can make your wishes known with an advance directive.

Advance Directives Entail the Wishes of the Dying

Advance directives are documents that state what your wishes are for certain medical treatments when you can no longer communicate those wishes. The "advance directive" is a general term for different types of documents that state what your wishes are for certain medical treatments when you can no longer tell those wishes to your caregivers. In addition to decisions about relieving symptoms at the end of life, it is also helpful to decide if and when you want certain treatments to stop. Advance directives make sure your wishes about treatments and life-saving procedures to keep you alive are known ahead of time. Without knowing your wishes, doctors will do everything medically possible to keep you alive, such as cardiopulmonary resuscitation (CPR) and the use of a ventilator (breathing machine).

Each state has its own laws for advance directives. Make sure your advance directives follow the laws of the state where you live and are being treated.

The following are types of documents that communicate your wishes in advance:

- **Living will:** A legal document that states whether you want certain life-saving medical treatments to be used or not used under certain circumstances. Some of the treatments covered by a living will include CPR, use of a ventilator (breathing machine), and tube-feeding.

- **Healthcare proxy (HCP):** A document in which you choose a person (called a "proxy") to make medical decisions if you become unable to do so. It is important that your proxy knows your values and wishes so that she or he can make the decisions you would make if you were able. You do not have to state specific decisions about individual treatments in the document, just state that the proxy will make medical decisions for you. HCP is also known as a "durable power of attorney for healthcare" (DPOAHC) or "medical power of attorney" (MPOA).

- **Do-not-resuscitate (DNR) order:** A document that tells medical staff in the hospital not to do cardiopulmonary resuscitation (CPR) if your heart or breathing stops. A DNR order is a decision only about CPR. It does not affect other treatments that may be used to keep you alive, such as medicine or food.

- **Out-of-hospital DNR order:** A document that tells emergency medical workers outside of a hospital that you do not wish to have CPR or other types of resuscitation. Each state has its own rules for a legal out-of-hospital DNR order, but it is usually signed by the patient, a witness, and the doctor. It is best to have several copies so one can quickly be given to emergency medical workers when needed.

- **Do-not-intubate (DNI) order:** A document that tells medical staff in a hospital or nursing facility that you do not wish to have a breathing tube inserted and to be put on a ventilator (breathing machine).

- **Physician Orders for Life-Sustaining Treatment (POLST):** A form that states what kind of medical treatment you want toward the end of your life. It is signed by you and your doctor.

- **Medical Orders for Life-Sustaining Treatment (MOLST):** A form that states the care you would like to receive if you are not able to communicate. This care includes CPR, intubation (breathing tubes), and other life-saving procedures. Under current law, the information in a MOLST form must be followed both in the home and hospital by all medical staff, including emergency medical workers.

Making Caregivers Aware of Advance Directives

All your caregivers need to have copies of your advance directives. Give copies of your advance directives to your doctors, caregivers, and family members. Advance directives need to move with you. If your doctors or your place of care changes, copies of your advance directives need to be given to your new caregivers. This will make sure that your wishes are known through all cancer stages and places of care. You can change or cancel an advance directive at any time.

The Transition to End-of-Life Care

The word transition can mean a passage from one place to another. The transition or change from looking toward recovery to receiving end-of-life care is not an easy one and there are important decisions to be made. If you become too sick before you have made your wishes known, others will make care and treatment decisions for you, without knowing what you would have wanted. It may be less stressful for everyone if you, your family, and your healthcare providers have planned ahead for this time.

The goal of end-of-life care is to prevent suffering and relieve symptoms. The right time to transition to end-of-life care is when this supports your changing condition and changing goals of care.

There are certain times when you may think about stopping treatment and transitioning to comfort care. These include:

- Finding out that the cancer is not responding to treatment and that more treatment is not likely to help

- Having poor QOL due to the side effects or complications of treatment

- Being unable to carry out daily activities when the disease progresses

Together with your doctor, you and your family members can share an understanding about treatment choices and when the transition to end-of-life care is the best choice. When you make the decisions and plans, doctors and family members can be sure they are doing what you want.

Chapter 19

HIV/AIDS and End-of-Life Issues

Preparing Patients and Families for Imminent Death
Eliciting and Addressing Patient and Family Caregiver Concerns

Perhaps the most helpful first step in preparing patients and families for imminent death is to elicit their concerns. It may be necessary to precede this discussion with a check on the patient and/or family member's understanding of the clinical situation. Asking patients and family members for their assessment of the clinical situation can be useful in starting a discussion about care for imminent death. Straightforward, open-ended questions are helpful, such as "What are your biggest concerns now?" In addition, it is often useful to specifically probe the following important domains:

• Optimizing physical comfort

• Maintaining a sense of continuity with one's self

• Maintaining and enhancing relationships

This chapter includes text excerpted from "A Clinical Guide to Supportive and Palliative Care for HIV/AIDS," Health Resources and Services Administration (HRSA), 2003. Reviewed September 2019.

- Making meaning of one's life and death

- Achieving a sense of control

- Confronting and preparing for death

Table 19.1 offers useful questions to help healthcare providers discuss these domains with patients and their family members.

Table 19.1. Useful Questions for Exploring Patient and/or Family Concerns

Domain	Question
Physical comfort	Tell me about your pain. Can you rate it on a 10-point scale?
	How much do you suffer from physical symptoms, such as shortness of breath, fatigue, or bowel problems?
Continuity with one's self	What makes life most worth living for you at this time?
	If you were to die sooner rather than later, what would be left undone?
Maintaining and enhancing relationships	How are your family (or loved ones) handling your illness?
	Have you had a chance to tell your family (or loved ones) how they are important to you?
Making meaning of life and death	What kind of legacy do you want to leave behind?
	What would allow you to feel that going through this illness has a purpose?
	Do you have spiritual beliefs that are important in how you deal with this illness?
Achieving a sense of control	How would you like your death to go?
Confronting and preparing for death	How much are you thinking about dying now?
	What are you thinking about it?

Neglect of problems in these domains can lead to depression and difficulty adjusting to the situation for both the patient and family members. The empirical demonstration of the importance of paying attention to these domains is just beginning.

Negotiating a Plan for Care and Contingency Plans for Complications

In addition to assessing the clinical situation, the clinician must also become familiar with patient and family concerns in order to discuss goals of care and develop a plan to meet them. The discussion of goals of care is an important step that should precede the discussion of "do-not-resuscitate" (DNR) orders, and this discussion should address the following issues:

- Physical symptoms, such as pain or dyspnea

- Psychological issues, such as depression or anxiety

- Social issues, such as family coping

- Practical logistics, including the expected place of death

- Spiritual or existential issues, such as chaplain support or sense of accomplishment in life

- Special goals for life closure, such as family quarrels to resolve

It is important to understand how patients and family members balance the quality of life (QOL) with a length of life. Patients and family members should be informed that a peaceful death can often be achieved with medical care that is not intrusive. Family members should further understand that their involvement in care is critical and that there are specific roles that they may play (e.g., physical care and medication administration; helping a patient with leaving a legacy; orchestrating visits from friends; helping with goodbye telephone calls; or, simply being present).

Table 19.2 presents information to help healthcare providers address some of the common concerns for family members of imminently dying patients.

Table 19.2. Common Family Concerns for Family Members of Imminently Dying Patients

Concern	Fact
Dying will be painful.	Most pain can be controlled to a degree that the patient finds acceptable with noninvasive pain medications.
Everything possible must be done.	Some invasive treatments aimed at sustaining life, such as cardiopulmonary resuscitation (CPR), are painful and ineffective for imminently dying patients.

Table 19.2. Continued

Concern	Fact
Do Not Resuscitate orders will mean that medical care will be limited in important ways.	DNR orders can actually allow medical staff and family to focus on issues that are more important for patients, including legacy-building and time for closure with important people.
More medical care will be available in the hospital than at home.	Spending one's last hours at home has a powerful importance for many patients, and most medical issues for dying patients can be handled at home. If complications arise, hospitalization or placement at a hospice facility may be possible.
End-of-life care with home hospice will mean losing contact with primary human immunodeficiency virus (HIV) clinicians.	Contact with important clinicians can still occur with phone calls. Home hospice is directed by the primary physician; it does not mean that they have to lose contact.

Discussions about DNR orders are best set into the larger context of the care plan. Once patients and families understand what medical care will provide, and how they can contribute to care, DNR orders are much less likely to become the focal point for a struggle around how to ensure that a patient is being cared for.

Encouraging Life Closure

Making sense of life is not something that a clinician can do for a patient, but clinicians can facilitate or encourage life review activities for patients and their families. These activities can include the following:

- Telling and sharing stories—events that were important, funny, worth remembering; storytelling can be audiotaped or videotaped for a more permanent kind of legacy

- Deciding what to do with one's things—giving a favorite sweater to a friend, or a treasured stamp collection to a nephew

- Planning the patient's memorial service—music, readings, people who will speak, someone to preside over the service, whether to have a religious service or nondenominational service

Some clinicians use a mnemonic of five important conversations to complete for a peaceful death. These five items themselves lack the context and richness of life, but they are helpful as brief reminders of the kinds of issues that patients may want to talk about with important people before death.

- "Thank you"

- "I forgive you"

- "Please forgive me"

- "I love you"

- "Goodbye"

Finally, most patients recognize some transcendent dimension to life, and addressing spiritual issues can be critical near death. It is helpful to remember that spirituality differs from religion; spirituality refers to an individual's relationship with the transcendent, whereas religion is a set of beliefs, practices, and language that characterize a community searching for transcendent meaning in a particular way. Even though many patients will feel alienated from particular religions, they may yet have a spirituality that can help them make sense of their life and their death. Psychosocial clinicians and chaplains with experience in end-of-life care can be particularly helpful if they are available.

Clinical Management of Imminently Dying Patients
Clinical Recognition of Imminent Death

It is important that the family and patient understand normal landmarks in the dying process and overcome common misperceptions regarding imminent death. One such misperception is the belief that lack of appetite and diminished oral intake are causing profound disability and that fluid and nutrition are required. The normal dying process includes the following changes:

- Loss of appetite

- Decreased oral fluid intake, and decreased thirst

- Increasing weakness and/or fatigue

- Decreasing blood perfusion, including decreased urine output, peripheral cyanosis, and cool extremities

- Neurologic dysfunction, including delirium, lethargy, and coma, and changes in respiratory patterns

- Loss of ability to close eyes

- Noisy breathing as pharyngeal muscles relax

In particular, neurologic dysfunction can sometimes result in terminal delirium which can include a mounting syndrome of confusion, hallucinations, delirium, myoclonic jerks, and seizures prior to death. Recognized early, this can be treated with neuroleptics, such as haloperidol or chlorpromazine.

When death occurs, the clinical signs include the following:

- Absence of heartbeat and respiration

- Fixed pupils

- Skin color turns to a waxen pallor and extremities may darken

- Body temperature drops

- Muscles and sphincters relax, sometimes resulting in the release of stool or urine

Preparation, which can involve the family, should include the following:

- Creating a peaceful environment to the patient's liking

- Preparing instructions about whom to call (usually not 911) when death occurs

- Taking time to witness what is happening

- Creating or using rituals that can help mark the occasion in a respectful way

When a death occurs, families should be encouraged to take whatever time they need to feel what has happened, and say their goodbyes. There is no need to rush the body to a funeral home, and some families want to stay with the body for a period of time after death.

Considering Withdrawal of Nutrition and Hydration

In every culture, giving nourishment is seen as an act of caring as well as a method for improving health. As a person approaches death, eating and drinking become more difficult as one must have adequate strength to chew and to maintain an upright position. The palliative care team must find other ways for the family to offer support and care without forcing a dying person to take in more substance than they can handle. As the energy requirements diminish, forcing fluids, in particular, may cause more difficulty than withholding liquids might. Excess fluid tends to localize in the pharynx causing a gurgling sound or "death rattle," which can be distressing to families. Fluids also accumulate in the lungs, the abdominal cavity, and the lower extremities. As the activity level of the patient decreases, this excess fluid will be reabsorbed by the patient, making the oral intake of fluids less crucial.

Table 19.3. Symptom Management at the End of Life

Symptom	Management
Fatigue and weakness	Turn patient from side to side, protecting bony prominences with hydrocolloid dressing to prevent formation of pressure ulcers.
Loss of thirst	Explain normal dying process; intravenous fluids can actually increase secretions, edema, and discomfort.
Dry mouth	Moisten oral mucosa with baking soda mouthwash (1 teaspoon salt, 1 teaspoon baking soda, 1 quart tepid water) or artificial saliva. Coat lips with petroleum jelly.
Pain	Watch for delirium or muscular fasciculations related to opioid metabolite accumulation as renal function declines; dosing interval may need to be decreased just before death.
Myoclonic jerks	Benzodiazepines, such as lorazepam 1–2 mg tablet dissolved in 1 ml water and administered to oral mucosa; may need hourly dosing.
Delirium	Haloperidol 0.5–2.0 mg IV, SQ, or rectally; chlorpromazine 10–25 mg q6 is more sedating; both may need titration.
Loss of ability to swallow	Stop oral intake to prevent aspiration; scopolamine 1–3 transdermal patches as frequently as needed or glycopyrrolate 0.2 mg sq, will reduce saliva.

The American Academy of Hospice and Palliative Medicine (AAHPM), the professional organization for physicians and other direct care providers in the field of palliative care, has issued a statement on the use of nutrition and hydration which recognizes dying as a natural process. It recognizes that clinical judgment and skill are necessary to determine when interventions regarding hydration and nutrition might be appropriate. The statement reads, in part, as follows:

"Hydration and nutrition are traditionally considered useful and necessary components of good medical care. They are provided with the primary intention of benefiting the patient. However, when a person is approaching death, the provision of artificial hydration and nutrition is potentially harmful and may provide little or no benefit to the patient and at times may make the period of dying more uncomfortable for both patient and family. For this reason, the AAHPM believes that the withholding of artificial hydration and nutrition near the end of life may be appropriate and beneficial medical care."

Ventilator Withdrawal for Intubated Patients

In instances such as fatal *Pneumocystis carinii* pneumonia, mechanical ventilation may be withdrawn in order to discontinue futile and invasive medical treatment. These decisions are complex and involve ethical principles of withdrawing life-sustaining treatments that are well established. In particular, it is important that clinicians establish with the family and, if possible, the patient, that the goal of withdrawing ventilator support is to remove a treatment that is no longer desired or does not provide comfort to the patient. Clinicians need to work to develop a consensus among the healthcare team in order to withdraw ventilatory support; it is seldom an emergency decision, and time should be taken to resolve disagreements and concerns among the team and family. This procedure requires informed consent discussions, especially to inform family members that patients may not die immediately after ventilation is withdrawn.

A protocol developed by experienced critical care physicians appears in Table 19.4.

Table 19.4. Protocol for Ventilator Withdrawal at the End of Life

Step	Specific Actions
Prepare the family and patient (if conscious)	Hear concerns, address fears, establish informed consent, explain procedure so they are prepared, give family a place at the patient's bedside if they wish.
Appropriate setting and monitoring	Provide privacy to the greatest degree possible in the intensive care unit (ICU) setting. Turn off all monitors. Remove tubes, drains, and associated machinery if possible without compromising comfort. Liberalize visitation as much as possible.

Table 19.4. Continued

Step	Specific Actions
Ensure adequate sedation	Establish continuous infusions of analgesia and antianxiety medications; provide wide latitude in drug dosing to nurses who have experience in evaluating suffering in patients who cannot talk.
Reduce inspired oxygen to 21% (air)	This should be done in steps, with adequate time to ensure that any dyspnea or air hunger is controlled with the morphine infusion; if the infusion is increased, bolus doses should be given to rapidly establish the new steady state.
Remove positive-end expiratory pressure (PEEP)	Air hunger must be relieved before proceeding with morphine.
Set ventilator to intermittent mandatory ventilation (IMV) or PS level to fully meet patient's ventilatory needs	This provides another period to establish patient comfort before proceeding.
Observe and modify sedatives while gradually reducing IMV rate or PS level to 5	This process may take 15 to 30 minutes. Family may wish to be present, but should be warned of the possibility of transient increases in agitation or respiratory rate as sedation is being titrated. Ventilator alarms must be disabled so they are not triggered by terminal hypoventilation.
Extubate or leave on humidified air by T-piece	Offer the family the possibility of private time with the patient if feasible, or support from any staff members they wish to have present. Rituals devised by the family or performed by clergy may have an important role.

Chapter 20

Ethics and Legal Issues in Palliative Care

The life expectancy of the American people has reached an all-time high, but along with the increased life expectancy is an increase in the number of people living with, and dying from, chronic debilitating diseases, such as heart disease, cancer, stroke, and chronic obstructive pulmonary disease. While the elderly with chronic illnesses comprise a group one might associate with end-of-life issues, there are other groups for whom these concerns are important. Examples extend across the life span including neonates in intensive care units, children with acquired immunodeficiency syndrome (AIDS), teens with cancer, and young adults with degenerative diseases. Coupled with this spectrum of individuals is the increased availability of technologies and treatments that can be used to prolong life and, in some cases, death. Defining when these technologies and treatments shift from life-saving interventions to burdensome and futile procedures that negatively impact the quality of life (QOL) has proved elusive. When these technologies and treatments become futile, the individuals'

This chapter contains text excerpted from the following sources: Text in this chapter begins with excerpts from "Quality of Life for Individuals at the End-of-Life," National Institutes of Health (NIH), August 2, 2000. Reviewed September 2019; Text under the heading "Legal Issues in End-of-Life Care" is excerpted from "Ethical Practices in End-of-Life Care," National Center for Ethics in Health Care (NCEHC), U.S. Department of Veterans Affairs (VA), December 9, 2013. Reviewed September 2019.

families and significant others may be involved in a difficult period of decision-making about how much aggressive treatment to try and when to stop. Conversely, there is widespread fear that the only alternative to aggressive treatment is abandonment and suffering.

For many Americans, end-of-life care is fragmented, painful, and emotionally distressing, with unnecessary transitions between healthcare institutions, community-based organizations, and home care settings. There are opportunities for healthcare providers to learn more about how to deliver optimal end-of-life care.

There are many national initiatives underway to improve the care of the dying. Significant efforts are being made to better train health professionals and to encourage public awareness of the issues. Yet important gaps in knowledge limit our ability to help individuals who are dying achieve the highest possible quality of life. "From the cellular to the social level, much remains to be learned about how people die and how reliably excellent and compassionate care can be achieved." Research is needed to better define what is meant by "end of life" to identify aspects of an optimal death experience within the cultural and ethnic context of the individual so that better palliative care can be provided, to facilitate communication and ethical decision-making among those involved in end-of-life decisions, and to support the development of a well-integrated healthcare system that includes the family and the multidisciplinary team.

More needs to be understood about the physical, emotional, social, cultural, and spiritual experiences of people who are dying and about the environmental context which influences the quality of the life remaining. Issues related to research methods are important to consider with an inquiry into dying. There are pressing needs to better define key concepts, identify and test appropriate measures, develop strategies to minimize subject burden, and devise methods for complex data analysis. Advances in understanding how to help individuals who are dying to attain the highest quality of life possible can be advanced with innovative, science-based research.

Legal Issues in End-of-Life Care

Historically, end-of-life care was shaped by a presumption in favor of curative medical interventions. Any decision not directed specifically at maximizing survival was understood negatively as "withdrawing," "withholding," or "refusing" treatment. With the evolution of hospice and palliative care, caregiving goals of comfort, relief of suffering, and a dignified death have come to be recognized as positive and appropriate for patients with advanced illness. To honor the range of end-of-life options available to patients, palliative care emphasizes shared decision-making that is based on explicitly identifying achievable and desired goals of care.

Your responsibility to provide respectful and clinically appropriate care at the end of life is based on four ethical obligations:

1. Your obligation to respect the patient's right to self-determination. This right, sometimes referred to as "autonomy," is well established in law and ethics, and best summarized in the words of Justice Benjamin Cardozo in the 1914 court case that gave legal recognition to the concept of informed consent: "Every human being of adult years and sound mind has a right to determine what shall be done with his own body."

2. Your obligation to prevent or remove harm and to promote the patient's good. This is also known as "beneficence."

3. Your obligation to refrain from causing harm or imposing unnecessary risk. This is also known as "nonmaleficence."

4. Your obligation to not abandon the patient. The healing relationship is distinguished by the vulnerability of the patient, the imbalance of knowledge and power between the healthcare provider and patient, and the expectation that healthcare providers will use their knowledge and skills to help the patient. Patients have a legitimate expectation that their welfare will be paramount and that they will not be abandoned by their healthcare providers.

Chapter 21

Last Days of Life

The end of life may be months, weeks, days, or hours. It is a time when many decisions about treatment and care are made for patients. It is important for families and healthcare providers to know the patient's wishes ahead of time and to talk with the patient openly about end-of-life plans. This will help make it easier for family members to make major decisions for the patient at the end of life.

When treatment choices and plans are discussed before the end of life, it can lower the stress on both the patient and the family. It is most helpful if end-of-life planning and decision-making begin soon after the life-threatening illness is diagnosed and continue during the course of the disease. Having these decisions in writing can make the patient's wishes clear to both the family and the healthcare team.

When a child is terminally ill, end-of-life discussions with the child's doctor may reduce the time the child spends in the hospital and help the parents feel more prepared. This chapter discusses care during the last days and the last hours of life, including the treatment of common symptoms and ethical questions that may come up. It may help patients and their families prepare for decisions that they need to make during this time.

This chapter includes text excerpted from "Last Days of Life (PDQ®)—Patient Version," National Cancer Institute (NCI), April 8, 2016. Reviewed September 2019.

Care in the Final Hours
Knowing What to Expect in the Final Days or Hours Helps Comfort the Family

Most people do not know the signs that show death is near. Knowing what to expect can help them get ready for the death of their loved ones and make this time less stressful and confusing. Healthcare providers can give family members information about the changes they may see in their loved ones in the final hours and how they may help their loved ones through this.

Patients May Not Want to Eat or Drink in the Final Days or Hours

In the final days to hours of life, patients often lose the desire to eat or drink, and may not want food and fluids that are offered to them. The family may give ice chips or swab the mouth and lips to keep them moist. Food and fluids should not be forced on the patient. This can make the patient uncomfortable or cause choking.

Patients near Death May Not Respond to Others

Patients may withdraw and spend more time sleeping. They may answer questions slowly or not at all, seem confused, and may not be interested in what is going on around them. Most patients are still able to hear after they are no longer able to speak. It may give some comfort if family members continue to touch and talk to the patient, even if the patient does not respond.

A Number of Physical Changes Are Common When the Patient Is near Death

Certain physical changes may occur in the patient at the end of life:

- The patient may feel tired or weak.

- The patient may pass less urine and it may be dark in color.

- The patient's hands and feet may become blotchy, cold, or blue. Caregivers can use blankets to keep the patient warm. Electric blankets or heating pads should not be used.

- The heart rate may go up or down and become irregular.

- Blood pressure usually goes down.

- Breathing may become irregular, with very shallow breathing, short periods of not breathing, or deep, rapid breathing.

However, these signs and changes do not always occur in everyone. For this reason, it may be hard to know when a patient is near death.

Patients and Their Families May Have Cultural or Religious Beliefs and Customs That Are Important at the Time of Death

After the patient dies, family members and caregivers may wish to stay with the patient a while. There may be certain customs or rituals that are important to the patient and family at this time. These might include rituals for coping with death, handling the patient's body, making final arrangements for the body, and honoring the death. The patient and family members should let the healthcare team know about any customs or rituals they want to be performed after the patient's death.

Healthcare providers, hospice staff, social workers, or spiritual leaders can explain the steps that need to be taken once death has occurred, including contacting a funeral home.

Symptoms during the Final Months, Weeks, and Days of Life

Delirium
Delirium Can Have Many Causes at the End of Life

Delirium is common during the final days of life. Most patients have a lower level of consciousness. They may be withdrawn, be less alert, and have less energy. Some patients may be agitated or restless, and have hallucinations (see or hear things that are not really there). Patients should be protected from having accidents or hurting themselves when they are confused or agitated.

Delirium can be caused by the direct effects of cancer, such as a growing tumor in the brain. Other causes include the following:

- A higher- or lower-than-normal amount of certain chemicals in the blood that keeps the heart, kidneys, nerves, and muscles working the way they should

- Side effects of drugs or drug interactions (changes in the way a drug acts in the body when taken with certain other drugs, herbal medicine, or foods)

- Stopping the use of certain drugs or alcohol
- Dehydration (the loss of needed water from the body)

Delirium May Be Controlled by Finding and Treating the Cause

Depending on the cause of the delirium, doctors may do the following:

- Give drugs to fix the level of certain chemicals in the blood.
- Stop or lower the dose of the drugs that are causing delirium, or are no longer useful at the end of life, such as drugs to lower cholesterol.
- Treat dehydration by putting fluids into the bloodstream.

For some patients in the last hours of life, the decision may be to treat only the symptoms of delirium and make the patient as comfortable as possible. There are drugs that work very well to relieve these symptoms.

Hallucinations That Are Not Related to Delirium Often Occur at the End of Life

It is common for dying patients to have hallucinations that include loved ones who have already died. It is normal for family members to feel distressed when these hallucinations occur. Speaking with clergy, the hospital chaplain, or other religious advisors may help.

Fatigue
Fatigue Is One of the Most Common Symptoms in the Last Days of Life

Fatigue (feeling very tired) is one of the most common symptoms in the last days of life. A patient's fatigue may become worse every day during this time. Drowsiness, weakness, and sleep problems may occur. Drugs that increase brain activity, alertness, and energy may be helpful.

Shortness of Breath
Feeling Short of Breath Is Common and May Get Worse during the Final Days or Weeks of Life

Shortness of breath or not being able to catch your breath is often caused by advanced cancer. Other causes include the following:

- Build-up of fluid in the abdomen

- Loss of muscle strength

- Hypoxemia (a condition in which there is not enough oxygen in the blood)

- Chronic obstructive pulmonary disease (COPD)

- Pneumonia

- Infection

The Use of Opioids and Other Methods Can Help the Patient Breathe More Easily

Opioids may relieve shortness of breath in patients. Some patients have spasms of the air passages in the lungs along with shortness of breath. Bronchodilators (drugs that open up small airways in the lungs) or steroid drugs (which relieve swelling and inflammation) may relieve these spasms.

Other ways to help patients who feel short of breath include the following:

- Give extra oxygen if shortness of breath is caused by hypoxemia.

- Aim a cool fan toward the patient's face.

- Have the patient sit up.

- Have the patient do breathing and relaxation exercises, if able.

- Give antibiotics if shortness of breath is caused by an infection.

In rare cases, shortness of breath may not be relieved by any of these treatments. Sedation with drugs may be needed, to help the patient feel more comfortable.

Pain
Pain Medicines Can Be Given in Several Ways

In the last days of life, a patient may not be able to swallow pain medicine. When patients cannot take medicines by mouth, the pain medicine may be given by placing it under the tongue or into the rectum, by injection or infusion, or by placing a patch on the skin. These methods can be used at home with a doctor's order.

Pain during the Final Hours of Life Can Usually Be Controlled

Opioid analgesics work very well to relieve pain and are commonly used at the end of life. Some patients and family members worry that the use of opioids may cause death to occur sooner, but studies have shown no link between opioid use and early death.

Cough
Cough at the End of Life Can Be Treated in Several Ways

Chronic cough at the end of life may add to a patient's discomfort. Repeated coughing can cause pain and loss of sleep, increase tiredness, and make shortness of breath worse. At the end of life, the decision may be to treat the symptoms of the cough rather than to find and treat the cause. The following types of drugs may be used to make the patient as comfortable as possible:

- Over-the-counter (OTC) cough medicines with expectorants to increase bronchial fluids and loosen mucus.
- Medicines to decrease mucus that can cause coughing in patients who have trouble swallowing.
- Opioids to stop the coughing.

Constipation
Constipation May Occur in the Last Days of Life

Patients with cancer may have constipation in the last days of life. Patients who have trouble swallowing may not be able to take laxatives by mouth. If needed, laxatives may be given rectally to treat constipation and make the patient comfortable.

Trouble Swallowing
Patients May Have Trouble Swallowing Food and Fluids at the End of Life

Patients with cancer may have trouble swallowing in the last days of life. Both fluids and food may be hard to swallow, causing a loss of appetite, weight loss and muscle wasting, and weakness. Small amounts of food that the patient enjoys may be given if they want to eat. Supplemental nutrition does not benefit patients in the last days of life and may increase the risk of aspiration and infections.

When the patient cannot swallow, the medicine may be given by placing it in the rectum, by injection or infusion, or by placing a patch on the skin.

Death Rattle
Rattle Occurs When Saliva or Other Fluids Collect in the Throat and Upper Airways

Rattle occurs when saliva or other fluids build up in the throat and airways in a patient who is too weak to clear the throat. There are two types of rattle. The death rattle is caused by saliva pooling at the back of the throat. The other kind of rattle is caused by fluid in the airways from an infection, a tumor, or extra fluid in the body tissues.

Drugs may be given to decrease the amount of saliva in the mouth or to dry the upper airway. Since most patients with rattle are unable to swallow, these drugs are usually given by infusion.

Nondrug Treatments for Rattle Include Changing the Patient's Position and Giving Less Fluid

Raising the head of the bed, propping the patient up with pillows, or turning the patient to either side may help relieve the rattle. If the rattle is caused by fluid at the back of the throat, the fluid may be gently removed from the mouth using a suction tube. If the rattle is caused by fluid in the airways, the fluid is usually not removed by suction, because it causes severe physical and mental stress on the patient. At the end of life, the body needs less food and fluid. Reducing food and fluids can lessen the extra fluid in the body and greatly relieve rattle.

Death Rattle Is a Sign That Death May Soon Occur

Death rattle is a sign that death may occur in hours or days. Rattle can be very upsetting for those at the bedside. It does not seem to be painful for the patient and is not the same as shortness of breath.

Myoclonic Jerking
Myoclonic Jerks May Be Caused by Taking Very High Doses of Opioids for a Long Time

Myoclonic jerks are sudden muscle twitches or jerks that cannot be controlled by the person having them. A hiccup is one type of myoclonic jerk. Brief, shock-like jerks can occur in one or more different muscle groups anywhere in the body. Taking very high doses of an opioid for a long time may cause this side effect, but it can have other causes as well.

When opioids are the cause of myoclonic jerking, changing to another opioid may help. Different patients respond to opioids in different ways and certain opioids may be more likely than others to cause myoclonic jerking in some people.

When the patient is very near death, medicine to stop the myoclonic jerking may be given instead of changing the opioid. When myoclonic jerking is severe, drugs may be used to calm the patient down, relieve anxiety, and help the patient sleep.

Fever
Fever May Be Caused by Infection, Medicines, or the Cancer Itself

Treatment of fever in the last days of life depends on whether it causes the patient distress or discomfort. Fever may be caused by infection, medicines, or cancer itself. While infections may be treated with antibiotics, patients near the end of life may choose not to treat the cause of the fever.

Hemorrhage
Sudden Hemorrhage (Heavy Bleeding) May Occur in Patients Who Have Certain Cancers or Disorders

Hemorrhage (heavy bleeding in a short time) is rare but may occur in the last hours or minutes of life. Blood vessels may be damaged by certain cancers or cancer treatments. Radiation therapy, for example, can weaken blood vessels in the area that was treated. Tumors can also damage blood vessels. Patients with the following conditions have an increased risk of hemorrhage:

- Advanced cancer, especially head and neck cancers

- Ulcers

- Mucositis caused by chemotherapy

- Blood clotting disorders

The patient and family should talk with the doctor about any concerns they have about the chance of hemorrhage.

Making the Patient Comfortable Is the Main Goal of Care during Hemorrhage at the End of Life

It is hard to know when hemorrhage might occur. When sudden bleeding occurs at the end of life, patients usually become unconscious and die soon afterward. Resuscitation (restarting the heart) usually will not work.

The main goal of care is to help the patient be comfortable and to support family members. If hemorrhage occurs, it can be very upsetting for family members. It is helpful if the family talks about the feelings these causes and asks questions about it.

Care Decisions in the Final Weeks, Days, and Hours of Life

Decisions about Chemotherapy

Decisions about whether to continue or stop chemotherapy are made by the patient and doctor together. About one-third of patients with advanced cancer continue to receive chemotherapy or other treatment near the end of life.

Treatment with chemotherapy at this time can result in the following:

- Serious side effects

- Spending more days in the hospital

- Spending the last days in an intensive care unit

However, some patients with cancer choose to continue chemotherapy because they feel it helps them to live in the present and focus on active treatment. Other patients choose palliative or comfort care to treat pain and other symptoms. These decisions are based on the patient's goals of care and the likely risks and benefits of treatment.

Decisions about Hospice

Hospice care is an important end-of-life option for patients with advanced cancer. Patients may feel that beginning hospice care means they have given up. Some patients fear losing their relationship with their oncologist. However, many patients and caregivers feel they receive important benefits from hospice care.

Patients who receive hospice care seem to have the following:

- Better mental outlook

- Better relief of symptoms

- Better communication

- Less stressful death (without causing death to happen sooner)

Hospice-related services include:

- Visiting nurse

- Chaplain

- Counselor

- Home health aide

- Respite care

Doctors, patients, and caregivers should discuss hospice care and when it should begin.

When hospice benefits are covered by Medicare, physicians are required to certify that patients are not expected to live more than 6 months and that patients are not being treated to be cured. Other policies may be different, depending on the hospice and the state.

Decisions about Place of Death

Many patients with advanced cancer wish to die at home. Patients who die at home with hospice services and support seem to have better symptom control and quality of life (QOL). They also feel better prepared for death than patients who die in a hospital or intensive care unit. Grieving caregivers have less trouble adjusting to their loss and feel they have honored the patient's wishes when their loved one dies at home.

Patients who get hospice care are more likely to be able to die at home. Hospice care can help control the patient's symptoms and give the caregiver the help they need.

However, not all patients choose to die at home. It is important for the patient, caregivers, and doctors to discuss where the patient wishes to die and the best way to fulfill the patient's decision.

Chapter 22

Termination of
Life-Sustaining Treatments

Decisions about Life-Sustaining Treatments in the
Last Days of Life
*In the Last Days of Life, Patients and Family Members
Are Faced with Making Decisions about Treatments to
Keep the Patient Alive*

Decisions about whether to use life-sustaining treatments that may
extend life in the final weeks or days cause a great deal of confusion
and anxiety. Some of these treatments are ventilator use, parenteral
nutrition, and dialysis.

Patients may be guided by their oncologist, but have the right to
make their own choices about life-sustaining treatments. The following
are some of the questions to discuss:

- What are the patient's goals of care?

- How would the possible benefits of life-sustaining treatments
  help reach the patient's goals of care, and how likely would this
  be?

This chapter includes text excerpted from "Last Days of Life (PDQ®)—Patient
Version," National Cancer Institute (NCI), April 8, 2016. Reviewed September
2019.

205

- How would the possible harms of life-sustaining treatments affect the patient's goals of care? Is the possible benefit worth the possible harm?

- Besides possible benefits and harms of life-sustaining treatments, what else can affect the decision?

- Are there other professionals, such as a chaplain or medical ethicist, who could help the patient or family decide about life-sustaining treatments?

Choices about Care and Treatment at the End of Life Should Be Made While the Patient Is Able to Make Them

A patient may wish to receive all possible treatments, only some treatments, or no treatment at all in the last days of life. These decisions may be written down ahead of time in an advance directive, such as a living will. An "advance directive" is a general term for different types of legal documents that describe the treatment or care a patient wishes to receive or not receive when she or he is no longer able to speak their wishes.

Studies have shown that cancer patients who have end-of-life discussions with their doctors choose to have fewer procedures, such as resuscitation or the use of a ventilator. They are also less likely to be in intensive care, and the cost of their healthcare is lower during their final week of life. Reports from their caregivers show that these patients live as long as patients who choose to have more procedures and that they have a better quality of life (QOL) in their last days.

Care That Supports a Patient's Spiritual Health May Improve Quality of Life

A spiritual assessment is a method or tool used by doctors to understand the role that religious and spiritual beliefs have in the patient's life. This may help the doctor understand how these beliefs affect the way the patient copes with cancer and makes decisions about cancer treatment.

Serious illnesses like cancer may cause patients or family caregivers to have doubts about their beliefs or religious values and cause spiritual distress. Some studies show that patients with cancer may feel anger at God or may have a loss of faith after being diagnosed. Other patients may have feelings of spiritual distress when coping with cancer. Spiritual distress may affect end-of-life decisions and increase depression.

Doctors and nurses, together with social workers and psychologists, may be able to offer care that supports a patient's spiritual health. They may encourage patients to meet with their spiritual or religious leaders or join a spiritual support group. This may improve patients' QOL and ability to cope. When patients with advanced cancer receive spiritual support from the medical team, they are more likely to choose hospice care and less aggressive treatment at the end of life.

Fluids
The Goals of Giving Fluids at the End of Life Should Be Discussed by Patient, Family, and Doctors

Fluids may be given when the patient can no longer eat or drink normally. Fluids may be given with an intravenous (IV) catheter or through a needle under the skin.

Decisions about giving fluids should be based on the patient's goals of care. Giving fluids has not been shown to help patients live longer or to improve QOL. However, the harms are minor and the family may feel there are benefits if the patient is less fatigued and more alert.

The family may also be able to give the patient sips of water or ice chips or swab the mouth and lips to keep them moist.

Nutrition Support
The Goals of Nutrition Support for Patients in the Last Days of Life Are Different from the Goals during Cancer Treatment

Nutrition support can improve health and boost healing during cancer treatment. The goals of nutrition therapy for patients during the last days of life are different from the goals for patients in active cancer treatment and recovery. In the final days of life, patients often lose the desire to eat or drink and may not want food or fluids that are offered to them. Also, procedures used to put in feeding tubes may be hard on a patient.

Making Plans for Nutrition Support in the Last Days Is Helpful

The goal of end-of-life care is to prevent suffering and relieve symptoms. If nutrition support causes the patient more discomfort than help, then nutrition support near the end of life may be stopped. The needs and best interests of each patient guide the decision to give nutrition support. When decisions and plans about nutrition support are made by the patient, doctors and family members can be sure they are doing what the patient wants.

Two Types of Nutrition Support Are Commonly Used

If the patient cannot swallow, two types of nutrition support are commonly used:

- **Enteral nutrition** uses a tube inserted into the stomach or intestine.

- **Parenteral nutrition** uses an intravenous (IV) catheter inserted into a vein.

Each type of nutrition support has benefits and risks.

Antibiotics
The Benefits of Using Antibiotics in the Last Days of Life Are Unclear

The use of antibiotics and other treatments for infection is common in patients in the last days of life, but it is hard to tell how well they work. It is also hard to tell if there are any benefits of using antibiotics at the end of life.

Overall, doctors want to make the patient comfortable in the last days of life rather than give treatments that may not help them live longer.

Transfusions
The Decision to Use Blood Transfusions in Advanced Cancer Depends on Goals of Care and Other Factors

Many patients with advanced cancer have anemia. Patients with advanced blood cancers may have thrombocytopenia (a condition in which there is a lower-than-normal number of platelets in the blood). Deciding whether to use blood transfusions for these conditions is based on the following:

- Goals of care

- How long the patient is expected to live

- The benefits and risks of the transfusion

208

The decision is hard to make since patients usually need to receive transfusions in a medical setting rather than at home.

Many patients are used to receiving blood transfusions during active treatment or supportive care and may want to continue transfusions to feel better. However, studies have not shown that transfusions are safe and effective at the end of life.

Resuscitation
Patients Should Decide Whether or Not They Want Cardiopulmonary Resuscitation

An important decision for the patient to make is whether to have cardiopulmonary resuscitation (CPR) (trying to restart the heart and breathing when it stops). It is best if patients talk with their family, doctors, and caregivers about their wishes for CPR as early as possible (for example, when being admitted to the hospital or when active cancer treatment is stopped). A do-not-resuscitate (DNR) order is written by a doctor to tell other health professionals not to perform CPR at the moment of death so that the natural process of death occurs. If the patient wishes, she or he can ask the doctor to write a DNR order. The patient can ask that the DNR order be changed or removed at any time.

Last Days in the Hospital or Intensive Care Unit
Choices about Whether to Use Intensive Care Should Be Discussed

Near the end of life, patients with advanced cancer may be admitted to a hospital or intensive care unit (ICU) if they have not made other choices for their care. In the ICU, patients or family members have to make hard decisions about whether to start, continue, or stop aggressive treatments that may make the patient live longer, but do not improve the patient's QOL. Families may be unsure of their feelings or have trouble deciding whether to limit or avoid treatments.

Sometimes, treatments like dialysis or blood transfusions may be tried for a short time. However, at any time, patients or families may talk with doctors about whether they want to continue with ICU care. They may choose instead to change over to comfort care in the final days.

Ventilator Use May Keep the Patient Alive after Normal Breathing Stops

A ventilator is a machine that helps patients breathe. Sometimes, using a ventilator will not improve the patient's condition, but will keep the patient alive longer. If the goal of care is to help the patient live longer, a ventilator may be used, according to the patient's wishes. If ventilator support stops helping the patient or is no longer what the patient wants, the patient, family, and healthcare team may decide to turn the ventilator off.

Before a Ventilator Is Turned Off, Family Members Will Be Given Information about What to Expect

Family members will be given information about how the patient may respond when the ventilator is removed and about pain relief or sedation to keep the patient comfortable. Family members will be given time to contact other loved ones who wish to be there. Chaplains or social workers may be called to give help and support to the family.

Suffering and Palliative Sedation at the End of Life
The Emotions of Patients and Caregivers Are Closely Connected

Patients and caregivers share the distress of cancer, with the caregiver's distress sometimes being greater than the patient's. Since caregiver suffering can affect the patient's well-being and the caregiver's adjustment to loss, early and constant support of the caregiver is very important.

Palliative Sedation Lowers the Level of Consciousness and Relieves Extreme Pain and Suffering

Palliative sedation uses special drugs called "sedatives" to relieve extreme suffering by making a patient calm and unaware.

The decision of whether to sedate a patient at the end of life is a hard one. Sedation may be considered for a patient's comfort or for a physical condition such as uncontrolled pain. Palliative sedation may be temporary. A patient's thoughts and feelings about end-of-life sedation may depend greatly on her or his own culture and beliefs. Some patients who become anxious facing the end of life may want to be sedated. Some patients and their families may wish to have a level of sedation that allows them to communicate with each other.

Other patients may wish to have no procedures, including sedation, just before death.

Studies have not shown that palliative sedation shortens life when used in the last days.

It is important for the patient to tell family members and healthcare providers of her or his wishes about sedation at the end of life. When patients make their wishes about sedation known ahead of time, doctors and family members can be sure they are doing what the patient would want. Families may need support from the healthcare team and mental-health counselors while palliative sedation is used.

Chapter 23

Organ Donation of the Deceased and Transplantation

What Is Organ Donation and Transplantation?

Organ transplantation is the surgical removal of an organ or tissues from one person (the donor) and placing it in another person (the recipient). Organ donation is when you allow your organs or tissues to be removed and given to someone else. Most donated organs and tissues are from people who have died. But, a living person can donate some organs. Blood, stem cells, and platelets can also be donated.

This chapter contains text excerpted from the following sources: Text under the heading "What Is Organ Donation and Transplantation?" is excerpted from "Organ Donation and Transplantation Fact Sheet," Office on Women's Health (OWH), U.S. Department of Health and Human Services (HHS), July 16, 2012. Reviewed September 2019; Text under the heading "What Is the Status of Organ Donation and Transplantation in the United States?" is excerpted from "Organ Donation Statistics," Organdonor.gov, Health Resources and Services Administration (HRSA), January 2019; Text under the heading "Frequently Asked Questions on Organ Donation" is excerpted from "Organ Donation FAQs," Organdonor. gov, Health Resources and Services Administration (HRSA), December 11, 2016. Reviewed September 2019; Text under the heading "The Deceased Donation Process" is excerpted from "The Deceased Donation Process," Organdonor.gov, Health Resources and Services Administration (HRSA), March 22, 2016. Reviewed September 2019.

What Is the Status of Organ Donation and Transplantation in the United States?

There are over 113,000 candidates for transplant on the U.S. national waiting list. Nearly 2 out of every 3 people on the waiting list are over the age of 50. Almost 2,000 children under 18 are on the waiting list. Almost 70,000 people (58%) on the list are ethnic minorities.

Frequently Asked Questions on Organ Donation

Who Can Become an Organ Donor?

All adults in the United States and in some states people under the age of 18 can indicate their commitment to a donation by signing up to be an organ donor. Whether someone is suitable for donation is determined at the time of death. Authorization by a parent or guardian is generally necessary for individuals under 18 who have died to become an actual donor.

Are There Age Limits for Donating Your Organs?

There are no age limitations on who can donate. Newborns, as well as senior citizens, have been organ donors. Whether or not you can donate depends on your physical condition and the condition of your organs, not age.

Can Nonresidents Donate and Receive Organs in the United States?

Nonresident aliens—people who do not live in the United States or are not citizens—can donate and receive organs in the United States. Organs are given to patients according to medical need, not citizenship.

However, only about 1 in 100 people who receive transplants are non-U.S. residents.

If I Have a Medical Condition, Can I Still Donate?

Do not rule yourself out from being an organ donor because you have a health condition. You are always encouraged to register. There are very few conditions that would prevent someone from being organ, eye, or tissue donors—such as human immunodeficiency virus (HIV) infection, active cancer, or systemic infection. Even with an illness, you may be able to donate your organs or tissues.

The transplant team will determine what can be used at the time of your death based on clinical evaluation, medical history, and other factors. Even if there is only one organ or tissue that can be used, that is one life saved or improved.

Can I Be an Organ and Tissue Donor, and Also Donate My Body to Medical Science?

Total body donation generally is not an option if you choose to be an organ and tissue donor. However, eye donors still may be accepted. There are also a few medical schools and research organizations that may accept an organ donor for research.

If you wish to donate your entire body, you should contact the medical organization of your choice directly and make arrangements. Medical schools, research facilities, and other agencies study bodies to understand how the disease affects human beings. This research is vital to saving and improving lives.

I Have an Organ Donor Card. Is That Enough?

No. There is no way of knowing if the card would be with you or if it would be examined in the event of your death. If you wish to be a donor, sign up in your state registry.

I Have My Organ Donor Status on My Driver's License. Is That Enough?

That is an important step, but it is also important to share your wishes with your family. Most families want to carry out the wishes of their loved one, so please be sure to tell them how you feel.

Can I Specify What I Want to Donate?

When registering online, most states give you the option to choose which organs and tissues you donate or to donate everything that can be used. Check with your state registry to learn more.

Can I Remove Myself from the Registered Donors List?

Yes, you can change your donor status at any time. Look for an option such as "updating your status" on your state's site.

If you have a donor designation on your driver's license, removing yourself from the registry will not change that. So, unless your state uses a removable sticker on the license to identify donors, you will likely need to change your license at your local motor vehicle office.

If I Register as a Donor, Will My Wishes Be Carried Out?

If you signed up as a deceased donor in your state registry and you are over 18, then you have legally authorized your donation and no one can overrule your consent. Signing a card is not enough. If you are under 18, your parents or legal guardian must authorize donation.

What Organs and Tissues Can Be Donated?

- Eight vital organs can be donated: heart, kidneys (2), pancreas, lungs (2), liver, and intestines. Hands and faces have also been added to the list.

- Tissue: cornea, skin, heart valves, bone, blood vessels, and connective tissue

- Bone marrow and stem cells, umbilical cord blood, peripheral blood stem cells (PBSC)

If I Am a Registered Donor, Will It Affect the Medical Care I Receive at the Hospital?

No! The medical team trying to save your life is separate from the transplant team. Every effort is made to save your life before donation becomes a possibility.

Will Donation Disfigure My Body? Can There Be an Open Casket Funeral?

Donation does not interfere with having an open casket service. Surgical techniques are used to retrieve organs and tissues, and all incisions are closed.

Are There Any Costs to My Family for Donation?

No. Your family pays for your medical care and funeral costs, but not for organ donation. Costs related to donation are paid by the recipient, usually through insurance, Medicare, or Medicaid.

Can I Sell My Organs?

No! The National Organ Transplant Act (Public Law 98-507) makes it illegal to sell human organs and tissues in the United States. Violators are subject to fines and imprisonment.

One reason Congress made this law was to make sure the wealthy do not have an unfair advantage for obtaining donated organs and tissues.

Can People of Different Races and Ethnicities Match Each Other?

Yes. People of different ethnicities frequently match each other.

How Are Donated Organs Distributed?

Organs are matched to patients based on a number of factors, including blood and tissue typing, medical need, time on the waiting list, and geographical location.

I Would like to Donate a Kidney to Someone. How Can I Be Tested to See If I Am a Match?

Within the United States, living donations of a kidney can be made to a family member, friend, or anyone on the waiting list. Living donations are arranged through many kidney transplant centers throughout the United States. They will test to see if you are a match and if you are healthy enough to safely undergo surgery.

Remember that there is a lot to do before you can be considered a living donor.

How Many People Are Currently Waiting for Organs?

The number of patients waiting for organs varies every day, but on average, the number is well over 120,000 and climbing. Every 10 minutes, another person is added to the waiting list.

The number of patients now on the waiting list and other data are available on the Organ Procurement and Transplantation Network (OPTN) website. The number of people requiring a lifesaving transplant continues to rise faster than the number of available donors. Approximately 300 new transplant candidates are added to the waiting list each month.

Why Do Minorities Have a Higher Need for Transplants?

More than half of all people on the transplant waiting list are from a racial or ethnic minority group. That is because some diseases that cause end-stage organ failure are more common in these populations than in the general population.

For example, African Americans, Asians, Native Hawaiians, and Pacific Islanders, and Hispanics/Latinxs are three times more likely than Whites to suffer from end-stage renal (kidney) disease, often as the result of high blood pressure.

Native Americans are four times more likely than Whites to suffer from diabetes. An organ transplant is sometimes the best—or only—option for saving a life.

Transplanting the Organs

The transplant operation takes place after the transport team arrives at the hospital with the new organ. The transplant recipient is typically waiting at the hospital and may already be in the operating room awaiting the arrival of the lifesaving organ. Surgical teams work around the clock as needed to transplant the new organs into the waiting recipients.

The Deceased Donation Process

Registering as a Donor

The process of donation most often begins with your consent to be a donor by registering in your state. Signing up does not guarantee you will be able to donate your organs, eyes, or tissues—and registering usually takes place many years before donation becomes possible. But it is the first step to being eligible to save lives.

Medical Care of Potential Donors

For someone to become a deceased donor, she or he has to die in very specific circumstances. Most often, a patient comes to a hospital because of illness or accident, such as severe head trauma, a brain aneurysm or stroke.

The patient is put on artificial or mechanical support, which keeps the blood with oxygen flowing to the organs. The medical team does everything possible to save the patient's life. At this point, whether or not the person is a registered donor is not considered.

Brain Death Testing

Even though the medical team members do everything they can to save the patient's life, sometimes the injuries are too severe and the patient dies.

If the patient is dead and is not responding, physicians will perform a series of tests to determine if brain death has occurred. A patient who is brain dead has no brain activity and cannot breathe on her or his own. Brain death is death and it is irreversible. Someone who is brain dead cannot recover.

Only after brain death has been confirmed and the time of death noted, can organ donation become a possibility.

Organ Procurement Organization

The hospital notifies the local Organ Procurement Organization (OPO) of every patient that has died or is nearing death. This is in keeping with federal regulations.

The hospital gives the OPO information about the deceased patient to confirm whether she or he has the potential to be a donor. If the person could be a candidate for donation, a representative from the OPO travels immediately to the hospital.

Authorizing Donation

The OPO representative searches to see if the deceased is registered as a donor on their state registry. If so, that will serve as legal consent for donation.

If the deceased has not registered, and there was no other legal consent for donation, such as a notation on the driver's license, the OPO will ask the next of kin for authorization.

After authorization, a medical evaluation takes place, including obtaining the deceased's complete medical and social history from the family.

The Matching Process

If the deceased person's evaluation allows donation, the OPO contacts the Organ Procurement and Transplantation Network (OPTN).

The OPTN operates the national database of all patients in the United States. waiting for a transplant. The OPO enters information about the deceased donor into the computer system and the search begins.

The computer system generates a list of patients who match the donor (by organ). Each available organ is offered to the transplant team of the best-matched patient.

The transplant surgeon determines whether the organ is medically suitable for that patient or may refuse the organ—for example, if the patient is too sick to be transplanted or cannot be reached in time.

Most organs go to patients in the area where the organs were recovered. The others are shared with patients in other regions of the country.

Recovering and Transporting Organs

While the search for matching recipients is underway, the deceased donor's organs are maintained on artificial support. Machines keep blood containing oxygen flowing to the organs. The condition of each organ is carefully monitored by the hospital medical staff and the OPO procurement coordinator.

A transplant surgical team replaces the medical team that treated the patient before death. (The medical team trying to save the patient's life and the transplant team are never the same team.)

The surgical team removes the organs and tissues from the donor's body in an operating room. First, organs are recovered, and then additional authorized tissues, such as bone, cornea, and skin. All incisions are surgically closed. Organ donation does not interfere with open-casket funerals.

Organs remain healthy only for a short period of time after removal from the donor, so minutes count. The OPO representative arranges the transportation of the organs to the hospitals of the intended recipients. Transportation depends on the distance involved and can include ambulances, helicopters, and commercial airplanes.

Transplanting the Organs

The transplant operation takes place after the transport team arrives at the hospital with the new organ. The transplant recipient is typically waiting at the hospital and may already be in the operating room awaiting the arrival of the lifesaving organ.

Surgical teams work around the clock as needed to transplant the new organs into the waiting recipients.

Chapter 24

Physician-Assisted Suicide and Euthanasia

Every patient longs for a life free of suffering. When suffering is prolonged, a patient sometimes reaches the point of being unwilling to go on. Patients in extreme duress and unremitting pain, and those aware of the ongoing medical costs associated with continuing a treatment that will not end in a cure but will likely leave surviving family members in considerable debt, may come to decide that death is preferable to life and continued treatment. Physician-assisted suicide (PAS) is suicide undertaken with the aid of a physician or other healthcare provider. Physician-assisted suicide can be accomplished in two ways. In the first method, the physician provides the patient with information and a humane means to end her or his life. In the second method, the physician not only provides the information and means to end life, but also takes co-responsibility to ensure the safe and effective execution of the act.

In recent years, "physician-assisted suicide" has replaced the term "physician-assisted death." PAS differs from "euthanasia," which refers to the act of assisting people to end their lives without the approval of a controlling legal authority.

"Physician-Assisted Suicide and Euthanasia," © 2020 Omnigraphics. Reviewed September 2019.

Understanding Euthanasia and Palliative Sedation

Also, called "mercy killing," euthanasia is generally defined as a deliberate intervention undertaken at a patient's request to end her or his life in order to relieve intractable suffering. While both euthanasia and palliative sedation address extreme suffering associated with painful terminal illnesses, euthanasia may have slightly different connotations in different countries. In euthanasia, the physician administers appropriate medication in the required lethal amount to ensure that the patient loses consciousness and ceases to breathe. This is followed by cardiac arrest and death. The patient's death signifies that the intervention was successful.

Palliative sedation, also called "terminal sedation," is defined as the administration of nonopioid drugs as an intervention to treat unremitting, refractory pain or other clinical symptoms that have failed to respond to symptom-specific palliative care. The practice aims to sedate a terminally ill patient to a lowered state of consciousness that limits the patient's awareness of suffering and pain. Interventions for safely achieving sedation are used in other medical contexts, such as surgery, and do not have a detrimental effect on life, nor do they hasten the end-of-life process.

Often used as a last resort, palliative sedation is not considered an isolated intervention, but rather a symptom-control strategy within the continuum of palliative care. That being said, death may or may not occur upon achieving symptom control. Palliative sedation differs from euthanasia in three aspects: the intervention itself; the intention; and the act. While euthanasia involves an explicit intention to aid the patient in ending life, palliative sedation involves providing relief from otherwise unmanageable symptoms.

Core Ethical Issues and Attitudes Regarding Physician-Assisted Suicide and Euthanasia

The ethical debate over personal control at life's end has generated serious discussion concerning the pros and cons of legalizing PAS and euthanasia. Mounting concern about the potential harm or abuse of legalizing the practices remains a huge deterrent to the legalization of these practices. One argument against PAS asserts that, while the practice may seem compatible with patient autonomy and self-determination, the manner in which the practice is applied in a medical setting would actually undermine patient autonomy.

Some argue that mental disorders such as major depression can prevent patients from making a rational choice and thereby raises serious concerns regarding the role of patient self-determination in the practice of PAS. Detractors also point out that a lack of viable alternatives for medical treatment or personal support can compel patients to choose PAS as a means of ending suffering, pain, and further medical expenses associated with end-of-life medical treatment. This lack of viable alternatives, they argue, also requires serious consideration of the rationale behind these practices.

The debate about PAS and euthanasia also raises complex questions about the goals of the medical profession and duties of physicians. While some hold that PAS may be considered ethically legitimate in exceptional cases, they also advocate that professional standards are necessary and that the legal system should not authorize such practices. Others advocate legalizing PAS, euthanasia, or both, for the terminally ill.

Opposition to Physician-Assisted Suicide

Some argue that the physician's role as a healer and obligation to respect human life is deeply established in the code of medical ethics and that the Hippocratic Oath is in total variance with PAS and euthanasia. Opponents of PAS also argue that the practice goes against the deep belief in the right to life.

Studies say that religion and spirituality deeply influence end-of-life decisions. Religious doctrines defend the sacredness of life, recognize a supreme being as the "giver" of life, and bestow upon this supreme being the right to judge when life should end. Both PAS and euthanasia are perceived as moral transgressions by most religious belief systems. Most religious systems, on the other hand, approve of the use of palliative care to manage pain when it is administered alongside spiritual care, which includes creative, narrative, and ritualistic work. Such practices have been widely used to improve quality of life in the short term while helping to manage both physical and spiritual suffering during the end of life.

References

1. "Physician-Assisted Suicide," American Medical Association (AMA), n.d.

2. "The Physician's Role in Physician-Assisted Suicide," National Center for Biotechnology Information (NCBI), August 8, 2012.

Part Four

End-of-Life Care Facilities

Chapter 25

Long-Term Care

Chapter Contents

Section 25.1—What Is Long-Term Care? 228

Section 25.2—Long-Term Care: Making the Right
Decision.. 235

Section 25.3—Choosing a Nursing Home 236

Section 25.1

What Is Long-Term Care?

This section contains text excerpted from the following sources: Text in this section begins with excerpts from "What Is Long-Term Care?" National Institute on Aging (NIA), National Institutes of Health (NIH), May 1, 2017; Text under the heading "Residential Facilities, Assisted Living, and Nursing Homes" is excerpted from "Residential Facilities, Assisted Living, and Nursing Homes," National Institute on Aging (NIA), National Institutes of Health (NIH), May 1, 2017; Text under the heading "What Are My Other Long-Term-Care Choices?" is excerpted from "What Are My Other Long-Term-Care Choices?" Centers for Medicare & Medicaid Services (CMS), August 18, 2012. Reviewed September 2019.

Long-term care involves a variety of services designed to meet a person's health or personal care needs during a short or long period of time. These services help people live as independently and safely as possible when they can no longer perform everyday activities on their own.

Long-term care is provided in different places by different caregivers, depending on a person's needs. Most long-term care is provided at home by unpaid family members and friends. It can also be given in a facility such as a nursing home or in the community, for example, in an adult daycare center.

The most common type of long-term care is personal care—help with everyday activities, also called "activities of daily living" (ADL). These activities include bathing, dressing, grooming, using the toilet, eating, and moving around—for example, getting out of bed and into a chair.

Long-term care also includes community services, such as meals, adult daycare, and transportation services. These services may be provided free or for a fee.

People often need long-term care when they have a serious, ongoing health condition or disability. The need for long-term care can arise suddenly, such as after a heart attack or stroke. Most often, however, it develops gradually, as people get older and frailer or as an illness or disability gets worse.

Home-Based Long-Term-Care Services

Home-based long-term care includes health, personal, and support services to help people stay at home and live as independently as possible. Most long-term care is provided either in the home of the person receiving services or at a family member's home. In-home services may be short-term—for someone who is recovering from an operation, for example—or long-term, for people who need ongoing help.

Most home-based services involve personal care, such as help with bathing, dressing, and taking medications, and supervision to make sure a person is safe. Unpaid family members, partners, friends, and neighbors provide most of this type of care.

Home-based long-term-care services can also be provided by paid caregivers, including caregivers found informally, and healthcare professionals, such as nurses, home healthcare aides, therapists, and homemakers, who are hired through home healthcare agencies. These services include home healthcare, homemaker services, friendly visitor/companion services, and emergency response systems.

Home Healthcare

Home healthcare involves part-time medical services ordered by a physician for a specific condition. These services may include nursing care to help a person recover from surgery, an accident, or illness. Home healthcare may also include physical, occupational, or speech therapy and temporary home health aide services. These services are provided by home healthcare agencies approved by Medicare, a government insurance program for people over age 65.

Homemaker Services

Home health agencies offer personal care and homemaker services that can be purchased without a physician's order. Personal care includes help with bathing and dressing. Homemaker services include help with meal preparation and household chores. Agencies do not have to be approved by Medicare to provide these kinds of services.

Friendly Visitor/Companion Services

Friendly visitor/companion services are usually staffed by volunteers who regularly pay short visits (less than 2 hours) to someone who is frail or living alone. You can also purchase these services from home health agencies.

Transportation Services

Transportation services help people get to and from medical appointments, shopping centers, and other places in the community.

Some senior housing complexes and community groups offer transportation services. Many public transit agencies have services for people with disabilities. Some services are free. Others charge a fee.

Emergency Response Systems

Emergency response systems automatically respond to medical and other emergencies via electronic monitors. The user wears a necklace or bracelet with a button to push in an emergency. Pushing the button summons emergency help to the home. This type of service is especially useful for people who live alone or are at risk of falling. A monthly fee is charged.

To find home-based services, contact Eldercare Locator at 800-677-1116 or visit www.eldercare.acl.gov. You can also call your local Area Agency on Aging (AAA), Aging and Disability Resource Center (ADRC), department of human services or aging, or a social service agency.

Residential Facilities, Assisted Living, and Nursing Homes

At some point, support from family, friends, and local programs may not be enough. People who require help full-time might move to a residential facility that provides many or all of the long-term-care services they need. Facility-based long-term-care services include board and care homes, assisted living facilities, nursing homes, and continuing care retirement communities. Some facilities have only housing and housekeeping, but many also provide personal care and medical services. Many facilities offer special programs for people with Alzheimer disease (AD) and other types of dementia.

Board and Care Homes

Board and care homes, also called "residential care facilities" or "group homes," are small private facilities, usually with 20 or fewer residents. Rooms may be private or shared. Residents receive personal care and meals and have staff available around the clock. Nursing and medical care usually are not provided on-site.

Assisted Living

Assisted living is for people who need help with daily care, but not as much help as a nursing home provides. Assisted living facilities range in size from as few as 25 residents to 120 or more. Typically, a few "levels of care" are offered, with residents paying more for higher levels of care.

Assisted living residents usually live in their own apartments or rooms and share common areas. They have access to many services, including up to three meals a day; assistance with personal care; help with medications, housekeeping, and laundry; 24-hour supervision, security, and on-site staff; and social and recreational activities. Exact arrangements vary from state to state.

Nursing Homes

Nursing homes, also called "skilled nursing facilities," provide a wide range of health and personal care services. Their services focus on medical care more than most assisted living facilities. These services typically include nursing care, 24-hour supervision, three meals a day, and assistance with everyday activities. Rehabilitation services, such as physical, occupational, and speech therapy, are also available.

Some people stay at a nursing home for a short time after being in the hospital. After they recover, they go home. However, most nursing home residents live there permanently because they have ongoing physical or mental conditions that require constant care and supervision.

What Are My Other Long-Term-Care Choices?

You may have other long-term-care options (besides nursing home care) available to you. Talk to your family, your doctor or other healthcare provider, a person-centered counselor, or a social worker for help deciding what kind of long-term care you need.

Before you make any decisions about long-term care, talk to someone you trust to understand more about other long-term-care services and supports such as the ones listed below. You might want to talk to:

- Your family

- Your doctor or other healthcare provider

- A person-centered counselor

- A social worker

If you are in a hospital, nursing home, or working with a Home Health Agency (HHA), you can get support to help you understand your options or help you arrange care. Talk to:

231

- A discharge planner

- A social worker

- An organization in a "No Wrong Door System," such as an ADRC, AAA, or Center for Independent Living (CIL)

American Indians and Alaska Natives can contact their local Indian healthcare providers for more information.

Some long-term-care options you can consider:

Home- and Community-Based Services

A variety of home- and community-based services may be available to help with your personal care and activities.

Medicaid may cover some services, including:

- Home care (such as cooking, cleaning, or help with other daily activities)

- Home health services (such as physical therapy or skilled nursing care)

- Transportation to medical care

- Personal care

- Respite care

- Hospice

- Case management

Medicaid programs vary from state to state. Medicaid may offer more services in your state. Call your Medicaid office for more information.

These types of services may also be available through other programs, such as the AAA, Medicare, or hospice programs.

Community sources, such as volunteer groups that help with things such as shopping or transportation, which may be free or low cost (or may ask for a voluntary donation) are another option. Examples of the services and programs that may be available in your community are:

- Adult day services

- Adult day healthcare (which offers nursing and therapy)

- Care coordination and case management (including transition services to leave a nursing home)

- Home care (such as cooking, cleaning, or help with other daily activities)

- Meal programs (such as Meals on Wheels)

- Senior centers

- Friendly visitor programs

- Help with shopping and transportation

- Help with legal questions, bill pay, and other financial matters

Accessory Dwelling Unit

An accessory dwelling unit (ADU) (sometimes called an "in-law apartment," "accessory apartment," or a "second unit") is a second living space within a home or on a lot. It has a separate living and sleeping area, a place to cook, and a bathroom. If you or a loved one owns a single-family home, adding an ADU to an existing home may help you keep your independence.

Space, such as an upper floor, basement, attic, or over a garage may be turned into an ADU. Family members may be interested in living in an ADU in your home, or you may want to move into an ADU at a family member's home.

Check with your local zoning office to be sure ADUs are allowed in your area and find out if there are any special rules. The cost of an ADU can vary widely, depending on many factors, like the size of the project.

Subsidized Senior Housing

There are state and federal programs that help pay for housing for some seniors with low to moderate incomes. Some of these housing programs also offer help with meals and other activities, such as housekeeping, shopping, and doing the laundry. Residents usually live in their own apartments within an apartment building. Rent payments are usually based on a percentage of a person's income.

Continuing Care Retirement Communities

Continuing care retirement communities (CCRCs) offer different kinds of housing and levels of care. In the same community, there may be:

- Individual homes or apartments (for residents who still live on their own)

- An assisted living facility (for people who need some help with daily care)

- A nursing home (for people who require higher levels of care)

Residents can move from one level to another based on their needs but usually stay within the CCRC. If you are considering a CCRC, be sure to check the quality of its nursing home and the inspection report (posted in the facility).

Group Living Arrangements

Residential care communities (sometimes called "adult foster/family homes" or "personal care homes") and assisted living communities are types of group living arrangements. In some states, residential care and assisted living communities mean the same thing. Both can help with some of the activities of daily living, such as bathing, dressing, using the bathroom and meals. Whether they offer nursing services or help with medications varies by state.

In most cases, residents of these communities pay a regular monthly rent and additional fees depending on the type of personal care services they get.

Program of All-Inclusive Care for the Elderly

The Program of All-inclusive Care for the Elderly (PACE) is a Medicare/Medicaid program that helps people meet healthcare needs in the community.

Section 25.2

Long-Term Care: Making the Right Decision

This section includes text excerpted from "Planning for Long-Term Care," National Institute on Aging (NIA), National Institutes of Health (NIH), May 1, 2017.

You can never know for sure if you will need long-term care. Maybe you will never need it. But an unexpected accident, illness, or injury can change your needs, sometimes suddenly. The best time to think about long-term care is before you need it. Planning for the possibility of long-term care gives you time to learn about services in your community and what they cost. It also allows you to make important decisions while you are still able. People with Alzheimer disease (AD) or other cognitive impairment should begin planning for long-term care as soon as possible.

Planning for Long-Term Care
Decisions about Housing

In thinking about long-term care, it is important to consider where you will live as you age and how your place of residence can best support your needs if you can no longer fully care for yourself.

Most people prefer to stay in their own home for as long as possible.

Decisions about Health

Begin by thinking about what would happen if you became seriously ill or disabled. Talk with your family, friends, and lawyer about who would provide care if you needed help for a long time. Read about how to prepare healthcare advance directives.

You might delay or prevent the need for long-term care by staying healthy and independent. Talk to your doctor about your medical and family history and lifestyle. She or he may suggest actions you can take to improve your health.

Healthy eating, regular physical activity, not smoking, and limited drinking of alcohol can help you stay healthy. So can an active social life, a safe home, and regular healthcare.

Decisions about Finances

Long-term care can be expensive. Americans spend billions of dollars a year on various services. How people pay for long-term care depends on their financial situation and the kinds of services they use. Often, they rely on a variety of payment sources, including:

- Personal funds, including pensions, savings, and income from stocks

- Government health insurance programs, such as Medicaid (Medicare does not cover long-term care but may cover some costs of short-term care in a nursing home after a hospital stay.)

- Private financing options, such as long-term-care insurance

- Veterans' benefits

- Services through the Older Americans Act (OAA, 1965)

Section 25.3

Choosing a Nursing Home

This section includes text excerpted from "Choosing a Nursing Home," National Institute on Aging (NIA), National Institutes of Health (NIH), May 1, 2017.

A nursing home, also known as a "skilled nursing facility," provides a wide range of health and personal care services.

These services typically include nursing care, 24-hour supervision, three meals a day, and assistance with everyday activities. Rehabilitation services, such as physical, occupational, and speech therapy, are also available.

Some people stay at a nursing home for a short time after being in the hospital. After they recover, they go home. However, most nursing home residents live there permanently because they have ongoing physical or mental conditions that require constant care and supervision.

How to Choose a Nursing Home?

If you need to go to a nursing home after a hospital stay, the hospital staff can help you find one that will provide the kind of care that is best for you. If you are looking for a nursing home, ask your doctor's office for recommendations. Once you know what choices you have, it is a good idea to:

- Consider what is important to you—nursing care, meals, physical therapy, a religious connection, hospice care, or special care units for dementia patients? Do you want a place close to family and friends so they can easily visit?

- Ask your friends, relatives, social workers, and religious groups to find out what places they suggest. Check with healthcare providers about which nursing homes they feel provide good care.

- Call and get in touch with each place on your list. Ask questions about how many people live there and what it costs. Find out about waiting lists.

- Visit and make plans to meet with the director and the nursing director.

- For example, look for:

  - Medicare and Medicaid certification

  - Handicap access

  - Residents who look well cared for

  - Warm interaction between staff and residents

- Talk and do not be afraid to ask questions. For example, ask the staff to explain any strong odors. Bad smells might indicate a problem; good ones might hide a problem. You might want to find out how long the director and heads of nursing, food, and social services departments have worked at the nursing home. If key members of the staff change often, that could mean there is something wrong.

- Make a second visit without calling ahead. Try another day of the week or time of day so you will meet other staff members and see different activities. Stop by at mealtime. Is the dining room attractive and clean? Does the food look tempting?

- Understand the contract once you select a nursing home by carefully reading the same. Question the director or assistant director about anything you do not understand. Ask a good friend or family member to read over the contract before you sign it.

237

The Centers for Medicare and Medicaid Services (CMS) requires each state to inspect any nursing home that gets money from the government. Homes that do not pass inspection are not certified. Ask to see the current inspection report and certification of any nursing home you are considering.

Chapter 26

Home Care for
Critically Ill Patients

Chapter Contents

Section 26.1—Home Care for Cancer Patients.......................... 240
Section 26.2—Home Healthcare for Critically Ill
and Older Adults.. 251
Section 26.3—Assistive Devices and Rehabilitative
Technologies for Patients with
Chronic Conditions... 254

Section 26.1

Home Care for Cancer Patients

This section includes text excerpted from "Family Caregivers in
Cancer (PDQ®)—Patient Version," National Cancer Institute (NCI),
July 14, 2015. Reviewed September 2019.

Who Is the Caregiver?

Family caregivers may be spouses, partners, children, relatives, or
friends who help the patient with activities of daily living and healthcare needs at home.

Many cancer patients today receive part of their care at home.
Hospital stays are shorter than they used to be, and there are now
more treatments that do not need an overnight hospital stay or can
be given outside of the hospital. People with cancer are living longer
and many patients want to be cared for at home as much as possible.
This care is often given by family caregivers. These caregivers may be
spouses, partners, children, relatives, or friends.

The family caregiver works with the healthcare team and has an
important role in improving the patient's health and quality of life
(QOL). Today, family caregivers do many things that used to be done
in the hospital or doctor's office by healthcare providers. Caregiving
includes everyday tasks, such as helping the patient with medicines,
doctor visits, meals, schedules, and health insurance matters. It also
includes giving emotional and spiritual support, such as helping the
patient deal with feelings and making hard decisions.

It is important that the family caregiver is a part of the team right
from the start. The family caregiver has the very important job of
watching for changes in the patient's medical condition while giving
long-term care at home. Family caregivers can help plan treatment,
make decisions, and carry out treatment plans all through the different
parts of treatment.

This summary is about adult family caregivers in cancer.

Caregiver's Point of View
Caregivers Need Help and Emotional Support

A caregiver responds in her or his own way to the cancer patient's
diagnosis and prognosis. The caregiver may feel emotions that are as
strong as or stronger than those felt by the patient. The caregiver's

need for information, help, and support is different from what is needed by the patient.

The life of a family caregiver changes in many ways when cancer is diagnosed. These changes affect most parts of life and continue after treatment ends.

Caregiver's Role Changes as the Patient's Needs Change

Key times when the caregiver's role changes and new challenges come up are at diagnosis, during treatment at the hospital, when the patient needs care at home, after treatment ends, and at the patient's end of life.

At Diagnosis

Family caregivers take an active role that begins when the cancer is being diagnosed. The caregiver has to learn about the kind of cancer the patient has and new medical terms. The caregiver also goes with the patient to new places for treatment and helps the patient make treatment decisions.

During Treatment at the Hospital

The patient may ask the caregiver to be the one to talk to the healthcare team and make important decisions. The relationship between the caregiver and the patient affects how well this works. Disagreements between the patient and caregiver can make important decisions harder to make and affect treatment choices. In addition to talking to the healthcare team, the caregiver may also do the following:

- Take on many of the patient's household duties.

- Schedule hospital visits and plan travel to and from the visits.

- Work through the healthcare system for the patient.

- Arrange for home care.

- Take care of insurance matters.

During the active treatment phase, a caregiver needs to meet the demands of supporting the patient as well as the demands of home, work, and family. This may be physically and emotionally exhausting.

During Care in the Home

When the patient moves from one care setting (such as the hospital) to another (such as the home), it can be stressful for the patient and the caregiver. The patient usually would rather be at home, which is a familiar and comforting place. The return home usually means more work for the caregiver.

In addition to hands-on patient care, the caregiver may also do the following:

• Be a companion to the patient.

• Continue doing many of the patient's household duties.

• Take care of medicines and meals.

• Schedule doctor visits, plan travel to and from the visits, and go with the patient to them.

• Arrange for home visits by therapists or other professionals.

• Deal with medical emergencies.

• Take care of insurance matters.

• Work through the healthcare system for the patient.

Caregivers worry about how they will be able to do all this and also take care of themselves. The caregiver sometimes has to give up social activities and miss work. This can all be very hard and very tiring in a physical and emotional way for both the caregiver and the patient. These demands can be especially hard on older caregivers.

After Treatment Ends

Some patients and caregivers expect life to go back to the way it was before the cancer was diagnosed and this may not happen. Caregiver stress may continue after the patient's treatment ends, as roles change once again. Some caregivers have problems adjusting for the first year after the end of treatment. Part of this is caused by a worry that the cancer will come back. When the caregiver is the partner or spouse of the cancer survivor, there may be sexual problems, also. Studies have shown that these adjustment problems usually do not last long. Problems with adjusting that can last a long time include the following:

• Problems in the relationship between the caregiver and the patient

- Poor communication between the caregiver and the patient

- Lack of social support

At the End of Life

Caring for a patient at home at the end of life brings a new set of challenges for the caregiver. The patient depends even more on the caregiver for physical and emotional support. The patient's symptoms also may be more difficult to manage. The caregiver may feel distressed by these new challenges and by not being able to take part in activities and interests that are important to her or him. The caregiver may feel even more distressed if the patient goes into hospice care. Studies have shown that caregivers have a lower quality of life and poorer health when giving the patient end-of-life care than they do during active treatment.

Some hospital or hospice programs offer end-of-life support services to improve the patient's quality of life and help both the caregiver and the patient. End-of-life support services include the following:

- A team approach helping the patient and family with their physical, emotional, social, spiritual, and economic needs in order to improve the quality of life of the patient and caregiver

- Including the caregiver in medical decisions and managing the patient's symptoms

- Watching the caregiver for signs of distress and work with her or him to get the kind of help they need

Roles for the Family Caregiver
The Family Caregiver Has Many Roles besides Giving the Patient Hands-On Care

Most people think first of the physical care given by a family caregiver, but a caregiver fills many other roles during the patient's cancer experience. In addition to hands-on care, the caregiver may also do the following:

- Manage the patient's medical care, insurance claims, and bill payments.

- Be a companion to the patient.

- Go with the patient to doctor appointments, run personal errands, cook, clean, and do other housekeeping chores.

- Find doctors and specialists needed and get information that may be hard to find.

- Help the patient connect with family, friends, neighbors, and community members.

A family caregiver faces the tough job of taking on new roles and challenges as the patient's needs change over time.

The Caregiver Takes on Different Roles

Caregivers may take on the roles of decision maker, patient advocate, and communicator.

Decision Maker

Doctors, caregivers, and patients are partners in making decisions. Making a decision involves getting the right information in a way that it can be understood. Cancer patients have many information needs. They want to know about staying healthy, tests and treatments, side effects and symptoms, and emotional issues.

In order to make treatment decisions, caregivers and patients often want more information and they may look for help and information from sources other than the doctor. It is common for patients and their families to do the following:

- Use the Internet to search for more information on the patient's cancer and its treatment.

- Check on the information given by the doctor.

- Look into other treatments or complementary or alternative medicine.

- Ask for advice from family and friends.

Information from outside sources is sometimes wrong or may be different from what the doctor said. It is important to get information that can be trusted and to talk to the doctor about it. Most libraries can help people find articles about cancer in medical journals and cancer information written for patients and the public. Good places to get information include government agencies, cancer centers, and cancer organizations.

Advocate

The family caregiver knows and understands the needs of the patient. The caregiver becomes an advocate for the patient by giving

244

this information to the healthcare team. Although a caregiver may not have a medical background, daily contact with the patient gives the caregiver important information that helps the healthcare team help the patient. Information about the patient's symptoms and problems can help the doctor make better treatment plans and improve the patient's chance of getting better.

As the patient's advocate, the family caregiver may do the following:

- Talk with the healthcare team about the patient's needs and wishes for the patient.

- Get information that may be hard to find.

- Find doctors and specialists needed.

- Watch the patient for changes and problems.

- Help the patient follow treatments.

- Tell the healthcare team about any new symptoms or side effects and ask for help to treat them.

- Help the patient make healthy changes and follow healthy behaviors.

- Pay the patient's bills and take care of insurance claims.

Communicator

Good communication between the doctor, patient, and caregiver can improve the patient's health and medical care. The family caregiver will often take on the role of speaking for the patient while keeping the patient included in decision making. Good communication helps both the doctor and the caregiver get the information they need to support the patient. Doctors need to hear about patients' concerns and caregivers need to understand the disease and treatment options. Poor communication may cause confusion about treatment. This can affect choices made about treatment and the patient's chance of getting better.

Cultural differences between the doctors and the caregiver or patient can affect communication. In some cultures, it is the custom to keep a life-threatening diagnosis a secret from the patient and avoid talking about the disease. Sometimes it is left to the caregiver to tell the patient the truth about a serious or terminal illness. This can be stressful for caregivers and increase their feelings of loneliness and responsibility. Caregivers should tell the healthcare team if they think cultural beliefs may affect how they talk about cancer and making treatment decisions.

Caregiver's Quality of Life
Caring for a Patient with Cancer Affects the Family Caregiver's Quality of Life

Family caregivers usually begin caregiving without training and are expected to meet many demands without much help. A caregiver often neglects her or his own quality of life by putting the patient's needs first. Today, many healthcare providers watch for signs of caregiver distress during the course of the patient's cancer treatment. When caregiver strain affects the quality of caregiving, the patient's well-being is also affected. Helping the caregiver also helps the patient.

Caregiver's Quality of Life in Many Areas

The caregiver's well-being is affected in many areas. These include psychological, physical, social, financial, and spiritual.

Psychological Issues

Psychological distress is the most common effect of caregiving on the caregiver's quality of life. Caring for a cancer patient is a difficult and stressful job. Caregiver distress comes from the practical demands of the caregiver role as well the emotional ones, such as seeing the patient suffer. Family members seeing a loved one with cancer may feel as much or more distress than the patient does. Distress is usually worse when the cancer is advanced and the patient is no longer being treated to cure the cancer.

Caregivers who have health problems of their own or demands from other parts of their lives may enter the caregiving role already overwhelmed. For an older adult caregiver, problems that are a part of aging may make caregiving harder to handle.

The caregiver's ability to cope with distress may be affected by her or his personality type. Someone who is usually hopeful and positive may cope better with problems of caregiving.

Physical Issues

Cancer patients often need a lot of physical help during their illness. This is physically demanding for the caregiver, who may need to help the patient with many activities during the day, such as:

- Use the toilet

- Eat

- Change position in bed

- Move from one place to another, such as from bed to toilet

- Use medical equipment

The amount of physical help a patient needs depends on the following:

- Whether the patient can do normal activities of daily living, such as dressing and walking

- The amount of fatigue the patient has

- The stage of the cancer

- The symptoms and how bad they are

- Side effects of the cancer and the cancer treatments

As caregivers try to meet the physical demands of caregiving, they may not get enough rest and may not take care of their own health. Healthy habits, such as exercise, a healthy diet, and regular medical checkups may be pushed to the side. Health problems the caregiver already has may become worse, or they may have new health problems.

Social Issues

Caregivers often have less time to spend with friends and in the community as their days are filled with caring for the cancer patient. If there are problems in the relationship between the caregiver and the patient, the caregiver may feel even more alone.

In the beginning, there may be a lot of support from friends. The caregiver may be able to continue working and keep up work relationships. When cancer care continues for a long time, the caregiver may need to stop working and friends may call or visit less often. As caregivers struggle to meet the ongoing demands of caregiving, they may want more help from family and friends. Caregivers can find support in other places, such as caregiver groups and cancer organizations, where they can talk with other families. Some caregivers find it helpful to join a support group or talk to a counselor, psychologist, or other mental health professional. Others also find it helpful to turn to a leader in their faith or spiritual community.

Money Issues

There are many financial costs of cancer. Families must pay insurance deductibles, copayments, and for services that are not covered by insurance, such as transportation and home care help. Some caregivers give up their jobs and income so they can stay home with the patient, which makes it harder to pay for everything.

Caregivers who work may have less distress if they are able to take leave from work under the Family and Medical Leave Act (FMLA). FMLA applies to businesses with at least 50 employees. It allows employees to take time off from work for their own illness or a relative's serious medical condition without losing their jobs or benefits. Caregivers may take up to 12 weeks of leave.

Spiritual Issues

Feelings of spiritual well-being may help lower the caregiver's stress. Keeping faith and finding meaning and hope have been shown to decrease the effect of caregiving stress on mental health. Spiritual well-being may help some caregivers be more hopeful, find meaning in the cancer experience, and be more accepting of what is.

Rewards of Caregiving

Caregivers become caregivers for many different reasons. Some feel it is natural to care for someone they love. Sometimes there are practical reasons, such as no insurance or money to pay for other help. Whatever the reasons, giving care and support during cancer is not easy, yet many caregivers find something positive from it.

Caring for a person with cancer causes many caregivers to look at life in new ways. They think about the purpose of life and they often focus on what they value most. For some caregivers, looking for meaning is a way to cope.

Some caregivers will have the following rewards:

• Find they can be strong during bad times

• Have a better sense of self-worth or personal growth

• Feel closer to the cancer patient

Getting support from healthcare professionals may help caregivers find more positive rewards.

Assessing Caregiver Needs
Caregiver Assessment Is Done to Find Out If the Caregiver Needs Support in the Caregiving Role

Caregiver assessment helps the healthcare team understand the caregiver's everyday life, recognize the many jobs done by the caregiver, and look for signs of caregiver strain. Caregiver strain occurs when caregivers are not comfortable in their roles or feel they cannot handle everything they need to do. Caregiver strain may lead to depression and general psychological distress. If the caregiver feels too much strain, caregiving is no longer healthy for either the caregiver or the patient.

A caregiver assessment should look at not only what the patient needs the caregiver to do, but also what the caregiver is willing and able to do. Caregiver strain may occur when the family caregiver does not have the knowledge needed to care for the patient. The healthcare team can support the caregiver in this area.

Family caregivers report many problems with their caregiving experiences. Assessment is done to find out what the problems are, in order to give the caregiver the right kind of support. Support services can help the caregiver stay healthy, learn caregiving skills, and remain in the caregiving role, all of which help the patient as well.

Some of the factors that affect caregiver strain:

- The number of hours spent caregiving

- How prepared the caregiver is for caregiving

- The types of care being given

- How much the patient is able to do without help (such as bathing and dressing)

Caregiver Well-Being Is Assessed in Several Areas to Find Out What Type of Help Is Needed

There is no standard tool for caregiver assessment. It may be different for each caregiver and family. Some of the factors assessed are culture, age, health, finances, and roles and relationships. Support services can then be chosen to help where the caregiver needs it.

Culture

Studies have shown that a family's culture affects how they handle the caregiver role. In some cultures, the family chooses not to get any outside help. Caregivers who have no outside help or help from other family members are usually more depressed than those who receive help from other sources.

Some of the reasons caregivers do not get outside help is that they:

- Do not want to share family matters with others

- Cannot find outside help

- Do not trust social service providers

- Do not know how hospice care can help them

Age and Health

Caregivers may have issues related to age and health that increase their risk for caregiver strain:

- For an older adult caregiver, issues that are a part of aging may make caregiving harder to handle. Older caregivers may have health problems, live on fixed incomes, and have little social support. As they try to meet the demands of caregiving, older caregivers may not take care of their own health. This can make their health worse or cause new health problems. Caregiver strain in older caregivers may lead to an earlier death than noncaregivers the same age.

- Middle-aged and younger caregivers who have jobs and children or other family members to care for are often strained by the caregiving role. These caregivers try to meet the needs of work and family and give up much of their social life while caring for the patient.

Costs of Care

Families with low household incomes may not be able to afford the costs of caregiving. When the family cannot pay for costs related to treatment, the patient's recovery may be affected. Caregiver distress increases.

Roles and Relationships

As the number of roles the caregiver must fill increases, the risk of caregiver strain also increases. Given too many roles to fill, the caregiver will not have the time and energy to do them all. For example, caregivers who have a job and also care for children report high levels of stress. However, working while caregiving can also be helpful. Time away from the caregiving role and the social support from coworkers can give the caregiver some relief.

Roles and relationships among family members can be affected by caregiving. A caregiver assessment looks at family relationships to see if there is a risk of caregiver strain.

Section 26.2

Home Healthcare for Critically Ill and Older Adults

This section includes text excerpted from "Home Healthcare," Administration for Community Living (ACL), October 17, 2015. Reviewed September 2019.

Home healthcare helps older adults live independently for as long as possible, even with an illness or injury. It covers a wide range of services and can often delay the need for long-term nursing home care.

Home healthcare may include occupational and physical therapy, speech therapy, and skilled nursing. It may involve helping older adults with activities of daily living, such as bathing, dressing, and eating. It can also include assistance with cooking, cleaning, other housekeeping, and monitoring one's medication regimen.

It is important to understand the difference between home healthcare and home care services. Although home healthcare may include some home care services, it is medical in nature. Home care services include chores and house cleaning, whereas home healthcare usually involves helping someone to recover from an illness or injury. Home healthcare professionals are often licensed practical nurses, therapists, or home health aides. Most of them work for home health agencies, hospitals, or public health departments licensed by the state.

Ensuring Quality Care in Home Healthcare Agencies

As with any important purchase, it is wise to talk with friends, neighbors, and your local Area Agency on Aging (AAA) to learn more about the home healthcare agencies in your community. Consider using the following questions to guide your search.

- How long has the agency served this community?

- Does the agency have a brochure describing services and costs? If so, take or download it.

- Is the agency an approved Medicare provider?

- Does a national accrediting body, such as the Joint Commission for the Accreditation of Healthcare Organizations (JCAHO), certify the quality of care?

- Does the agency have a current license to practice (if required by the state)?

- Does the agency offer a "Bill of Rights" that describes the rights and responsibilities of both the agency and the person receiving care?

- Does the agency prepare a care plan for the patient (with input from the patient, her or his doctor, and family members)? Will the agency update the plan as necessary?

- How closely do supervisors oversee care to ensure quality?

- Are agency staff members available around the clock, seven days a week, if necessary?

- Does the agency have a nursing supervisor available for on-call assistance at all times?

- Whom does the agency call if the home healthcare worker cannot come when scheduled?

- How does the agency ensure patient confidentiality?

- How are agency caregivers hired and trained?

- How does the agency screen prospective employees?

- Will the agency provide a list of references for its caregivers?

- What is the procedure for resolving problems, if they occur? Whom can I call with questions or complaints?

- Is there a sliding fee schedule based on ability to pay, and is financial assistance available to pay for services?

When purchasing home healthcare directly from an individual provider (instead of an agency), it is even more important to conduct thorough screening. This should include an interview with the home health caregiver. You should also request references. Prepare for the interview by making a list of the older adult's special needs. For example, the patient may require help getting into or out of a wheelchair. If so, the caregiver must be able to provide appropriate assistance.

Whether you arrange for home healthcare through an agency or hire an independent aide, it helps to spend time preparing the person who will provide care. Ideally, you will spend a day with the caregiver, before the job formally begins, to discuss what is involved in the daily routine. At a minimum, inform the caregiver (verbally and in writing) of the following things that she or he should know.

- Health conditions, including illnesses and injuries

- Signs of an emergency medical situation

- General likes and dislikes

- Medication, including how and when each must be taken

- Need for dentures, eyeglasses, canes, walkers, hearing aids, etc.

- Possible behavior problems and how best to handle them

- Mobility issues (trouble walking, getting into or out of a wheelchair, etc.)

- Allergies, special diets, or other nutritional needs

- Therapeutic exercises with detailed instructions

A Word of Caution

Although most states require home healthcare agencies to perform criminal background checks on their workers and carefully screen applicants, actual regulations will vary depending on where you live. Therefore, before contacting a home healthcare agency, you may want to call your local area agency on aging or department of public health to learn what laws apply in your state.

Paying for Care

The cost of home healthcare varies across and within states. In addition, costs will fluctuate based on the type of healthcare professional required. Home care services can be paid directly by patients and their families or through a variety of public and private sources. Sources for home healthcare funding include Medicare, Medicaid, the Older Americans Act (OAA), the Veterans Administration, and private insurance.

Section 26.3

Assistive Devices and Rehabilitative Technologies for Patients with Chronic Conditions

This section includes text excerpted from "What Are Some Types of Assistive Devices and How Are They Used?" *Eunice Kennedy Shriver* National Institute of Child Health and Human Development (NICHD), October 24, 2018.

Assistive Devices and Their Use

Some examples of assistive technologies are:

- Mobility aids, such as wheelchairs, scooters, walkers, canes, crutches, prosthetic devices, and orthotic devices

- Hearing aids to help people hear or hear more clearly

- Cognitive aids, including computer or electrical assistive devices, to help people with memory, attention, or other challenges in their thinking skills

- Computer software and hardware, such as voice recognition programs, screen readers, and screen enlargement applications, to help people with mobility and sensory impairments use computers and mobile devices

- Tools, such as automatic page turners, book holders, and adapted pencil grips to help learners with disabilities participate in educational activities

- Closed captioning to allow people with hearing problems to watch movies, television programs, and other digital media

- Physical modifications in the built environment, including ramps, grab bars, and wider doorways to enable access to buildings, businesses, and workplaces

- Lightweight, high-performance mobility devices that enable persons with disabilities to play sports and be physically active

- Adaptive switches and utensils to allow those with limited motor skills to eat, play games, and accomplish other activities

- Devices and features of devices to help perform tasks, such as cooking, dressing, and grooming; specialized handles and grips, devices that extend reach, and lights on telephones and doorbells are a few examples

Rehabilitative Technologies and Their Use

Rehabilitative technologies and techniques help people recover or improve function after injury or illness. Examples include the following:

- **Robotics.** Specialized robots help people regain and improve function in arms or legs after a stroke.

- **Virtual reality.** People who are recovering from injury can retrain themselves to perform motions within a virtual environment.

- **Musculoskeletal modeling and simulations.** These computer simulations of the human body can pinpoint underlying mechanical problems in a person with a movement-related disability. This technique can help improve assistive aids or physical therapies.

- **Transcranial magnetic stimulation (TMS).** TMS sends magnetic impulses through the skull to stimulate the brain. This system can help people who have had a stroke recover movement and brain function.

- **Transcranial direct current stimulation (tDCS).** In tDCS, a mild electrical current travels through the skull and stimulates the brain. This can help recover movement in patients recovering from stroke or other conditions.

- **Motion analysis.** Motion analysis captures video of human motion with specialized computer software that analyzes the motion in detail. The technique gives healthcare providers a detailed picture of a person's specific movement challenges to guide proper therapy.

Some devices incorporate multiple types of technologies and techniques to help users regain or improve function. For example, the BrainGate project, which was partially funded by *Eunice Kennedy Shriver* National Institute of Child Health and Human Development (NICHD) through the National Center for Medical Rehabilitation Research (NCMRR), relied on tiny sensors being implanted in the brain. The user could then think about moving their arm, and a robotic arm would carry out the thought.

Chapter 27

Palliative Care and Hospice Care: Comforting the Terminally Ill

Many Americans die in facilities such as hospitals or nursing homes receiving care that is not consistent with their wishes. To make sure that does not happen, older people need to know what their end-of-life care options are and state their preferences to their caregivers in advance. For example, if an older person wants to die at home, receiving end-of-life care for pain and other symptoms, and makes this known to healthcare providers and family, it is less likely she or he will die in a hospital receiving unwanted treatments.

Caregivers have several factors to consider when choosing end-of-life care, including the older person's desire to pursue life-extending or curative treatments, how long she or he has left to live, and the preferred setting for care.

Understanding Palliative Care

Doctors can provide treatment to seriously ill patients in the hopes of a cure for as long as possible. These patients may also receive

This chapter includes text excerpted from "What Are Palliative Care and Hospice Care?" National Institute on Aging (NIA), National Institutes of Health (NIH), May 17, 2017.

medical care for their symptoms, or palliative care, along with curative treatment.

A palliative care consultation team is a multidisciplinary team that works with the patient, family, and the patient's other doctors to provide medical, social, emotional, and practical support. The team is made of palliative care specialist doctors and nurses, and includes others, such as social workers, nutritionists, and chaplains.

Palliative care can be provided in hospitals, nursing homes, outpatient palliative care clinics, and certain other specialized clinics, or at home. Medicare, Medicaid, and insurance policies may cover palliative care. Veterans may be eligible for palliative care through the U.S. Department of Veterans Affairs (VA). Private health insurance might pay for some services. Health insurance providers can answer questions about what they will cover. Check to see if insurance will cover your particular situation.

In palliative care, you do not have to give up treatment that might cure a serious illness. Palliative care can be provided along with curative treatment and may begin at the time of diagnosis. Over time, if the doctor or the palliative care team believes ongoing treatment is no longer helping, there are two possibilities. Palliative care could transition to hospice care if the doctor believes the person is likely to die within six months. Or, the palliative care team could continue to help with increasing emphasis on comfort care.

Who Can Benefit from Palliative Care?

Palliative care is a resource for anyone living with a serious illness, such as heart failure, chronic obstructive pulmonary disease (COPD), cancer, dementia, Parkinson disease (PD), and many others. Palliative care can be helpful at any stage of illness and is best provided from the point of diagnosis.

In addition to improving quality of life and helping with symptoms, palliative care can help patients understand their choices for medical treatment. The organized services available through palliative care may be helpful to any older person having a lot of general discomfort and disability very late in life. Palliative care can be provided along with curative treatment and does not depend on prognosis.

Understanding Hospice Care

Increasingly, people are choosing hospice care at the end of life. Hospice can be provided in any setting—home, nursing home, assisted living facility, or inpatient hospital.

At some point, it may not be possible to cure a serious illness, or a patient may choose not to undergo certain treatments. Hospice is designed for this situation. The patient beginning hospice care understands that her or his illness is not responding to medical attempts to cure it or to slow the disease's progress.

Like palliative care, hospice provides comprehensive comfort care as well as support for the family, but, in hospice, attempts to cure the person's illness are stopped. Hospice is provided for a person with a terminal illness whose doctor believes she or he has 6 months or less to live if the illness runs its natural course.

Hospice is an approach to care, so it is not tied to a specific place. It can be offered in two types of settings—at home or in a facility, such as a nursing home, hospital, or even in a separate hospice center.

Hospice care brings together a team of people with special skills—among them nurses, doctors, social workers, spiritual advisors, and trained volunteers. Everyone works together with the person who is dying, the caregiver, and/or the family to provide the medical, emotional, and spiritual support needed.

A member of the hospice team visits regularly, and someone is always available by phone—24 hours a day, 7 days a week. Hospice may be covered by Medicare and other insurance companies; check to see if insurance will cover your particular situation.

It is important to remember that stopping treatment aimed at curing an illness does not mean discontinuing all treatment. A good example is an older person with cancer. If the doctor determines that the cancer is not responding to chemotherapy and the patient chooses to enter into hospice care, then the chemotherapy will stop. Other medical care may continue as long as it is helpful. For example, if the person has high blood pressure, she or he will still get medicine for that.

Although hospice provides a lot of support, the day-to-day care of a person dying at home is provided by family and friends. The hospice team coaches family members on how to care for the dying person and even provides respite care when caregivers need a break. Respite care can be for as short as a few hours or for as long as several weeks.

Families of people who received care through a hospice program are more satisfied with end-of-life care than are those of people who did not have hospice services. Also, hospice recipients are more likely to have their pain controlled and less likely to undergo tests or be given medicines they do not need, compared with people who do not use hospice care.

259

What Does the Hospice Six-Month Requirement Mean?

Some people misinterpret their doctors' suggestion to consider hospice. They think it means death is very near. But, that is not always the case. Sometimes, people do not begin hospice care soon enough to take full advantage of the help it offers. Perhaps they wait too long to begin hospice; they are too close to death. Or, some people are not eligible for hospice care soon enough to receive its full benefit.

In the United States, people enrolled in Medicare can receive hospice care if their healthcare provider thinks they have less than 6 months to live should the disease take its usual course. Doctors have a hard time predicting how long an older, sick person will live. Health often declines slowly, and some people might need a lot of help with daily living for more than 6 months before they die.

Talk to the doctor if you think a hospice program might be helpful. If she or he agrees, but thinks it is too soon for Medicare to cover the services, then you can investigate how to pay for the services that are needed.

What Does Happen If Someone Under Hospice Care Live Longer than Six Months?

If the doctor continues to certify that that person is still close to dying, Medicare can continue to pay for hospice services. It is also possible to leave hospice care for a while and then later return if the healthcare provider still believes that the patient has less than 6 months to live.

Chapter 28

End-of-Life Care Settings

Decades ago, most people died at home, but medical advances have changed that. Most Americans are in hospitals or nursing homes at the end of their lives. Some people enter the hospital to get treated for an illness. Some may already be living in a nursing home.

There is no right place to die. And, of course, where we die is not always something we get to decide. But, if given the choice, each person and/or her or his family should consider which type of care makes the most sense, where that kind of care can be provided, whether family and friends are available to help, and how they will pay for it.

End-of-Life Care in Hospitals

In a hospital setting, medical professionals are available who know what needs to be done for someone who is dying. This can be very reassuring. In addition to the regular care team, some hospitals may have palliative care teams that can assist with managing uncomfortable symptoms and making medical decisions for patients who may or may not be at the end of life.

This chapter includes text excerpted from "Where Can I Find Care for a Dying Relative?" National Institute on Aging (NIA), National Institutes of Health (NIH), May 17, 2017.

The Doctor Wants to Move My Relative to the Intensive Care Unit. What Can We Expect?

The intensive care unit (ICU) and coronary care unit (CCU) are types of critical care units. These units are parts of a hospital where seriously ill patients can benefit from specially trained staff who have quick access to advanced equipment. The medical staff in ICUs and CCUs closely monitor and care for a small number of patients. Doctors who work in these units are called "intensivists."

Patients in the ICU or CCU are often connected to monitors that check breathing, heart rate, pulse, blood pressure, and oxygen levels. An intravenous (IV) tube may supply medicines, fluids, and/or nutrition. Another tube called a "Foley catheter" may take the urine out of the body. A tube through the nose or stomach area may provide nutrition and remove unwanted fluids. A breathing tube may be attached to a ventilator or respirator to help with breathing.

Often, these external supports—designed to be used for a short time—will maintain vital functions while the body heals. But sometimes, even with intensive care, the body cannot heal, and organs start to fail. When this happens, survival is unlikely. In this case, the healthcare team might talk to the family—and the patient if she or he is conscious—about considering whether or not to continue intensive treatment.

End-of-Life Care in Nursing Homes

More and more people are in nursing homes at the end of life. In a nursing home, nursing staff are always present. Unlike a hospital, a doctor is not in the facility all the time, but maybe available by phone. Plans for end-of-life care can be arranged ahead of time, so when the time comes, care can be provided as needed without first consulting a doctor.

If the person has lived in the nursing home for a while, the staff and family probably already have a relationship. This can make the care feel more personalized than in a hospital. Additionally, if the person is enrolled in hospice, the hospice team will be available to assist nursing facility staff with end-of-life care.

As in a hospital, privacy may be an issue in nursing homes. You can ask if arrangements can be made to give your family more time alone when needed.

End-of-Life Care at Home

Home is likely the most familiar setting for someone who needs end-of-life care. Family and friends can come and go freely. Care at home can be a big job for family and friends—physically, emotionally, and financially. But, there are benefits too, and it is often a job caregivers are willing to take on. Hiring a home nurse is an option for people who need additional help and have financial resources.

Talk with your healthcare provider about the kind of care needed. Frequently, this care does not require a nurse but can be provided by nursing assistants or family and friends without medical training.

To make comfort care available at home, you will have to arrange for services (such as visiting nurses) and special equipment (such as a hospital bed or bedside commode). Health insurance might only cover these services or equipment if they have been ordered by a doctor; make sure you check with your insurance company before ordering.

Work with the doctor to decide what is needed to support comfort care at home. If the seriously ill person is returning home from the hospital, sometimes a hospital discharge planner, often a social worker, can help with the planning. Your local Area Agency on Aging (AAA) might be able to recommend other sources of help.

A doctor has to be available to oversee the patient's care at home— she or he will arrange for new services, adjust treatment, and order medicines as needed. It is important to follow the doctor's plan in order to make the dying person as comfortable as possible. Talk with the doctor if you think a treatment is no longer helping. Hospice is frequently used to care for people who are home at the end of life.

Chapter 29

Insurance for End-of-Life Care

Chapter Contents

Section 29.1—Insurance Coverage for Hospice 266

Section 29.2—Long-Term-Care Insurance 270

Section 29.1

Insurance Coverage for Hospice

This section includes text excerpted from "Hospice Toolkit—An Overview of the Medicaid Hospice Benefit," Centers for Medicare & Medicaid Services (CMS), February 2016. Reviewed September 2019.

Where Is Hospice Care Received?

Hospice care is usually provided in your home. If you live in a facility, such as a nursing home, Medicaid considers the facility to be your home. There are also other locations, such as assisted living facilities, rehabilitation centers, or hospitals, where hospice services can be covered. Check with your state Medicaid agency (SMA) for other facilities that may be considered your home under the Medicaid hospice benefit. In June 2013, Medicare and Medicaid set rules about coordination between hospice and long-term-care facilities. The reason for the change in the rules is to:

- Improve the quality of care you receive, and
- Improve communication between nursing homes and hospice providers

Communication among your various healthcare providers is important. Communication is also necessary so you, your providers, and your family members can stay informed. If you live in a nursing home or other facility and you are not sure about something, you should ask questions.

What Does the Medicaid Hospice Program Cover?

Hospice services are covered as part of your Medicaid benefits. Services are provided by a team to meet your needs. The hospice team may include you, your family, and others who can help meet your physical, psychosocial, spiritual, and emotional needs. Your needs are written in a plan of care (POC), also called a "plan."

The benefits listed below are examples of hospice services you may receive:

- Physician services provided by the hospice agency
- Nursing care
- Medical equipment

- Medical supplies

- Drugs for symptom control and pain relief

- Hospice aide and homemaker services

- Physical therapy

- Occupational therapy

- Speech-language pathology services

- Social worker services

- Dietary counseling

- Short-term inpatient care for pain control, symptom management, and respite care

Hospice benefits may also include anything needed to manage your terminal illness and related conditions that are normally covered by Medicaid. The following hospice services must be provided directly by hospice employees:

- Nursing care

- Physician services

- Medical social services

- Counseling

Other hospice services may be provided, such as visits by a physician who specializes in your illness. Hospice benefits may be different in each state. Check with your SMA about hospice benefits in the area.

Are You Receiving Quality Care?

If you are receiving hospice services, you have a right to quality care. Some examples of quality care are:

- Care is focused on you and your family

- Information is provided to you and your family so you can make decisions

- Staff members respect decisions made by you and your family

- Care addresses your total needs

- You are not denied access to care because of your race, gender, religion, or sexual orientation

- Staff members are trained in how to care for you and your family

- Care is coordinated between your medical team and hospice agency

If you feel you are not getting quality care, you should tell the hospice provider who helped you enroll in hospice. You can also call the following agencies:

- Adult Protective Services (APS) agency

- Your SMA, or

- The long-term-care ombudsman's office, if you live in a nursing home

What Can You Do to Help?

You play an important role in protecting the quality of care you receive and the Medicaid program. By knowing the Medicaid rules, you can ask the right questions about the services you are receiving. You should also report things that do not seem right. Here are some things you can do to help:

- Talk to your physician to see if you are eligible for hospice care. Your physician must certify that you have a reduced life expectancy resulting from your condition(s).

- Check with your SMA about what services may be covered under hospice.

- Remember, the choice to get the hospice benefit is up to you. If you are too ill, a representative can.

- Complete and sign the forms. No one should pressure you to enroll. Never sign a blank form without.

- Ask questions.

- Ask the hospice agency about the type of care you receive.

- Ask the hospice agency or SMA about what services you will receive and which services will no longer be covered after you elect hospice.

- Ask questions about bills you receive or services you are getting.

- Be careful to whom you give your Medicaid, Medicare, or Social Security number (SSN).

Where Should You Report Concerns Related to Hospice Care?

Report any acts of physical abuse or suspected fraud to your state Medicaid Fraud Control Unit (MFCU) or SMA. If you are receiving hospice care or are being pressured to enroll in hospice care, but believe hospice care may not be appropriate for you, report it. If hospice services were billed but were not provided to you, report it. Information on contacting your SMA or MFCU is available at www.cms.gov/medicare-medicaid-coordination/fraud-prevention/fraudabuseforconsumers/report_fraud_and_suspected_fraud.html on the Centers for Medicare & Medicaid Services (CMS) website, or contact the U.S. Department of Health and Human Services (HHS), Office of Inspector General (HHS-OIG). Toll-free: 800-HHS-TIPS (800-447-8477).

You play an important role in protecting the quality of care you receive and the Medicaid program. Discussing end-of-life care and choosing services that will help make you comfortable may be difficult and confusing. It is best to learn about hospice care and understand what Medicaid covers in the early stages of an illness. This helps make the decision to choose hospice easier if you become terminally ill.

You should talk to your physician to see if you are eligible for hospice care. Ask questions and stay informed. Report mistakes to your SMA. By knowing the answers to the questions discussed in this booklet, you can help protect yourself (and the Medicaid program) from fraud and abuse.

Section 29.2

Long-Term-Care Insurance

This section includes text excerpted from "Costs and How to Pay," LongTermCare.gov, Administration for Community Living (ACL), October 10, 2017.

What Is Long-Term-Care Insurance?

Unlike traditional health insurance, long-term-care insurance is designed to cover long-term services and supports, including personal and custodial care in a variety of settings, such as your home, a community organization, or other facilities.

Long-term-care insurance policies reimburse policyholders a daily amount (up to a preselected limit) for services to assist them with activities of daily living, such as bathing, dressing, or eating. You can select a range of care options and benefits that allow you to get the services you need, where you need them.

The cost of your long-term-care policy is based on:

• How old you are when you buy the policy

• The maximum amount that a policy will pay per day

• The maximum number of days (years) that a policy will pay

• The maximum amount per day times the number of days determines the lifetime maximum amount that the policy will pay

• Any optional benefits you choose, such as benefits that increase with inflation

If you are in poor health or already receiving long-term-care services, you may not qualify for long-term-care insurance as most individual policies require medical underwriting. In some cases, you may be able to buy a limited amount of coverage, or coverage at a higher "nonstandard" rate. Some group policies do not require underwriting.

What Long-Term-Care Insurance Covers

Most policies sold are comprehensive. They typically allow you to use your daily benefit in a variety of settings, including:

• Your home

- Adult day service centers

- Hospice care

- Respite care

- Assisted living facilities (also called "residential care facilities" or "alternate care facilities")

- Alzheimer special care facilities

- Nursing homes

In the home setting, comprehensive polices generally cover these services:

- Skilled nursing care

- Occupational, speech, physical, and rehabilitation therapy

- Help with personal care, such as bathing and dressing

Receiving Long-Term-Care Insurance Benefits

In order to receive benefits from your long-term-care insurance policy, you meet two criteria: the Benefit Trigger and the Elimination Period.

Benefit triggers are the criteria that an insurance company will use to determine if you are eligible for benefits. Most companies use a specific assessment form that will be filled out by a nurse/social worker team. Benefit triggers:

- Are the criteria insurance policies use to determine if you are eligible for long-term-care benefits

- Are determined through a company-sponsored nurse/social worker assessment of your condition

- Usually, are defined in terms of activities of daily living (ADLs) or cognitive impairments

- Most policies pay benefits when you need help with two or more of six ADLs or when you have a cognitive impairment

- Once you have been assessed, your care manager from the insurance company will approve a Plan of Care that outlines the benefits for which you are eligible

The "elimination period" is the amount of time that must pass after a benefit trigger occurs but before you start receiving payment for services. An elimination period:

271

- Is like the deductible you have on car insurance, except it is measured in time rather than by dollar amount

- Most policies allow you to choose an elimination period of 30, 60, or 90 days at the time you purchased your policy.

- During the period, you must cover the cost of any services you receive.

- Some policies specify that in order to satisfy an elimination period, you must receive paid care or pay for services during that time.

Once your benefits begin:

- Most policies pay your costs up to a preset daily limit until the lifetime maximum is reached.

- Other policies pay a preset cash amount for each day that you meet the benefit trigger, whether you receive paid long-term-care services on those days or not.

- These "cash disability" policies offer more flexibility but are potentially more expensive.

Buying Long-Term-Care Insurance

People with certain conditions may not qualify for long-term-care insurance. Since standards vary between different insurance companies, if one company denies you, it is possible that another company will accept you. Common reasons why you might not be able to buy long-term-care insurance include:

- You currently use long-term-care services

- You already need help with activities of daily living (ADL)

- You have acquired immunodeficiency syndrome (AIDS) or AIDS-Related Complex (ARC)

- You have Alzheimer disease or any form of dementia or cognitive dysfunction

- You have a progressive neurological condition such as multiple sclerosis (MS) or Parkinson disease

- You had a stroke within the past year to two years or a history of strokes

- You have metastatic cancer (cancer that has spread beyond its original site)

Insurance companies also consider other health conditions when determining your eligibility. If you buy your long-term-care insurance before you develop one of the health conditions listed above, then your policy will cover the care you need for that condition.

Before You Buy

You should consider a number of things before purchasing long-term-care insurance:

- Do not buy more insurance than you think you may need. You may have enough income to pay a portion of your care costs and you may only need a small policy for the remainder. You also may have family members willing and able to supplement your care needs.

- Do not buy too little insurance. That will only delay the use of your own assets or income to pay for care. Think about how you feel about having care costs that are not covered. While you can usually decrease your coverage, it is more difficult to increase coverage, especially if your health has declined.

- Look carefully at each policy. There is no "one-size-fits-all" policy.

- If you choose a policy that only pays for room and board in a facility, plan for other expenses, such as supplies, medications, linens, and other items and services that your policy may not cover.

- It costs less to buy coverage when you are younger. The average age of people buying long-term-care insurance is about 60. The average age of those purchasing policies offered at work is about 50.

- Make sure that you can afford the long-term-care insurance policy over time, as your monthly income may change.

- Research and consider different options and talk with a professional before finalizing your decision.

- Do not feel pressured into making a decision.

Where to Look for Long-Term-Care Insurance
Insurance Specialist

Most people buy long-term-care insurance directly from an insurance agent, a financial planner, or a broker. Some important points:

- States regulate which companies can sell long-term-care insurance.

- States regulate the products that companies can sell.

- There are more than 100 companies offering long-term-care insurance nationally, but 15 to 20 insurers sell most policies.

- The best way to find out which insurance companies offer long-term-care coverage in your state is to contact your state's Department of Insurance.

State Partnership Programs

Residents of some states may be able to find long-term-care coverage through a state Partnership Program that links special Partnership-qualified (PQ) long-term policies provided by private insurance companies with Medicaid. These PQ policies:

- Help people purchase shorter-term, more complete long-term-care insurance

- Include inflation protection, so the dollar amount of benefits you receive can be higher than the amount of insurance coverage you purchased

- All you to apply for Medicaid under modified eligibility rules if you continue to need long-term care and your policy maximum is reached

- Include a special "asset disregard" feature that allows you to keep assets like personal savings above the usual $2,000 Medicaid limit

Since Partnership-qualified policies must include inflation protection, the amount of the benefits you receive can be higher than the amount of insurance protection you purchased. For example, if you have a Partnership-qualified long-term-care insurance policy and receive $100,000 in benefits from it, you can apply for Medicaid and, if eligible, retain $100,000 worth of assets over and above the state's Medicaid asset threshold. In most states, the asset limit is $2,000 for a single person. Asset limits for married couples are often higher.

States must certify that partnership policies meet the specific requirements for their partnership program, including that those who sell partnership policies are trained and understand how these policies relate to public and private coverage options. To find out more about your state's program, including which insurance agents are selling partnership policies, or to find out if your state offers a partnership program, contact your state's Department of Insurance (DOI) (www.usa.gov/state-consumer).

Employer

Many private and public employers, including the federal government and a growing number of state governments, offer group long-term-care programs as a voluntary benefit, and generally:

- Employers do not typically contribute to the premium cost (as they do with health insurance), but they often negotiate a favorable group rate.

- If you are currently employed, it may be easier to qualify for long-term-care insurance through your employer than it is to purchase a policy on your own.

- You should check with your benefit or pensions office to see if your employer offers long-term-care insurance.

Long-Term-Care Insurance Costs

If you have a long-term-care insurance policy, the buyer pays a preset premium. The policy then pays for the services you need, when you need them (up to its coverage limits). On occasion, if the assumptions used to price the policy prove wrong, the insurance company can increase your premiums beyond the preset amount. Typically, you are not expected to pay premiums while you receive long-term care.

The cost of a long-term-care policy varies greatly based on:

- Your age at the time of purchase

- The policy type

- The coverage you select

In 2007, the average long-term-care insurance policy:

- Cost about $2,207 per year

- Covered 4.8 years of benefits, excluding the 20 percent of people who elected lifetime coverage

- Had a daily benefit amount of $160
- Was a comprehensive policy covering both facility and at-home care
- Included some form of automatic inflation protection

Part Five

End-of-Life Caregiving

Chapter 30

Communications among Patients, Families, and Providers

Chapter Contents

Section 30.1—Effective Communication for
　　　　Effective Care 280

Section 30.2—Talk about End-of-Life Wishes 281

Section 30.3—Communication in Cancer Care 283

Section 30.1

Effective Communication for Effective Care

This section includes text excerpted from "Effective Communication
in Caring for Older Adults," National Institute on Aging (NIA),
National Institutes of Health (NIH), May 17, 2017.

Good communication is an important part of the healing process.
Effective doctor–patient communication has research-proven benefits: Patients are more likely to adhere to treatment and have better
outcomes, they express greater satisfaction with their treatment, and
they are less likely to file malpractice suits.

Studies show that good communication is a teachable skill. Medical
students who receive communication training improve dramatically
in talking with, assessing, and building relationships with patients.
Time management skills also improve.

Interpersonal communication skills are considered so important
that they are a core competency identified by the Accreditation Council
on Graduate Medical Education (ACGME) and the American Board of
Medical Specialties (ABMS).

Learning—and using—effective communication techniques may
help you build more satisfying relationships with older patients and
become even more skilled at managing their care.

Special Communication Needs

With older patients, communication can involve special issues, such
as:

• How can you effectively interact with patients facing multiple
  illnesses and/or hearing and vision impairments?

• What is the best way to approach sensitive topics, such as
  driving abilities or end of life?

• Are there best practices to help older patients who are
  experiencing confusion or memory loss?

Three Tips for Communication with the Aged

• Stereotypes about aging and old age can lead patients and
  healthcare professionals alike to dismiss or minimize problems
  as an inevitable decline of aging. What we are learning from the

research is that aging alone does not cause illness nor does it automatically mean having to live with pain and discomfort.

- Many suggestions may appear at first glance to be time-consuming; however, an initial investment of time can lead to long-term gains for clinicians. You may get to know your patient's life history over the course of several visits rather than trying to get it all in one session, for example.

- Older patients are not all the same. You may see frail 60-year-olds and relatively healthy 80-year-olds. Your patients probably are culturally diverse, with varying socioeconomic and educational backgrounds. Some are quite active, while others may be sedentary. You are encouraged to view all older people as individuals who have a wide range of healthcare needs and questions.

Section 30.2

Talk about End-of-Life Wishes

This section includes text excerpted from "End of Life: Helping with Comfort and Care," National Institute on Aging (NIA), National Institutes of Health (NIH), July 2016. Reviewed September 2019.

Because of advances in medicine, each of us, as well as our families and friends, may face many decisions about the dying process. As hard as it might be to face the idea of your own death, you might take time to consider how your individual values relate to your wishes for end-of-life care.

By deciding what end-of-life care best suits your needs when you are healthy, you can help those close to you make the right choices when the time comes. This not only respects your values but also may give your loved one's comfort.

There are several ways to make sure others know the kind of care you want when dying.

The simplest, but not always the easiest, way is to talk about end-of-life care before an illness. Discussing your thoughts, values, and desires about end-of-life care before you become sick will help people who are close to you to know what care you want. You could discuss how you feel about using life-prolonging measures (for example, CPR or a ventilator) or where you would like to be cared for (for example, home or nursing home). Doctors should be told about these wishes as well.

For some people, it makes sense to bring this up at a small family gathering. Some may find that telling their family they have made a will (or have updated an existing one) provides an opportunity to bring up this subject with other family members. As hard as it might be to talk about your end-of-life wishes, knowing your preferences ahead of time can make decision-making easier for your family. You may also have some comfort knowing that your family can choose what you want.

On the other hand, if your parents (or another close relative or friend) are aging and you are unsure about what they want, you might introduce the subject. You can try to explain that having this conversation will help you care for them and do what they want. You might start by talking about what you think their values are, instead of talking about specific treatments. Try saying something like, "When Uncle Isaiah had a stroke, I thought you seemed upset that his kids wanted to put him on a respirator." Or, "I've always wondered why Grandpa did not die at home. Do you know?"

Encourage your parents to share the type of care they would choose to have at the end of life, rather than what they do not want. There is no right or wrong plan, only what they would like. If they are reluctant to have this conversation, do not force it, but try to bring it up again at a later time.

Section 30.3

Communication in Cancer Care

This section includes text excerpted from "Communication in Cancer Care (PDQ®)—Patient Version," National Cancer Institute (NCI), March 27, 2015. Reviewed September 2019.

Cancer Care Communication: An Overview
Good Communication Is Vital in Cancer Care

Good communication between patients, family caregivers, and the healthcare team is very important in cancer care. It helps improve patients' well-being and quality of life. Communicating about concerns and decision-making is important during all phases of treatment and supportive care for cancer.

The goals of good communication in cancer care are to:

- Build a trusting relationship between the patient, family caregivers, and the healthcare team

- Help the patient, family caregivers, and the healthcare team share information with each other

- Help the patient and family talk about feelings and concerns

Cancer Patients' Communication Needs

Patients with cancer have special communication needs. Patients, their families, and their healthcare team face many issues when cancer is diagnosed. Cancer is a life-threatening illness, even though advances in treatments have increased the chances of a cure or remission. A patient who is diagnosed with cancer may feel fear and anxiety about treatments that are often difficult, expensive, and complicated. Decisions about the patient's care can be very hard to make. Good communication can help patients, families, and doctors make these decisions together and improve the patient's well-being and quality of life.

Studies show that when patients and doctors communicate well during cancer care, there are many positive results. Patients are usually:

- More satisfied with the care and feel more in control

- More likely to follow through with treatment

- More informed

- More likely to take part in a clinical trial

- Better able to make the change from the care that is given to treat the cancer to palliative care

Patients and Families Need Much Information for Decision-Making

Some patients and families want a lot of information and choose to make decisions about care. Patients and their families should let the healthcare team know how much information they want about the cancer and its treatment. Some patients and families want a lot of detailed information. Others want less detail. Also, the need for information may change as the patient moves through diagnosis and treatment. Some patients with advanced disease want less information about their condition.

There may be differences in how involved patients and families want to be in making decisions about cancer care. Some patients and families may want to be very involved and make their own decisions about cancer care. Others may want to leave decisions to the doctor.

Communication Is Vital throughout Treatment

Communication is important throughout cancer care, but especially when important decisions are to be made. These important decision times include:

- When the patient is first diagnosed

- Any time new decisions about treatment need to be made

- After treatment, when discussing how well it worked

- Whenever the goal of care changes

- When the patient makes her or his wishes known about advance directives, such as a living will

Effective End-of-Life Discussions Lead to Better Caregiving

End-of-life discussions with the healthcare team may lead to fewer procedures and a better quality of life. Studies have shown that cancer patients who have end-of-life discussions with their doctors choose to have fewer procedures, such as resuscitation or the use of a ventilator. They are also less likely to be in intensive care, and the cost of their healthcare is lower during their final week of life. Reports from their caregivers show that these patients live as long as patients who choose to have more procedures and that they have a better quality of life in their last days.

Role of Family Caregivers
Family Caregivers Are Communication Partners

Families can help patients make better decisions about their cancer care. Patients and their family members can join together as partners to communicate with the doctor and healthcare team. When possible, patients should decide how much help they want from family members when making decisions. Communication between family caregivers and the healthcare team should continue throughout cancer care. It should include information about the goals of treatment, plans for the patient's care, and what to expect over time.

Benefits of Communication with Doctor

Communication with the doctor helps caregivers as well as patients. Communication that includes the patient and family is called "family-centered communication." Family-centered communication with the doctor helps the family understand its role in caregiving. Family caregivers who get specific and practical direction from the healthcare team are more confident about giving care. When caregivers receive this help, they can give the patient better care.

Language–Culture Influence on Communication

Language and culture can affect communication. Communication can be more difficult if the doctor does not speak the same language as the patient and family, or if there are cultural differences. Every patient with cancer has the right to get clear information about the diagnosis and treatment so she or he can take a full part in making decisions. Most medical centers have trained interpreters or have other ways to help with language differences.

If cultural beliefs will affect decisions about treatment and care, the healthcare team should be told about these beliefs. For example, a common Western belief is that an informed patient should make the final decision about cancer care.

Problems That Hinder Doctor–Patient Communication

There are many things that can block communication between the patient and doctor. This can happen if:

- The patient does not fully understand all the facts about treatment.

- The medical information is not given in a way the patient can understand.

- The patient believes the doctor will tell them the important facts about treatment and does not ask questions.

- The patient is afraid to ask too many questions.

- The patient is afraid to take too much of the doctor's time and does not ask questions.

Family caregivers can sometimes help when communication problems come up.

Role of Parents
Children Fear Less When Informed

Children with cancer need information that is right for their age. Studies show that children with cancer want to know about their illness and how they will be treated. The amount of information a child wants depends in part on her or his age. Most children worry about how their illness and treatment will affect their daily lives and the people around them. Studies also show that children have less doubt and fear when they are given information about their illness, even if it is bad news.

Communicating about Cancer to Your Child

There are many ways for parents to communicate with their children. When a child is seriously ill, parents may find that communication is better when they:

- Talk with the doctor at the beginning of cancer care about open communication with their child and other family members. Parents should discuss how the family feels about sharing medical information with their child and talk about any concerns they have.

- Talk with their child and share information throughout the course of the illness.

- Find out what their child already knows and wants to know about the illness. This will help clear up any confusion their child may have about the medical facts.

- Explain medical information according to what is right for their child's age and needs.

- Are sensitive to their child's emotions and reactions.

- Encourage their child by promising they will be there to listen to and protect her or him.

Talking with the Healthcare Team
Getting Ready for Medical Appointments

Patients and family caregivers can get ready for medical appointments. It is helpful for patients and caregivers to plan ahead for doctor visits. The following may help you get the most out of these visits:

- Keep a file or notebook of the patient's medical information that includes test and procedure dates, test results, and other records. Bring this file with you to the medical appointment.

- Keep a list of names and doses of medicines and how often they are taken. Bring this list with you.

- Use only trusted sources, such as government and national organizations, if you do research about a medical condition. Bring this research with you to discuss it with the doctor.

- Make a list of questions and concerns. List your most important questions first.

- If you have a lot to discuss with the doctor, ask if you can:

  - Schedule a longer appointment.

  - Ask questions by phone or e-mail.

  - Talk with a nurse or other members of the healthcare team. Nurses are an important part of the healthcare team and can share information with you and your doctor.

  - Bring a tape recorder or take notes so that later on you can listen to or review what you discussed.

  - Bring a family caregiver or friend to the doctor's visit so they can help you remember important information after the visit.

Patients and family caregivers should talk before the appointment to help get ready for possible bad news or information that is different than expected.

Patient–Caregiver Checklist on Cancer Treatment

Patients and caregivers can make a checklist of specific questions about treatment. When talking with the doctor, ask specific questions about any concerns you have. If an answer is not clear to you, ask the doctor to explain it in a way that you can understand. Include the following questions about the patient's treatment:

- What medical records should the patient bring to treatment?

- What can the patient do ahead of time to get ready for treatment?

- How long will the treatment take?

- Can the patient go to and from treatment alone? Should someone else go along?

- Can a family member be with the patient during treatment?

- What can be done to help the patient feel more comfortable during treatment?

- What are the side effects of treatment?

- After treatment, what problems should be watched for? When should a doctor be called?

- Who can help with questions about filing insurance claims?

Chapter 31

Long-Distance Caregiving

Who Is a Long-Distance Caregiver?

Anyone anywhere can be a long-distance caregiver, no matter your gender, income, age, social status, or employment. If you are living an hour or more away from a person who needs your help, you are probably a long-distance caregiver. Anyone who is caring for an aging friend, relative or parent from afar can be considered a long-distance caregiver.

What Can a Caregiver Really Do from Afar?

Long-distance caregivers take on different roles. You may:

- Help with finances, money management, or bill paying

- Arrange for in-home care—hire professional caregivers or home health or nursing aides and help get needed durable medical equipment

---

This chapter contains text excerpted from the following sources: Text beginning with the heading "Who Is a Long-Distance Caregiver?" is excerpted from "Getting Started with Long-Distance Caregiving," National Institute on Aging (NIA), National Institutes of Health (NIH), May 2, 2017; Text beginning with the heading "Know What You Need to Know as a Long-Distance Caregiver" is excerpted from "8 Tips for Long-Distance Caregiving," National Institute on Aging (NIA), National Institutes of Health (NIH), May 16, 2017.

- Locate care in an assisted living facility or nursing home (also known as a "skilled nursing facility")

- Provide emotional support and occasional respite care for a primary caregiver, the person who takes on most of the everyday caregiving responsibilities

- Serve as an information coordinator—research health problems or medicines, help navigate through a maze of new needs and clarify insurance benefits and claims

- Keep family and friends updated and informed

- Create a plan and get the paperwork in order in case of an emergency

- Evaluate the house and make sure it is safe for the older person's needs

Over time, as your family member's needs change, so will your role as a long-distance caregiver.

First Steps for New Long-Distance Caregivers

To get started:

- Ask the primary caregiver, if there is one, and the care recipient how you can be most helpful

- Talk to friends who are caregivers to see if they have suggestions about ways to help

- Find out more about local resources that might be useful

- Develop a good understanding of the person's health issues and other needs

- Visit as often as you can; not only might you notice something that needs to be done and can be taken care of from a distance, but you can also relieve a primary caregiver for a short time

Many of us do not automatically have a lot of caregiver skills. Information about training opportunities is available. Some local chapters of the American Red Cross might offer courses, as do some nonprofit organizations focused on caregiving. Medicare and Medicaid will sometimes pay for this training.

What Do Caregivers Need to Know about Their Family Member's Health?

Learn as much as you can about your family member's condition and any treatment. This can help you understand what is going on, anticipate the course of an illness, prevent crises, and assist in healthcare management. It can also make talking with the doctor easier.

Get written permission, as needed under the Health Insurance Portability and Accountability Act of 1996 (HIPAA) Privacy Rule, to receive medical and financial information. To the extent possible, the family member with permission should be the one to talk with all healthcare providers. Try putting together a notebook, on paper or online, that includes all the vital information about medical care, social services, contact numbers, financial issues, and so on. Make copies for other caregivers, and keep it up-to-date.

Making the Most out of Visits with Aging Parents or Relatives

Talk to the care recipient ahead of time and find out what she or he would like to do during your visit. Also, check with the primary caregiver, if appropriate, to learn what she or he needs, such as handling some caregiving responsibilities while you are in town. This may help you set clear-cut and realistic goals for the visit. Decide on the priorities and leave other tasks to another visit.

Remember to actually spend time visiting with your family member. Try to make time to do things unrelated to being a caregiver, such as watching a movie, playing a game, or taking a drive. Finding time to do something simple and relaxing can help everyone—it can be fun and build family memories. And, try to let outside distractions wait until you are home again.

How Can I Stay Connected with an Aging Parent or Relative from Far Away?

Try to find people who live near your loved one and can provide a realistic view of what is going on. This may be your other parent. A social worker may be able to provide updates and help with making decisions. Many families schedule conference calls with doctors, the assisted living facility team, or nursing home staff so that several relatives can be in one conversation and get the same up-to-date information about health and progress.

Do not underestimate the value of a phone and e-mail contact list. It is a simple way to keep everyone updated on your parents' needs.

You may also want to give the person you care for a cell phone (and make sure she or he knows how to use it). Or, if your family member lives in a nursing home, consider having a private phone line installed in her or his room. Program telephone numbers of doctors, friends, family members, and yourself into the phone, and perhaps provide a list of the speed-dial numbers to keep with the phone. Such simple strategies can be a lifeline. But, try to be prepared should you find yourself inundated with calls from your parents.

Long-distance caregiving presents unique challenges. If you find yourself in the long-distance caregiving role, here is a summary of things to keep in mind.

Know What You Need to Know as a Long-Distance Caregiver

Experienced caregivers recommend that you learn as much as you can about your family member or friend's illness, medicines, and resources that might be available. Information can help you understand what is going on, anticipate the course of an illness, prevent crises, and assist in healthcare management. It can also make talking with the doctor easier. Make sure at least one family member has written permission to receive medical and financial information. To the extent possible, one family member should handle conversations with all healthcare providers. Try putting all the vital information in one place—perhaps in a notebook or in a shared, secure online document. This includes all the important information about medical care, social services, contact numbers, financial issues, and so on. Make copies for other caregivers, and keep the information up to date.

Plan Your Visits with an Aging Parent or Relative

When visiting your loved one, you may feel that there is just too much to do in the time that you have. You can get more done and feel less stressed by talking to your family member or friend ahead of time and finding out what she or he would like to do. Also, check with the primary caregiver, if appropriate, to learn what she or he needs, such as handling some caregiving responsibilities while you are in town. This may help you set clear-cut and realistic goals for the visit. For instance, does your mother need to get some new winter clothes or visit another family member? Could your father use help in fixing things around the house? Would you like to talk to your mother's physician? Decide on the priorities and leave other tasks for another visit.

Activities to Do When Visiting an Aging Parent or Relative

Try to make time to do things unrelated to being a caregiver. Maybe you could find a movie to watch with your relatives, or plan a visit with old friends or other family members. Perhaps they would like to attend worship services. Offer to play a game of cards or a board game. Take a drive, or go to the library together. Finding a little bit of time to do something simple and relaxing can help everyone, and it builds more family memories. And keep in mind that your friend or relative is the focus of your trip—try to let outside distractions wait until you are home again.

Get in Touch and Stay in Touch

Many families schedule conference calls with doctors, the assisted living facility team, or nursing home staff so several relatives can participate in one conversation and get up-to-date information about a relative's health and progress. If your family member is in a nursing home, you can request occasional teleconferences with the facility's staff. Sometimes a social worker is good to talk to for updates as well as for help in making decisions. You might also talk with a family member or friend in the community who can provide a realistic view of what is going on. In some cases, this will be your other parent. Do not underestimate the value of a phone and e-mail contact list. It is a simple way to keep everyone updated on your parents' needs.

Help an Aging Parent Stay in Contact from Afar

For one family, having a private phone line installed in their father's nursing home room allowed him to stay in touch. For another family, giving Grandma a cell phone (and then teaching her how to use it) gave everyone some peace of mind. These simple strategies can be a lifeline. But be prepared—you may find you are inundated with calls or text messages. It is good to think in advance about a workable approach for coping with numerous calls.

Organize Paperwork for an Aging Parent

Organizing paperwork is one way that a long-distance caregiver can be a big help. An important part of effective caregiving depends on keeping a great deal of information in order and up to date. Often, long-distance caregivers will need access to a parent's or relative's personal, health, financial, and legal records.

Getting all this material together is a lot of work at first, and from far away it can seem even more challenging. But, once you have gathered everything together, many other caregiving tasks will be easier. Maintaining current information about your parent's health and medical care, as well as finances, homeownership, and other legal issues, lets you get a handle on what is going on and allows you to respond more quickly if there is a crisis.

As you are getting started, try to focus on gathering the essentials first, and fill in the blanks as you go along. Talk with the older person and the primary caregiver about any missing information or documentation and how you might help to organize the records. It is also a good idea to make sure that all financial matters, including wills and life insurance policies, are in order. It will also help if someone has a durable power of attorney (the legal document naming one person to handle financial and property issues for another).

Your family member or friend may be reluctant to share personal information with you. Explain that you are not trying to invade their privacy or take over their personal lives—you are only trying to assemble what will be needed in the event of an emergency. Assure them that you will respect their privacy, and then keep your promise. If they are still uncomfortable, ask if they would be willing to work with an attorney (some lawyers specialize in elder affairs) or perhaps with another trusted family member or friend.

Additional Tips for Caregiving

Whether you are the primary caregiver or a long-distance caregiver, getting some caregiving training can be helpful. As with a lot of things in life, many of us do not automatically have a lot of caregiver skills. For example, training can teach you how to safely move someone from a bed to a chair, how to help someone bathe, and how to prevent and treat bedsores, as well as basic first aid. Information about training opportunities is available online. Some local chapters of the American Red Cross might offer courses, as do some nonprofit organizations focused on caregiving. Medicare and Medicaid will sometimes pay for this training.

Chapter 32

Take Care of Yourself While Caring for Others

Chapter Contents

Section 32.1—How to Share Caregiving
Responsibilities with Family
Members 296

Section 32.2—Tips for Caregiver Self-Care 299

Section 32.3—Coping with Caregiving 301

Section 32.1

How to Share Caregiving Responsibilities with Family Members

This section includes text excerpted from "How to Share Caregiving Responsibilities with Family Members," National Institute on Aging (NIA), National Institutes of Health (NIH), May 9, 2017.

Caring for an older family member often requires teamwork. While one sibling might be local and take on most of the everyday caregiving responsibilities, a long-distance caregiver can also have an important role. As a long-distance caregiver, you can provide important respite to the primary caregiver and support to the aging family member.

Talk about Caregiving Responsibilities

First, try to define the caregiving responsibilities. You could start by setting up a family meeting and, if it makes sense, include the care recipient in the discussion. This is best done when there is not an emergency. A calm conversation about what kind of care is wanted and needed now, and what might be needed in the future, can help avoid a lot of confusion.

Decide who will be responsible for which tasks. Many families find the best first step is to name a primary caregiver, even if one is not needed immediately. That way the primary caregiver can step in if there is a crisis.

Agree in advance how each of your efforts can complement one another so that you can be an effective team. Ideally, each of you will be able to take on tasks best suited to your skills or interests.

Consider Your Strengths When Sharing Caregiving Responsibilities

When thinking about who should be responsible for what, start with your strengths. Consider what you are particularly good at and how those skills might help in the current situation:

- Are you good at finding information, keeping people up-to-date on changing conditions, and offering cheer, whether on the phone or with a computer?

- Are you good at supervising and leading others?

- Are you comfortable speaking with medical staff and interpreting what they say to others?

- Is your strongest suit doing the numbers—paying bills, keeping track of bank statements, and reviewing insurance policies and reimbursement reports?

- Are you the one in the family who can fix anything, while no one else knows the difference between pliers and a wrench?

Consider Your Limits When Sharing Caregiving Responsibilities

When thinking about who should be responsible for what, consider your limits. Ask yourself the following:

- How often, both mentally and financially, can you afford to travel?

- Are you emotionally prepared to take on what may feel like a reversal of roles between you and your parents—taking care of your parent instead of your parents taking care of you? Can you continue to respect your parent's independence?

- Can you be both calm and assertive when communicating from a distance?

- How will your decision to take on caregiving responsibilities affect your work and home life?

Be realistic about how much you can do and what you are willing to do. Think about your schedule and how it might be adapted to give respite to a primary caregiver. For example, you might try to coordinate holiday and vacation times. Remember that over time responsibilities may need to be revised to reflect changes in the situation, your care recipient's needs, and each family member's abilities and limitations.

How to Support a Local Caregiver from Far Away

A spouse or sibling who lives closest to an aging parent often becomes the primary caregiver. Long-distance caregivers can help by providing emotional support and occasional respite to the primary caregiver. Ask the primary caregiver what you can do to help. Staying in contact with your parents by phone or e-mail might also take some pressure off your parents or siblings. Just listening may not sound like much help, but often it is.

Long-distance caregivers can also play a part in arranging for professional caregivers, hiring home health and nursing aides, or locating care in an assisted living facility or nursing home (also known as a "skilled nursing facility").

Long-distance caregivers may find they can be helpful by handling things online—for example, researching health problems or medicines, paying bills, or keeping family and friends updated. Some long-distance caregivers help a parent pay for care; others step in to manage finances.

How to Help a Parent Who Is the Primary Caregiver

A primary caregiver—especially a spouse—may be hesitant to ask for help or a break. Be sure to acknowledge how important the caregiver has been for the care recipient. Also, discuss the physical and emotional effects caregiving can have on people. Although caregiving can be satisfying, it also can be very hard work.

Offer to arrange for respite care. Respite care will give your parents a break from caregiving responsibilities. It can be arranged for an afternoon or for several days. Care can be provided in the family home, through an adult day services program, or at a skilled nursing facility.

The Access to Respite Care and Help (ARCH) National Respite Locator Service can help you find services in your parents' community. You might suggest contacting the Well Spouse Association. It offers support to the wives, husbands, and partners of chronically ill or disabled people and has a nationwide listing of local support groups.

Your parents may need more help from home-based care to continue to live in their own homes. Some people find it hard to have paid caregivers in the house, but most also say that the assistance is invaluable. If the primary caregiver is reluctant, point out that with an in-home aide, she may have more energy to devote to caregiving and some time for herself. Suggest she tries it for a short time, and then decide.

In time, the person receiving care may have to move to assisted living or a nursing home. If that happens, the primary caregiver will need your support. You can help select a facility. The primary caregiver may need help adjusting to the person's absence or to living alone at home. Just listening may not sound like much help, but often it is.

Section 32.2

Tips for Caregiver Self-Care

This section contains text excerpted from the following sources:
Text in this section begins with excerpts from "3 Tips for Caregiver
Self-Care," National Cancer Institute (NCI), February 8, 2019;
Text under the heading "Make Yourself a Priority!" is excerpted
from "Make Yourself a Priority, Too: Tips for Caregivers," National
Institute on Aging (NIA), National Institutes of Health (NIH),
November 10, 2016. Reviewed September 2019.

Being a caregiver to a patient with a brain or spine tumor is an
important and challenging role. Caregivers are so often focused on the
medical, physical, and emotional needs of their loved one, they forget
to care for themselves. But caregivers, your health and wellness are
important, too.

It is time to make caregiver self-care a priority. Doing so can help
you as a caregiver manage your needs in a healthy way to avoid stress,
burn-out, sickness, and fatigue. It will also ensure you find a good
balance between caring for your loved one and yourself.

Here are self-care tips for caregivers of patients with a brain or
spine tumor. You may follow these tips to stay healthy.

Schedule Self-Care Time

Each day or week make time to focus on your needs. Make it a priority by scheduling a recurring one-hour appointment with yourself.
Your self-care time should include an activity you enjoy or an event
that provides comfort. Exercise, go shopping, meditate, have coffee
with a friend, or take a nap. The scheduled time will rejuvenate you
and help you make your physical and mental health a priority. Your
loved one needs you healthy, too.

- For any of the activities that you incorporate into a consistent
  routine, make sure you stay in the moment and enjoy yourself.
  You can think about anything you need to get done after you
  have taken this time for you.

Write Down Your Positive Qualities

Show yourself self-love by writing down the qualities that make you
a great caregiver and person. This can help build your self-esteem and
help you stay motivated. Here is an activity to try:

299

- Write the letters of the alphabet. Find one positive quality about yourself for each letter. Write it next to the letter. Keep this list handy and refer to it when you need a mental boost.

Make a Self-Care Emergency Plan

Having a plan can help you when you feel overwhelmed. In these moments, it can be difficult to think of things to do for yourself. The plan keeps you ready with a list of things you can do to stay calm and in control of how you feel. You can also include things to avoid that might make you feel worse. And keep this plan in a place where you see it consistently. Your plan should include:

- A list of activities that help you relax. For example, take a 30-minute walk or meditate for 10 minutes. Include activities that boost your mood and tips to remind you to stay calm and in the moment. And remember to breathe.

- A list of people to reach out to for help or support, such as a friend or loved one that can provide comfort or distraction, or groups to attend to meet other caregivers.

- Positive messages to say to yourself to keep you motivated.

Caregivers, remember, your health and wellness are as important as your loved one. And your loved one wants and needs you healthy, too. So, take care of yourself today and every day.

Make Yourself a Priority!

Nearly 15 million Americans provide unpaid care to an older adult. Caregivers who provide substantial care are more likely to have physical and emotional health problems. You will find tips in this section on how to make your needs become part of your priorities when you are so caught up with your duties and responsibilities as a caregiver. Caregiving can be rewarding, but difficult. Learn how you can put yourself back on the priority list:

- Caring for yourself is one of the most important things you can do as a caregiver.

- Ask for help when you need it.

- Spend time with friends.

- Join a support group either in person or online.

- Take breaks each day.
- Keep up with hobbies.
- Take care of yourself.

Section 32.3

Coping with Caregiving

This section includes text excerpted from "Coping with Caregiving," *NIH News in Health*, National Institutes of Health (NIH), December 2015. Reviewed September 2019.

It can be a labor of love, and sometimes a job of necessity. A total of about 43 million U.S. adults provide unpaid care for someone with a serious health condition each year. These often-unsung heroes provide hours of assistance to others. Yet the stress and strain of caregiving can take a toll on their own health. National Institutes of Health (NIH)-funded researchers are working to understand the risks these caregivers face. And scientists are seeking better ways to protect caregivers' health.

Many of us will end up becoming a caregiver at some point in our lives. Chances are we will be helping out older family members who cannot fully care for themselves. Such caregiving can include everyday tasks, such as helping with meals, schedules, and bathing and dressing. It can also include managing medicines, doctor visits, health insurance, and money. Caregivers often give emotional support as well.

People who provide unpaid care for an elderly, ill or disabled family member or friend in the home are called "informal caregivers." Most are middle-aged. Roughly two-thirds are women. Nearly half of informal caregivers assist someone who is age 75 or older. As the elderly population continues to grow nationwide, so will the need for informal caregivers.

Studies have shown that some people can thrive when caring for others. Caregiving may help to strengthen connections to a loved one. Some find joy or fulfillment in looking after others. But for many, the strain of caregiving can become overwhelming. Friends and family often take on the caregiving role without any training. They are

301

expected to meet many complex demands without much help. Most care-givers hold down a full-time job in addition to the hours of unpaid help they give to someone else.

"With all of its rewards, there is a substantial cost to caregiving—financially, physically, and emotionally," says Dr. Richard J. Hodes, director of NIH's National Institute on Aging (NIA). "One important insight from our research is that because of the stress and time demands placed on caregivers, they are less likely to find time to address their own health problems."

Caregivers' Health Risks Depend on the Health of the Person Being Caring For

Informal caregivers, for example, maybe less likely to fill a needed prescription for themselves or get a screening test for breast cancer. "Caregivers also tend to report lower levels of physical activity, poorer nutrition, and poorer sleep or sleep disturbance," says Dr. Erin Kent, an NIH expert on cancer caregiving.

Studies have linked informal caregiving to a variety of long-term health problems. Caregivers are more likely to have heart disease, cancer, diabetes, arthritis, and excess weight. Caregivers are also at risk for depression or anxiety. And they are more likely to have problems with memory and paying attention.

"Caregivers may even suffer from physical health problems related to caregiving tasks, such as back or muscle injuries from lifting patients," Kent adds.

Caregivers may face different challenges and risks depending on the health of the person they are caring for. Taking care of loved ones with cancer or dementia can be especially demanding. Research suggests that these caregivers bear greater levels of physical and mental burdens than caregivers of the frail elderly or people with diabetes.

"Cancer caregivers often spend more hours per day providing more intensive care over a shorter period of time," Kent says. "The health of cancer patients can deteriorate quickly, which can cause heightened stress for caregivers. And aggressive cancer treatments can leave patients greatly weakened. They may need extra care, and their medications may need to be monitored more often."

Cancer survivorship, too, can bring intense levels of uncertainty and anxiety. "A hallmark of cancer is that it may return months or even years later," Kent says. "Both cancer survivors and their caregivers may struggle to live with the ongoing fear and stress of a cancer recurrence."

Dementia can also create unique challenges for caregivers. The healthcare costs alone can take an enormous toll. A study found that out-of-pocket spending for families of dementia patients during the last five years of life averaged $61,522, which was 81 percent higher than for older people who died from other causes.

Research has found that caregivers for people with dementia have particularly high levels of potentially harmful stress hormones. Caregivers and care recipients often struggle with the problems related to dementia, such as agitation, aggression, trouble sleeping, wandering, and confusion. These caregivers spend more days sick with an infectious disease, have a weaker immune response to the flu vaccine, and have slower wound healing.

The Resources for Enhancing Alzheimer's Caregiver Health Program

One major successful and expanding effort to help ease caregiver stress is known as "REACH—Resources for Enhancing Alzheimer's Caregiver Health." Nearly a decade ago, NIH-funded researchers showed that a supportive, educational program for dementia caregivers could greatly improve their quality of life and reduce rates of clinical depression. As part of the program, trained staff connected with caregivers over 6 months by making several home visits, telephone calls, and structured telephone support sessions.

"REACH showed that what caregivers need is support. They need to know that there are people out there and resources available to help them," says Dr. John Haaga, who oversees NIH's behavioral and social research related to aging.

The REACH program is now being more widely employed. It has been adapted for use in free community-based programs, such as in local Area Agencies on Aging. It is also being used by the U.S. Department of Veterans Affairs and by the Indian Health Service, in collaboration with the Administration for Community Living.

"We know how to support families caring for an older adult. But, that knowledge is not easily accessible to the families who need it," says Dr. Laura Gitlin, a coauthor of the REACH study and an expert on caregiving and aging at Johns Hopkins University. "Caregivers need to know it is not only acceptable but recommended, that they find time to care for themselves. They should consider joining a caregiver's support group, taking breaks each day, and keeping up with their own hobbies and interests."

Chapter 33

Things to Look out for as Death Approaches

Caregivers Can Make a Person Comfortable as Death Approaches

In this chapter, we can read about the signs when death is approaching, and what the caregiver can do to make a person comfortable during this time.

Certain symptoms can help a caregiver anticipate when death is near. However, each person's experience at the end of life is different. What may happen to one person may not happen for another. Also, the presence of one or more of these symptoms does not necessarily mean that the patient is close to death. A member of the healthcare team can give family members and caregivers more information about what to expect. Here are some things to look out for as death approaches.

Withdrawal from Friends and Family

- People often focus on inward during the last weeks of life. This does not necessarily mean that patients are angry or depressed or that they do not love their caregivers. It could be caused by decreased oxygen to the brain, decreased blood flow, and/or mental preparation for dying.

This chapter includes text excerpted from "End-of-Life Care for People Who Have Cancer," National Cancer Institute (NCI), May 10, 2012. Reviewed September 2019.

- They may lose interest in things they used to enjoy, such as favorite TV shows, friends, or pets.

- Caregivers can let the patient know they are there for support. The person may be aware and able to hear, even if they are unable to respond. Experts advise that giving them permission to "let go" may be helpful. If they do feel like talking, they may want to reminisce about the joys and sorrows or tie up loose ends.

Sleep Changes

- People may have drowsiness, increased sleep, intermittent sleep, or confusion when they first wake up.

- Worries or concerns may keep patients up at night. Caregivers can ask them if they would like to sit in the room with them while they fall asleep.

- Patients may sleep more and more as time passes. Caregivers should continue to talk to them, even if they are unconscious, for the patient may still hear them.

Hard-to-Control Pain

- It may become harder to control pain as cancer gets worse. It is important to provide pain medication regularly. Caregivers should ask to see a palliative care doctor or a pain specialist for advice on the correct medicines and doses. It may be helpful to explore other pain control methods such as massage and relaxation techniques.

Increasing Weakness

- Weakness and fatigue will increase over time. The patient may have good days and bad days, so they may need more help with daily personal care and getting around.

- Caregivers can help patients save energy for the things that are most important to them.

Appetite Changes

- As the body naturally shuts down, the person with cancer will often need and want less food. The loss of appetite is caused by the body's need to conserve energy and its decreasing ability to use food and fluids properly.

- Patients should be allowed to choose whether and when to eat or drink. Caregivers can offer small amounts of the foods the patient enjoys. Since chewing takes energy, they may prefer milkshakes, ice cream, or pudding. If the patient does not have trouble with swallowing, offer sips of fluids and use a flexible straw if they cannot sit up. If a person can no longer swallow, offer ice chips. Keep their lips moist with lip balm and their mouth clean with a soft, damp cloth.

Awareness

- Near the end of life, people often have episodes of confusion or waking dreams. They may get confused about time, place, and the identity of loved ones. Caregivers can gently remind patients where they are and who is with them. They should be calm and reassuring. But, if the patient is agitated, they should not attempt to restrain them. Let the healthcare providers know if significant agitation occurs, as there are treatments available to help control or reverse it.

- Sometimes patients report seeing or speaking with loved ones who have died. They may talk about going on a trip, seeing lights, butterflies, or other symbols of reality we cannot see. As long as these things are not disturbing to the patient, caregivers can ask them to say more. They can let them share their visions and dreams, not trying to talk them out of what they believe they see.

The Dying Process

- There may be a loss of bladder or bowel control due to the muscles relaxing in the pelvis. Caregivers should continue to provide clean, dry bedding and gentle personal care. They can place disposable pads on the bed under the patient and remove them when soiled. Also, due to a slowing of kidney function and/or decreased fluid intake, there may be a decrease in the amount of urine. It may be dark and smell strong.

- Breathing patterns may become slower or faster, in cycles. The patient may not notice, but caregivers should let the doctor know if they are worried about the changes. There may be rattling or gurgling sounds that are caused by saliva and fluids collecting in the throat and upper airways. Although this can be very disturbing for caregivers, at this stage the patient is generally not experiencing any distress. Breathing may be easier if a person's body is turned to the side and pillows are placed behind the back and beneath the head. Caregivers can also ask the healthcare team about using a humidifier or external source of oxygen to make it easier for the patient to breathe if the patient is short of breath.

- Skin may become bluish in color and feel cool as blood flow slows down. This is not painful or uncomfortable for the patient. Caregivers should avoid warming the patient with electric blankets or heating pads, which can cause burns. However, they may keep the patient covered with a light blanket.

Chapter 34

What to Do When Death Occurs

When death comes suddenly, there is little time to prepare. In contrast, watching an older person become increasingly frail may mean that it is hard to know when the end of life begins because changes can happen so slowly. But, if you do know death is approaching and understand what will happen, then you do have a chance to plan.

Listen carefully to what doctors and nurses are saying. They may be suggesting that death could be soon. You might also ask—how much time do you think my loved one has left, based on your experience with other patients in this condition?

What Happens When Someone Dies

Just as each life is unique, so is each death. But, there are some common experiences very near the end:

- Shortness of breath, known as "dyspnea"

- Depression

This chapter contains text excerpted from the following sources: Text in this chapter begins with excerpts from "What Happens When Someone Dies?" National Institute on Aging (NIA), National Institutes of Health (NIH), May 17, 2017; Text under the heading "After Death" is excerpted from "What to Do after Someone Dies," National Institute on Aging (NIA), National Institutes of Health (NIH), May 17, 2017.

- Anxiety

- Tiredness and sleepiness

- Mental confusion or reduced alertness

- Refusal to eat or drink

- Each of these symptoms, taken alone, is not a sign of death. But, for someone with a serious illness or declining health, these might suggest that the person is nearing the end of life.

In addition, when a person is closer to death, the hands, arms, feet, or legs may be cool to the touch. Some parts of the body may become darker or blue-colored. Breathing and heart rates may slow. In fact, there may be times when a person's breathing becomes abnormal, known as "Cheyne-Stokes breathing." Some people hear a death rattle, noisy breathing that makes a gurgling or rattling sound. The chest stops moving, no air comes out of the nose, and there is no pulse. Eyes that are open can seem glassy.

After death, there may still be a few shudders or movements of the arms or legs. There could even be an uncontrolled cry because of muscle movement in the voice box. Sometimes there will be a release of urine or stool, but usually, only a small amount since so little has probably been eaten in the last days of life.

Should There Always Be Someone in the Room with a Dying Person?

Staying close to someone who is dying is often called "keeping a vigil." It can be comforting for the caregiver to always be there, but it can also be tiring and stressful. Unless your cultural or religious traditions require it, do not feel that you must stay with the person all the time. If there are other family members or friends around, try taking turns sitting in the room. Some people almost seem to prefer to die alone. They appear to slip away just after visitors leave.

After Death

Nothing has to be done immediately after a person's death. Take the time you need. Some people want to stay in the room with the body; others prefer to leave. You might want to have someone make sure the body is lying flat before the joints become stiff and cannot be moved. This rigor mortis begins sometime during the first few hours after death.

310

After death, how long you can stay with the body may depend on where death happens. If it happens at home, there is no need to move the body right away. This is the time for any special religious, ethnic, or cultural customs that are performed soon after death.

If the death seems likely to happen in a facility, such as a hospital or nursing home, discuss any important customs or rituals with the staff early on, if possible. That will allow them to plan so you can have the appropriate time with the body.

Some families want time to sit quietly with the body, console each other, and maybe share memories. You could ask a member of your religious community or a spiritual counselor to come. If you have a list of people to notify, this is the time to call those who might want to come and see the body before it is moved.

As soon as possible, the death must be officially pronounced by someone in authority such as a doctor in a hospital or nursing facility or a hospice nurse. This person also fills out the forms certifying the cause, time, and place of death. These steps will make it possible for an official death certificate to be prepared. This legal form is necessary for many reasons, including life insurance and financial and property issues.

If hospice is helping, a plan for what happens after death is already in place. If the death happens at home without hospice, try to talk with the doctor, local medical examiner (coroner), your local health department, or a funeral home representative in advance about how to proceed.

Arrangements should be made to pick up the body as soon as the family is ready and according to local laws. Usually, this is done by a funeral home. The hospital or nursing facility, if that is where the death took place, may call the funeral home for you. If at home, you will need to contact the funeral home directly or ask a friend or family member to do that for you.

The doctor may ask if you want an autopsy. This is a medical procedure conducted by a specially trained physician to learn more about what caused the death. For example, if the person who died was believed to have Alzheimer disease, a brain autopsy will allow for a definitive diagnosis. If your religion or culture objects to autopsies, talk to the doctor. Some people planning a funeral with a viewing worry about having an autopsy, but the physical signs of an autopsy are usually hidden by clothing.

Part Six

Death and Children:
Information for Parents

Chapter 35

When a Child Has Cancer

When a child has cancer, every member of the family needs support. Parents often feel shocked and overwhelmed following their child's cancer diagnosis. Honest and calm conversations build trust as you talk with your child and her or his siblings. Taking care of yourself during this difficult time is important; it is not selfish. As you dig deep for strength, reach out and let others support you.

Tips are shared to help you talk with children of all ages about cancer. Answers to commonly asked questions from parents and children are also included.

Talking with Your Child about Cancer

As you talk with your child, begin with the knowledge that you know your child best. Your child depends on you for helpful, accurate, and truthful information. Your child will learn a lot from your tone of voice and facial expressions, so stay calm when you talk with your child. Work to be gentle, open, and honest—so your child will trust and confide in you.

The age-related suggestions below may be helpful, as you work with the healthcare team so your child knows what to expect during treatment, copes well with procedures, and feels supported.

This chapter includes text excerpted from "Support for Families When a Child Has Cancer," National Cancer Institute (NCI), October 15, 2018.

If your child is less than 1 year old: Comfort your baby by holding and gently touching her. Skin to skin contact is ideal. Bring familiar items from home, such as toys or a blanket. Talk or sing to your child, since the sound of your voice is soothing. Try to keep up feeding and bedtime routines as much as possible.

If your child is 1 to 2 years old: Very young children understand things they can see and touch. Toddlers like to play, so find safe ways to let your child play. Toddlers also like to start making choices, so let your child choose a sticker or a flavor of medicine when possible. Prepare your child ahead of time if something will hurt. Not doing so may cause your child to become fearful and anxious.

If your child is 3 to 5 years old: To help your child understand his treatment better, ask the doctor if he can touch the models, machines, or supplies (tubes, bandages, or ports) ahead of time. If a procedure will hurt, prepare your child in advance. You can help to distract your child by reading a story or giving her a stuffed animal to hold.

If your child is 6 to 12 years old: School-aged children understand that medicines and treatment help them get better. They are able to co-operate with treatment but want to know what to expect. Children this age often have many questions, so be ready to answer them or to find the answers together. Relationships are important, so help your child to stay in touch with friends and family.

If your child is a teenager: Teens often focus on how cancer changes their lives—their friendships, their appearance, and their activities. They may be scared and angry about how cancer has isolated them from their friends. Look for ways to help your teen stay connected to friends. Give your teen some of the space and freedom he had before treatment and include him in treatment decisions.

Questions from Parents Whose Child Has Cancer

Talk with your child's healthcare team to get your questions answered. You may also find the suggestions below to be helpful:

Who Should Tell My Child?

Many parents receive their child's diagnosis from the doctor at the same time that their child learns of it. However, if you choose to be the

316

one to tell your child, the doctor or nurse can help you decide what to say and how to answer her questions.

When Should My Child Be Told?

Your child should be told as soon as possible. This will help build trust between you and your child. It does not mean that your child needs to hear everything all at once.

What Should I Tell My Child?

The information you share with your child depends on his age and what he can understand. Children of all ages need clear, simple information that makes sense to them. As much as possible, help him know what to expect by using ideas and words that he understands. Tell your child how treatment will make him feel and when something will hurt. Explain that strong medicine and treatments have helped other children.

How Much Should I Tell My Child?

Help your child to understand the basic facts about the illness, the treatment, and what to expect. It may be hard for many children to process too many details or information given too far in advance. Start with small amounts of information that your child can understand. Children often use their imaginations to make up answers to unanswered questions and may fear the worst. Answering questions honestly and having ongoing conversations can help your child. Telling untruths can cause your child to distrust you or people on their healthcare team.

How Might My Child React?

Each child is different. Some worry. Others get upset or become quiet, afraid, or defiant. Some express their feelings in words, others in actions. Some children regress to behaviors they had when they were younger. These are normal reactions to changes in life as they know it. Their schedule, the way they look and feel, and their friendships may all be changing. Expect that some days will be rough, and others will be easier. Tell your child, and find ways to show her, that you will always be there for her.

317

What Can I Do to Help My Child Cope?

Children take cues from their parents, so being calm and hopeful can help your child. Show your love. Think about how your child and family have handled difficult times in the past. Some children feel better after talking. Others prefer to draw, write, play games, or listen to music.

Questions That a Child with Cancer May Have

Talk with your child's healthcare team about how to answer questions your child may have. You may also find these suggestions helpful:

What Is Cancer?

When talking about cancer with your child, start with simple words and concepts. Explain that cancer is not contagious—it is not an illness children catch from someone or they can give to someone else. Young children may understand that they have a lump (tumor) that is making them sick or that their blood is not working the way it should.

Why Did I Get Cancer?

Some children think they did something bad or wrong to cause the cancer. Others wonder why they got sick. Tell your child that nothing he—or anyone else—did caused the cancer, and that doctors are working to learn more about what causes cancer in children.

- **You may tell your child:** I do not know. Not even doctors know exactly why one child gets cancer and another does not. We do know that you did not do anything wrong, you did not catch it from someone, and you cannot give it to anyone.

Will I Get Better?

Being in the hospital or having many medical appointments can be scary for a child. Some children may know or have heard about a person who has died from cancer. Your child may wonder if she will get better.

- **You may tell your child:** Cancer is a serious illness, and your doctors and nurses are giving you treatments that have helped other children. We are going to do whatever we can to help you get better. Let us talk with your doctor and nurse to learn more.

How Will I Feel during Treatment?

Your child may wonder how he may feel during treatment. Children with cancer often see others who have lost their hair or are very sick. Talk with the nurse or social worker to learn how your child's treatment may affect how your child looks and feels.

- **You may tell your child:** Even when two children have the same type of cancer, what happens to one child may not happen to the other one. Your doctors and I will talk with you and explain what we know and what to expect. We will all work together to help you feel as good as possible during treatment.

Helping Your Child with Cancer to Cope with Changes

Treatment brings many changes to a child's life and outlook. You can help your child by letting her live as normal a life as possible. Talk with the healthcare team to learn what changes your child may experience so you can prepare for them in advance.

Changes in Appearance

Children can be sensitive about how they look and how others respond to them. Here are some ways to help your child:

- **Prepare for hair loss.** If treatment will cause your child's hair to fall out, let your child pick out a fun cap, scarf, and/or wig ahead of time.

- **Be aware of weight and other physical changes.** Some treatments may cause weight loss and others may cause weight gain. Get advice from a dietician so you know what to expect and can help your child prepare for and cope with physical changes.

- **Be creative.** You and your child may shop for outfits that your child likes. Sometimes a cool t-shirt or fun hat may help to lift your child's spirits.

- **Help your child know how to respond.** Sometimes people will stare, mistake your child's gender, or ask personal questions. Talk with your child and come up with an approach that works. Your child may choose to respond or to ignore comments.

Changes in Friendships

Your child's friendships are tested and may change during a long and serious illness. Sometimes it may seem as though your child's old friends are no longer "there for them" or that they do not care anymore. It may help if your child takes the first step and reaches out to friends. The good news is that your child may make new friends through this experience. Here are some steps you can take with your child:

- **Help your child stay in touch with friends.** You can encourage and help your child to connect with friends through texts, e-mails, video chats, phone calls, and/or social media sites.

- **Get tips and advice.** A social worker or child life specialist can help your child think through what they would like to share with friends. If possible and when your child is up to it, friends may be able to visit.

Changes in Feelings

Although over time many children with cancer cope well, your child may feel anxious, sad, stressed, scared, or become withdrawn from time to time. Talk with your child about what she is feeling and help her find ways to cope. You and your child can also meet with a social worker, child life specialist, or psychologist about feelings that do not have easy solutions or seem to be getting worse over time. Try these tips to help your child cope with difficult emotions:

- **Find ways to distract or entertain your child.** Playing video games or watching movies can help your child to relax. Integrative medicine practices, such as muscle relaxation, guided imagery, and biofeedback may also help.

- **Stay calm but do not hide your feelings.** Your child can feel your emotions. If you often feel sad or anxious, talk with your child's healthcare team and your doctor about the best way to manage these emotions. However, if you often hide your feelings, your child may also hide their feelings from you.

- **Get help if you see signs of depression in your child.** It is normal for your child to feel down or sad sometimes, but if these feelings last for too long and happen on most days, they may be a sign of depression. Talk with the doctor about emotional changes you notice in your child.

Changes in Schedule

Your child may spend more time at the hospital and less time at school during treatment. Here are some ways to help your child cope with long stays at the hospital and time away from school.

- **Hospital stays.** Being in the hospital can be difficult for anyone, especially children. Photos, posters, games, and music can help cheer up your child. And if sports are off-limits, learn about other activities, such as music, games, or writing that may capture your child's interest.

- **Missing school.** Most children with cancer miss school during treatment. Some children are able to attend from time to time, whereas others need to take a leave of absence. Here are some ways to get the academic support your child needs during treatment:

  - Meet with your child's doctor to find out how treatment may affect your child's energy level and ability to do schoolwork. Ask the doctor to write a letter to your child's teachers that describes your child's medical situation, limitations, and how much school your child is likely to miss.

  - Keep your child's teachers updated. Tell your child's teachers and principal about your child's medical situation. Share the letter from your child's doctor. Learn what schoolwork your child will miss and ways for your child to keep up, as they are able.

  - Learn about assistance from the hospital and your child's school. Some hospitals have education coordinators, and others have nurses who can tell you about education-related resources and assistance. Ask about an individualized education plan (IEP) for your child.

Supporting Brothers and Sisters Whose Sibling Has Cancer

As a parent, you want to be there for all of your children, but this can be hard when one of your children is being treated for cancer. You may notice that your other children are having a difficult time but are not sure of what to do. These suggestions have helped others:

- **Listen to and talk with your other children.** Set aside sometime every day, even if it is just a few minutes, to spend with your other children. Ask how they are feeling, even if you

321

do not have an easy solution. It is still important to connect with them and to listen to them.

- **Keep them informed and involved.** Talk with your other children about their sibling's cancer and tell them what to expect during treatment. If possible, find ways to include them in visits to the hospital. If you are far from home, connect through e-mail, texts, and calls.

- **Keep things as normal as you can.** Arrange to keep your other children involved in school-related events and other activities that are important to them. Ask key people in your family's life to give siblings extra support. Most people want to help and will appreciate being asked.

Tips to Help Parents Cope
Work to Keep Relationships Strong

Relationships are strained and under pressure when a child has cancer. However, many marriages grow stronger during this time. Working to keep your marriage strong can also help your children. Here is what other parents said helped:

- **Keep lines of communication open.** Talk about how you each deal best with stress. Make time to connect, even when time is limited.

- **Remember that no two people cope the same way.** Couples often have different coping strategies. If your spouse or partner does not seem as distraught as you, it does not mean she or he is suffering any less than you are.

- **Make time.** Even a quick call, text message, or handwritten note to your spouse and other children can go a long way to making their day a good one.

Get Support

Research shows what you most likely already know—that help from others strengthens and encourages your child and your family. Let others help during this difficult time. Family and friends may want to assist, but might not know what you need.

You may want to:

- **Find an easy way to update family and friends.** You may want to use a social media site to update people and organize help from people in your community.

- **Tell people how they can help.** Keep a list of things that others can do for your family. For example, people can cook, clean, shop, or drive siblings to their activities.

- **Join a support group.** Some groups meet in person, whereas others meet online. Many parents benefit from the experiences and information shared by other parents.

- **Seek professional help.** If you are not sleeping well or are depressed, talk with your primary care doctor or people on your child's healthcare team. Ask them to recommend a mental health specialist, such as a psychiatrist, psychologist, counselor, or social worker.

Make Time to Renew Your Mind and Body

It can be tempting to put your own needs on hold and to focus solely on your child. But, it is important to take time for yourself so you have the energy to care for your child. Here are tips to get you started:

- **Find ways to relax and lower stress.** Some parents try something new, such as a yoga or deep-breathing class at the hospital. Others are refreshed by being outdoors, even for short periods. Whatever the method or place, find one that feels peaceful to you.

- **Stay physically active to sleep better and stay calm.** Try to walk, jog, go to the gym, or follow an exercise DVD. If it is hard to stay physically active at the hospital, try walking up and down the stairs or around the hospital or unit.

- **Fill waiting time.** Pick a few activities that you enjoy and can do in your child's room, such as playing a game, reading a book or magazine, writing, or listening to music.

Working with Your Child's Healthcare Team

These suggestions can help you and your child to establish strong and effective relationships with your child's healthcare team.

- **Build strong partnerships.** Give and expect to receive respect from the people on your child's healthcare team. Open and honest communication will also make it easier for you to ask questions, discuss options, and feel confident that your child is in good hands.

- **Take advantage of the many specialists who can help your child.** Work with them to help your child learn about cancer, how it will be treated, prepare for tests, manage side effects, and cope.

- **If you get information online, make sure the source is credible.** It is important to get accurate information that you understand and can use to make decisions. Share what you find with the healthcare team to confirm that it applies to your child.

- **Make sure you understand what your child's healthcare team tells you.** Speak up when something is confusing or unclear, especially when decisions need to be made. Ask to see pictures or videos to help understand new medical information.

- **Keep your child's pediatrician updated.** Ask for updates to be sent to your child's regular pediatrician.

Chapter 36

Pediatric Palliative Care

Palliative Care Provides Comfort and Support to Your Child and Family

When a child is seriously ill, each person in the family is affected differently. That is why it is important that you, your child, and your family get the support and care you need during this difficult time. A special type of care called "palliative" care can help. Palliative care is a key part of care for children living with a serious illness. It is also an important source of support for their families. The information in this brochure will help you understand how your child and family can benefit from this type of care.

What Is Palliative Care?

Palliative care can ease the symptoms, discomfort, and stress of serious illness for your child and family. Palliative care can help with your child's illness and give support to your family. It can:

- Ease your child's pain and other symptoms of illness

- Provide emotional and social support that respects your family's cultural values

This chapter includes text excerpted from "Palliative Care for Children," National Institute of Nursing Research (NINR), July 2015. Reviewed September 2019.

- Help your child's healthcare providers work together and communicate with one another to support your goals

Start open discussions with you, your child, and your healthcare team about options for care.

Palliative Care Provides Comfort for Your Child

Palliative care can help children and teenagers living with many serious illnesses, including genetic disorders, cancer, neurologic disorders, heart and lung conditions, and others. Palliative care is important for children at any age or stage of serious illness. It can begin as soon as you learn about your child's illness. Palliative care can help prevent symptoms and give relief from much more than physical pain. It can also enhance your child's quality of life.

Palliative Care Gives You and Your Family an Added Layer of Support

Serious illness in a child affects everyone in the family, including parents and siblings of all ages. Palliative care gives extra support for your whole family. It can ease the stress on all of your children, your spouse, and you during a hard time.

Palliative Care Surrounds Your Family with a Team of Experts Who Work Together to Support All of You

It is a partnership between your child, your family, and the healthcare team. This team listens to your preferences and helps you think through the care options for your family. They will work with you and your child to make a care plan for your family. They can also help when your child moves from one care setting (e.g., the hospital) to another (e.g., outpatient care or care at home).

Does Accepting Palliative Care Mean Our Family Is Giving up on Other Treatments?

No. The purpose of palliative care is to ease your child's pain and other symptoms and provide emotional and other support to your entire family. Palliative care can help children, from newborns to young adults, and their families—at any stage of a serious illness. Palliative care works alongside other treatments your child may be receiving. In fact, your child can start getting palliative care as soon as you learn about your child's illness.

How Is Palliative Care Different from Hospice Care

Your child does not need to be in hospice to get palliative care. Your child can get palliative care wherever they receive care: in the hospital, during clinic visits, or at home. Hospice care focuses on a person's final months of life, but palliative care is available to your child at any time during a serious illness. Some children receive palliative care for many years. Some hospice programs require that patients are no longer getting treatments to cure their illness, but palliative care is different—it can be given at the same time as other treatments for your child's illness

Palliative Care Helps Your Child Live a More Comfortable Life

Palliative care can provide direct support for your child by providing relief from distressing symptoms, such as:

* Pain

* Shortness of breath

* Fatigue

* Depression

* Anxiety

* Nausea

* Loss of appetite

* Problems with sleep

Palliative care can help your child deal with the side effects of medicines and treatments. Perhaps most important, palliative care can help enhance your child's quality of life. For example, helping to cope with concerns about school and friends might be very valuable to your child.

Palliative care may also include direct support for families such as assistance with:

* Including siblings in conversations

* Providing respite care for parents to be able to spend time with their other children

* Locating community resources for services such as counseling and support groups

Palliative care is effective. Scientists have studied how palliative care can help children living with serious illnesses. Studies show that patients who get palliative care say that it helps with:

• Pain and other distressing symptoms, such as nausea or shortness of breath

• Communication between healthcare providers and family members

• Emotional support

Other studies show that palliative care:

• It helps patients get the kinds of care they want.

• It meets the emotional, developmental, and spiritual needs of patients.

Palliative Care Focuses on the Needs of Your Child and Family

How Do You Know If Your Child or Family Needs Palliative Care?

Children living with a serious illness often experience physical and emotional distress related to their disease. Emotional distress is also common among their parents, siblings, and other family members. If your child has a genetic disorder, cancer, neurologic disorder, heart or lung condition, or another serious illness, palliative care may help reduce pain and enhance the quality of life.

Ask your child's healthcare provider about palliative care if your child or any member of your family (including you):

• Suffers from pain or other symptoms due to serious illness

• Experiences physical pain or emotional distress that is NOT under control

• Need help understanding your child's health condition

• Needs support coordinating your child's care

The Palliative Care Team Works with You, Your Child, and Your Care Team

Together with your child's healthcare providers, palliative care professionals will work with you and your child to make a care plan that is right for your child, your family, and you. The team will help you and your child include pain and other symptom management into every part of your child's care.

Palliative care experts spend as much time with you and your family as it takes to help you fully understand your child's condition, care options, and other needs. They also make sure your child experiences a smooth transition between the hospital and other services, such as getting care at home.

Your team will listen to your preferences and work with you and your child to plan care for all of your child's symptoms throughout the illness. This will include care for your child's current needs and flexibility for future changes.

Your Child's Palliative Care Team Is Unique

Every palliative care team is different. Your child's palliative care team may include:

- Doctors

- Nurses

- Social workers

- Pharmacists

- Chaplains

- Counselors

- Child life specialists

- Nutritionists

- Art and music therapists

How Can Our Family Get Palliative Care?

The palliative care process can begin when your child's healthcare provider refers you to palliative care services. Or, you or your child can ask your provider for a referral if you feel that palliative care would be helpful for your child, your family, or yourself. The palliative care process can begin when your child's healthcare provider refers you to palliative care services. Or, you or your child can ask your provider for a referral if you feel that palliative care would be helpful for your child, your family, or yourself.

If We Start Palliative Care, Can My Child Still See the Same Primary Healthcare Provider?

Yes. Your child does not have to change to a new primary healthcare provider when starting palliative care. The palliative care team and your child's healthcare provider work together to help you and your child decide the best care plan for your child.

What If My Child's Healthcare Provider Is Unsure about Referring Us?

Some parents are afraid they might offend their child's current healthcare providers by asking about palliative care, but this is unlikely. Most healthcare providers appreciate the extra time and information the palliative care team provides to their patients. Occasionally, a clinician may not refer a patient for palliative care services. If this happens, ask for an explanation. Let your child's healthcare provider know why you think palliative care could help your family.

Who Pays for Palliative Care?

Many insurance plans cover palliative care. If you have questions or concerns about costs, you can ask your healthcare team to put you in touch with a social worker, care manager, or financial advisor at your hospital or clinic to look at payment options.

Palliative Care Can Begin at Any Time and Be Provided Alongside Other Treatments Your Child May Be Receiving
Where Can My Child Get Palliative Care?

Your palliative care team will help you to know what services are available in your community. Your child and family may receive palliative care in a hospital, during clinic visits, or at home. You and your child will likely first meet with your palliative care team in the hospital or at a clinic. After the first visit, some visits may still occur in the clinic or hospital. But, many palliative care programs offer services at home and in the community. Home services can occur through telephone calls or home visits.

If palliative care starts in the hospital, your care team can help your child make a successful move to your home or other healthcare setting.

A home may feel most comfortable and safe for you and your child. Depending on your child's condition and treatment, the palliative care team may be able to help you find a nursing agency or community care agency to support palliative care for your child at home.

How Can My Child's Pain Be Managed?

The palliative care team can bring your child comfort in many ways. Treating pain often involves medication, but there are also other methods to address a child's discomfort. Your child may feel better with changes, such as low lighting, comfortable room temperatures, pleasant smells, guided relaxation, and deep breathing techniques. Your child may welcome additional activities, such as video chats, social media, soothing music, and massage and art therapy that may help decrease pain and anxiety.

If your child has an illness that causes pain that is not relieved by drugs, such as acetaminophen (Tylenol®) or ibuprofen (Motrin® or Advil®), your child's palliative care team may recommend trying stronger medicines. There is no reason to wait before beginning these medications. Should your child's pain increase, the dose may be safely increased over time to provide relief.

Pain relief can be offered in a hospital, at home, or in other healthcare settings. Your palliative care team will partner with you and your child to learn what is causing discomfort and how best to handle it.

Do Not Wait to Get Your Child and Family the Extra Support They Deserve
Talk to Your Loved Ones and Healthcare Team about Palliative Care

If your child wants palliative care, or if you think palliative care could be helpful to any member of your family, ask for it now. Talk with your child's healthcare provider about palliative care.

To see whether a hospital in your area offers a palliative care program, visit the Palliative Care Provider Directory of Hospitals at getpalliativecare.org.

Chapter 37

Sudden Infant Death Syndrome

Sudden infant death syndrome (SIDS) is the sudden, unexplained death of an infant younger than one year of age that remains unexplained after a complete investigation. This investigation can include an autopsy, a review of the death scene, and complete family and medical histories.

A diagnosis of SIDS is made by collecting information, conducting scientific or forensic tests, and talking with parents, other caregivers, and healthcare providers. If, after this process is complete, there is still no identifiable cause of death, the infant's death might be labeled as SIDS.

How Many Infants Die from Sudden Infant Death Syndrome or Are at Risk for It?

Data from the Centers for Disease Control and Prevention (CDC) show that 1,545 infants died from sudden infant death syndrome (SIDS) in 2014 (the most recent year for which data are available). SIDS was the leading cause of death in children between 1 month and

This chapter includes text excerpted from "Sudden Infant Death Syndrome (SIDS)," *Eunice Kennedy Shriver* National Institute of Child Health and Human Development (NICHD), January 31, 2017.

1 year of age in 2013. The majority (90%) of SIDS deaths occur before a child is 6 months old, with most happening between 1 month and 4 months of age.

What Factors Increase the Risk of Sudden Infant Death Syndrome?

Currently, there is no known way to prevent SIDS, but there are ways to reduce the risk. Several factors present during pregnancy, at birth, and throughout the first year after birth can impact SIDS risk. Many of these factors can be controlled or changed to reduce the risk, but some cannot be controlled or changed.

One of the most effective actions that parents and caregivers can take to lower SIDS risk is to place their baby to sleep on her or his back for all sleep times.

Research shows that:

- Back sleeping carries the lowest risk for SIDS and is recommended.

- Stomach sleeping carries the highest risk for SIDS—between 1.7 and 12.9 times the risk of back sleeping. It is not recommended.

- The side-lying position also increases the risk. It is unstable and babies can easily roll to their stomachs. It is not recommended.

Other known risk factors for SIDS include the following:

- **Preterm birth.** Infants born before 37 weeks in the womb are at higher risk for SIDS than are infants born at full term.

- **Smoking.** Maternal smoking during pregnancy and smoke in the infant's environment increase the risk of SIDS.

- **Race/ethnic origin.** African American and American Indian/Alaska Native infants are at higher risk for SIDS than are white, Hispanic American, or Asian/Pacific Islander American infants.

What Causes Sudden Infant Death Syndrome

Healthcare providers and researchers do not know the exact cause, but there are many theories.

More and more research evidence suggests that infants who die from sudden infant death syndrome (SIDS) are born with brain abnormalities or defects. These defects are typically found within a network of nerve cells that rely on a chemical called "serotonin" that allows one nerve cell to send a signal to another nerve cell. The cells are located in the part of the brain that probably controls breathing, heart rate, blood pressure, temperature, and waking from sleep.

But, scientists believe that brain defects alone may not be enough to cause a SIDS death. Evidence suggests that other events must also occur for an infant to die from SIDS. Researchers use the Triple-Risk Model to explain this concept. In this model, all three factors have to occur for an infant to die from SIDS. Having only one of these factors may not be enough to cause death from SIDS, but when all three combine, the chances of SIDS are high.

These factors are:

- **At-risk infant.** An infant has an unknown problem—such as a genetic change or a brain defect—that puts her or him at risk for SIDS. Healthcare providers, parents, and caregivers do not know about these problems, so they do not know the infant is at risk.

- **Important time in infant's development.** During the first 6 months after birth, infants go through many quick phases of growth that can change how well the body controls or regulates itself. Also, infant's bodies are learning how to respond to their environment.

- **Stressors in the environment.** All infants have stressors in their environments—sometimes called "external stressors" because they are outside the body. Being placed to sleep on the stomach, overheating during sleep, and exposure to cigarette smoke are all examples of external stressors. Infants who have no problems like those explained above can usually correct or overcome external stressors to survive and thrive. But, an infant who has an unknown problem and whose body systems are immature and unstable might not be able to overcome these stressors.

According to the Triple-Risk Model, all three things have to be present for SIDS to occur.

Removing one of these factors—such as external stressors—may tip the balance in favor of the infant's survival. Because the first two situations ca not be seen or pinpointed, the most effective way to reduce the risk of SIDS is to remove or reduce environmental stressors. Strategies to remove these stressors form the basis of the Safe to Sleep® campaign messages.

How Can I Reduce the Risk of Sudden Infant Death Syndrome?

Research shows that there are several ways to reduce the risk of SIDS and other sleep-related causes of infant death.

* **Always place baby on her or his back to sleep, for naps and at night, to reduce the risk of SIDS.** The back sleep position is the safest position for all babies, until they are 1 year old. Babies who are used to sleeping on their backs, but who are then placed to sleep on their stomachs, like for a nap, are at very high risk for SIDS. Preemies (infants born preterm) should be placed on their backs to sleep as soon as possible after birth.

* **Use a firm and flat sleep surface, such as a mattress in a safety-approved crib, covered by a fitted sheet with no other bedding or soft items in the sleep area.** Never place baby to sleep on soft surfaces, such as on a couch, sofa, waterbed, pillow, quilt, sheepskin, or blanket. These surfaces can be very dangerous for babies. Do not use a car seat, stroller, swing, infant carrier, infant sling or similar products as baby's regular sleep area. Following these recommendations reduces the risk of SIDS and death or injury from suffocation, entrapment, and strangulation.

* **Breastfeed your baby to reduce the risk of SIDS.** Breastfeeding has many health benefits for mother and baby. Babies who breastfeed, or are fed breastmilk, are at lower risk for SIDS than are babies who were never fed breastmilk. Longer duration of exclusive breastfeeding leads to lower risk.

  If you bring a baby into your bed for feeding, put her or him back in a separate sleep area when finished. This sleep area should be made for infants, such as a crib or bassinet, and close to your bed. If you fall asleep while feeding or comforting baby in an adult bed, place her or him back in a separate sleep area as soon as you wake up. Evidence shows that the longer a parent and an infant bed share, the higher the risk for sleep-related causes of infant death, such as suffocation.

* **Share your room with baby.** Keep baby in your room close to your bed, but on a separate surface designed for infants, ideally for baby's first year, but at least for the first 6 months. Room sharing reduces the risk of SIDS. Baby should not sleep

in an adult bed, on a couch, or on a chair alone, with you, or with anyone else, including siblings or pets. Having a separate safe sleep surface for the baby reduces the risk of SIDS and the chance of suffocation, strangulation, and entrapment. If you bring your baby into your bed for feeding or comforting, remove all soft items and bedding from the area. When finished, put the baby back in a separate sleep area made for infants, like a crib or bassinet, and close to your bed. Couches and armchairs can also be very dangerous for babies if adults fall asleep as they feed, comfort, or bond with baby while on these surfaces. Parents and other caregivers should be mindful of how tired they are during these times. There is no evidence for or against devices or products that claim to make bed-sharing "safer."

- **Do not put soft objects, toys, crib bumpers, or loose bedding under baby, over baby, or anywhere in baby's sleep area.** Keeping these items out of the baby's sleep area reduces the risk of SIDS and suffocation, entrapment, and strangulation. Because the evidence does not support using them to prevent injury, crib bumpers are not recommended. Crib bumpers are linked to serious injuries and deaths from suffocation, entrapment, and strangulation. Keeping these and other soft objects out of the baby's sleep area are the best way to avoid these dangers.

- To reduce the risk of SIDS, women should:

  - Get regular prenatal care during pregnancy

  - Avoid smoking, drinking alcohol, and using marijuana or illegal drugs during pregnancy or after the baby is born

  - Do not smoke during pregnancy, and do not smoke or allow smoking around your baby

- **Think about giving your baby a pacifier for naps and nighttime sleep to reduce the risk of SIDS.** Do not attach the pacifier to anything—such as a string, clothing, stuffed toy, or blanket—that carries a risk for suffocation, choking, or strangulation. Wait until breastfeeding is well established (often by 3 to 4 weeks) before offering a pacifier. Or, if you are not breastfeeding, offer the pacifier as soon as you want. Do not force the baby to use it. If the pacifier falls out of the baby's mouth during sleep, there is no need to put the pacifier back in. Pacifiers reduce the risk of SIDS for all babies, including breastfed babies.

- **Do not let your baby get too hot during sleep.** Dress your baby in sleep clothing, such as a wearable blanket designed to keep her or him warm without the need for loose blankets in the sleeping area. Dress baby appropriately for the environment, and do not over bundle. Parents and caregivers should watch for signs of overheating, such as sweating or the baby's chest feeling hot to the touch. Keep the baby's face and head uncovered during sleep.

- **Follow guidance from your healthcare provider on your baby's vaccines and regular health checkups.** Vaccines not only protect the baby's health, but research shows that vaccinated babies are at lower risk for SIDS.

- **Avoid products that go against safe sleep recommendations, especially those that claim to prevent or reduce the risk for SIDS.** There is currently no known way to prevent SIDS. Evidence does not support the safety or effectiveness of wedges, positioners, or other products that claim to keep infants in a specific position or to reduce the risk of SIDS, suffocation, or reflux. In fact, many of these products are associated with injury and death, especially when used in the baby's sleep area.

- **Do not use heart or breathing monitors in the home to reduce the risk of SIDS.** If you have questions about using these monitors for other health conditions, talk with your baby's healthcare provider, and always follow safe sleep recommendations.

- **Give your baby plenty of tummy time when she or he is awake and someone is watching.** Supervised Tummy Time helps strengthen your baby's neck, shoulder, and arm muscles. It also helps to prevent flat spots on the back of your baby's head. Limiting the time spent in car seats, once the baby is out of the car, and changing the direction the infant lays in the sleep area from week to week also can help to prevent these flat spots.

Make sure everyone who cares for your baby knows the ways to reduce the risk of SIDS and other sleep-related causes of infant death.

Chapter 38

Stillbirth, Miscarriage, and Infant Death

Chapter Contents

Section 38.1—Stillbirth 340

Section 38.2—Miscarriage 344

Section 38.3—Infant Death 349

Section 38.1

Stillbirth

This section includes text excerpted from "What Is Stillbirth?"
Centers for Disease Control and Prevention (CDC), August 29, 2019.

What Is Stillbirth?

The loss of a baby due to stillbirth remains a sad reality for many
families and takes a serious toll on families' health and well-being. A
stillbirth is the death or loss of a baby before or during delivery. Both
miscarriage and stillbirth describe pregnancy loss, but they differ
according to when the loss occurs. In the United States, a miscarriage
is usually defined as loss of a baby before the 20th week of pregnancy,
and a stillbirth is loss of a baby after 20 weeks of pregnancy.
Stillbirth is further classified as either early, late, or term.

• An early stillbirth is a fetal death occurring between 20 and 27
  completed weeks of pregnancy

• A late stillbirth occurs between 28 and 36 completed pregnancy
  weeks

• A term stillbirth occurs between 37 or more completed
  pregnancy weeks

How Many Babies Are Stillborn?

Stillbirth affects about 1 percent of all pregnancies, and each year
about 24,000 babies are stillborn in the United States. That is about
the same number of babies that die during the first year of life and it
is more than 10 times as many deaths as the number that occur from
Sudden Infant Death Syndrome (SIDS).

Because of advances in medical technology over the last 30 years,
prenatal care (medical care during pregnancy) has improved, which
has dramatically reduced the number of late and term stillbirth. However, the rate of early stillbirth has remained about the same over time.

What Increases the Risk of Stillbirth?

Stillbirth with an unknown cause is called "unexplained stillbirth."
Having an unexplained stillbirth is more likely to occur the further

along a woman is in her pregnancy. Having an autopsy on the baby and other laboratory tests is important in trying to understand why the baby died before birth. Your healthcare provider can share more information about this.

Stillbirth occurs in families of all races, ethnicities, and income levels, and to women of all ages. However, stillbirth occurs more commonly among certain groups of people including women who:

- Are of black race

- Are 35 years of age or older

- Are of low socioeconomic status

- Smoke cigarettes during pregnancy

- Have certain medical conditions, such as high blood pressure, diabetes and obesity

- Have multiple pregnancies such as triplets or quadruplets

- Have had a previous pregnancy loss

This does not mean that every individual of black race or older age is at higher risk of having a stillbirth. It simply means that overall as a group, more stillbirths occur among all mothers of black race or older age when compared to White mothers and mothers under 35 years of age. Differences in factors, such as maternal health, income, access to quality healthcare, stress, social and emotional support resources and cultural factors may explain how these factors are related to having a stillbirth. More research is needed to determine the underlying cause of stillbirths in these populations.

These factors are also associated with other poor pregnancy outcomes, such as preterm birth.

State laws require the reporting of fetal deaths, and federal law supports national collection and publication of fetal death data. The National Vital Statistics System (NVSS) released the first ever report on cause of fetal death using national data in 2016.

Data and Statistics

Stillbirth is more common than people realize, and some factors can increase the risk for stillbirth to occur. Read below for some significant research findings on stillbirth.

Occurrence

• In 2014, approximately 24,000 stillbirths were reported in the United States.

• Since the 1940s, improvements in maternity care resulted in a dramatic reduction in the occurrence of stillbirth; however, more recently, the decline has slowed or halted.

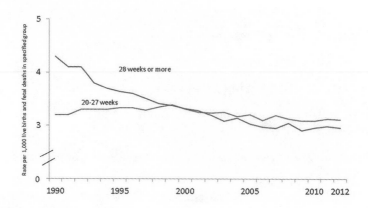

Figure 38.1. *Rate of Stillbirth Over Time by the Number of Completed Weeks of Pregnancy: United States, 2000 to 2013.* (Source: Centers for Disease Control and Prevention (CDC)/National Center for Health Statistics (NCHS), National Vital Statistics System (NVSS).)

This graph shows the rate of stillbirth over time by the number of completed weeks of pregnancy in the United States from 1990 through 2012. A blue line shows the rate of early stillbirth, meaning at 20 to 27 completed weeks, which was pretty stable from 1990 to 2005, declined 3 percent between 2005 to 2006, and then stabilized again from 2006 through 2012. A red line shows the rate of late stillbirth, meaning at 28 or more completed weeks of pregnancy. The rate of late stillbirth declined 28 percent from 1990 to 2003, increased slightly in 2004, and then declined another 4 percent from 2004 to 2005. The rate of late stillbirth then stabilized was essentially unchanged from 2005 through 2012.

Factors That Might Increase the Risk of Stillbirth

In high-income countries,

• Being obese or overweight during pregnancy contributes to about 8,000 stillbirths each year

- Advanced maternal age (greater than 35 years) contributes to about 4,200 stillbirths each year

- Smoking during pregnancy contributes to about 2,800 stillbirths each year

Racial/Ethnic Differences

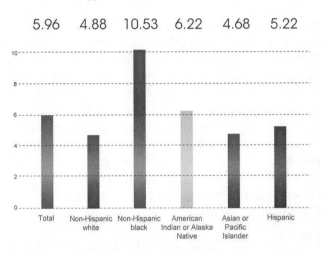

Figure 38.2. *Stillbirth (Fetal Death) Rates, by Race and Hispanic Origin of Mother: United States, 2013.* (Source: Centers for Disease Control and Prevention (CDC)/National Center for Health Statistics (NCHS), National Vital Statistics System (NVSS).)

This figure shows that the rate of stillbirth varies considerably by race and Hispanic origin of the mother. The rate for non-Hispanic White women was 4.88 per 1,000 live births and stillbirths. This rate is similar to that for Asian or Pacific Islander women, who had a stillbirth rate of 4.68. In stark contrast, the rate of stillbirth for non-Hispanic Black women was 10.53, more than twice the rate for non-Hispanic White women. The rate for American Indian or Alaska Native women was 6.22, which was 27 percent higher than non-Hispanic White women. The rate for Hispanic women was 5.22, which was about 7 percent higher than the rate for non-Hispanic White women.

Section 38.2

Miscarriage

This section includes text excerpted from "Pregnancy Loss (Before 20 Weeks of Pregnancy)," *Eunice Kennedy Shriver* National Institute of Child Health and Human Development (NICHD), September 1, 2017.

Pregnancy loss is the unexpected loss of a fetus before the 20th week of pregnancy. It is sometimes called "miscarriage," "early pregnancy loss," "mid-trimester pregnancy loss," "fetal demise," or "spontaneous abortion." Healthcare providers use a different term—"stillbirth"—to describe the loss of a fetus after 20 weeks of pregnancy.

Pregnancy loss may occur so early that a woman may not know she was pregnant. Researchers can only estimate the number of women who experience pregnancy loss, because some losses occur before a woman's pregnancy is confirmed by a healthcare provider or pregnancy test. But the American College of Obstetricians and Gynecologists estimates that early pregnancy loss is common, occurring in about 10 percent of confirmed pregnancies.

What Are the Symptoms of Pregnancy Loss (Before 20 Weeks of Pregnancy)?

Symptoms of pregnancy loss may include:

- Bleeding from the vagina

- Pain or cramps in the lower stomach area (abdomen)

- Low back pain

- Fluid, tissue, or clot-like material coming out of the vagina

However, bleeding from the vagina during pregnancy does not always mean a miscarriage. Many pregnant women have spotting and cramping in early pregnancy but do not miscarry. Your healthcare provider might call this pregnancy "threatened." In any case, pregnant women who have any of the symptoms of miscarriage should contact their healthcare provider immediately.

Some women do not experience any symptoms of pregnancy loss.

Although this is rare in the United States, some women who have a miscarriage may get an infection in the uterus, which can be life threatening. Women who have the following symptoms for more than 24 hours after a should call 911:

- A fever higher than 100.4 degrees Fahrenheit on more than two occasions

- Severe pain in the lower abdomen

- Bloody discharge from the vagina (which can include pus and be foul smelling)

Research has also found that morning sickness—nausea and vomiting during pregnancy—is linked to lower risk of pregnancy loss. *Eunice Kennedy Shriver* National Institute of Child Health and Human Development (NICHD) researchers are continuing to look for other factors that may indicate lower risk of pregnancy loss.

What Are the Causes and Risks of Pregnancy Loss (Before 20 Weeks of Pregnancy)?

Pregnancy loss may occur for many reasons, and sometimes the cause remains unknown even after additional tests are completed.

Possible Causes

Pregnancy loss often happens when a pregnancy does not develop normally.

In many cases, miscarriages result from a problem with the chromosomes in the fetus. The number of chromosomes the fetus has—too many or too few—can affect survival.

Other possible causes of pregnancy loss include:

- Being exposed to toxins in the environment

- Problems of the placenta, cervix, or uterus

- Problems with the father's sperm

In many cases, though, healthcare providers cannot identify a cause or causes for pregnancy loss.

Risk Factors

Problems with chromosomes happen more often in the fetuses of older parents, particularly among women who are older than 35 For this reason, risk of pregnancy loss increases as the parents age; it is much higher at age 45 than at age 35.

Women who have had previous miscarriages are also at a higher risk of pregnancy loss.

345

Health issues, such as chronic diseases, in the mother that can also increase risk of pregnancy loss include:

- Chronic diseases, such as high blood pressure, diabetes, thyroid disease, or polycystic ovary syndrome (PCOS)

- Problems with the immune system, such as an autoimmune disorder

- Infections (such as untreated gonorrhea or Zika)

- Hormone problems

- Extremes in weight, such as obesity or being too thin

- Lifestyle factors, such as using drugs or alcohol, smoking, or consuming more than 200 milligrams of caffeine per day (equal to about one 12-ounce cup of coffee)

Findings from the NICHD study suggest that women who are at higher risk of pregnancy loss because of two or more previous losses may increase their chances of carrying the pregnancy to term by taking a low-dose aspirin every day if they have high levels of inflammation.

Recent research has also found that morning sickness—nausea and vomiting during pregnancy—is linked to lower risk of pregnancy loss. The NICHD researchers are continuing their research to find other factors that may indicate lower risk of pregnancy loss.

How Do Healthcare Providers Diagnose and Treat Pregnancy Loss (Before 20 Weeks of Pregnancy)?

If a pregnant woman has any of the symptoms of pregnancy loss, such as abdominal cramps, back pain, light spotting, or bleeding, she should contact her healthcare provider immediately. Remember that vaginal bleeding during pregnancy does not definitely mean a pregnancy loss is occurring.

Diagnosing Pregnancy Loss

Depending on how far along the pregnancy is, healthcare providers may use different methods to determine whether a pregnancy loss has occurred:

- A blood test to check the level of human chorionic gonadotropin (hCG), the pregnancy hormone

- A pelvic exam to see whether the woman's cervix is dilated or thinned, which can be a sign of pregnancy loss

- An ultrasound test, which allows the provider to look at the pregnancy, uterus, and placenta1

If a woman has had more than one miscarriage, she may want to have a healthcare provider check her blood for chromosome problems, hormone problems, or immune system disorders that may be contributing to pregnancy loss.

Treating Pregnancy Loss

Treatments for pregnancy loss focus on ensuring that the nonviable pregnancy leaves the woman's body safely and completely. Women going through pregnancy loss are at risk for bleeding, pain, and infection, especially if some of the pregnancy tissue remains behind in the uterus.

The specific treatment used depends on how far along the pregnancy was, the woman's overall health, her age, and other factors.

In many cases, pregnancy loss before 20 weeks may not require any special treatment. The bleeding that occurs with pregnancy loss empties the uterus without any further problems.

Women who have heavy bleeding during pregnancy loss should contact a healthcare provider immediately. For reference, heavy bleeding refers to soaking at least two maxi pads an hour for at least 2 hours in a row.

Some women may need a surgical procedure called a "dilation and curettage" (D&C) to remove any pregnancy tissue that is still in the uterus. A D&C is recommended if a woman is bleeding heavily or if an ultrasound shows pregnancy tissue is still in the uterus. D&C may also be used if a woman has any signs of infection, such as a fever, or if she has other health problems, such as cardiovascular disease or a bleeding disorder.

Some women are treated with a medication called "misoprostol," which helps the tissue pass out of the uterus and controls the resulting bleeding. Research shows that misoprostol is safe and effective in most cases.

Women who lose a pregnancy may also need other treatments to control mild to moderate bleeding, prevent infection, relieve pain, and help with emotional support.

Is There a Way to Prevent Pregnancy Loss (Before 20 Weeks of Pregnancy)?

There is currently no known way to prevent pregnancy loss before 20 weeks from occurring, nor is there a way to stop pregnancy loss once it has started.

There are ways to lower the risk of general pregnancy complications, but none of them definitely prevent pregnancy loss. Some ways to lower overall risk include:

- Staying in good health before becoming pregnant and getting regular care during pregnancy

- Diagnosing any health conditions, such as diabetes or thyroid disorders, and taking steps to manage or treat the condition before getting pregnant

- Avoiding environmental hazards, such as exposure to radiation, pollution, or toxic chemicals

- Avoiding alcohol and drugs, including high levels of caffeine in both partners

- Protecting yourself from certain infections by not traveling to certain areas and by preventing mosquito bites

An NICHD study found that women who are at higher risk of pregnancy loss because of two or more previous losses may increase their chances of carrying the pregnancy to term by taking a low-dose aspirin every day if they have high levels of inflammation.

Section 38.3

Infant Death

This section contains text excerpted from the following sources: Text in this section begins with excerpts from "Infant Mortality," Centers for Disease Control and Prevention (CDC), March 27, 2019; Text under the heading "Prevention of Infant Mortality" is excerpted from "Are There Ways to Reduce the Risk of Infant Mortality?" *Eunice Kennedy Shriver* National Institute of Child Health and Human Development (NICHD), December 1, 2016. Reviewed September 2019.

Infant mortality is the death of an infant before her or his first birthday. The infant mortality rate is the number of infant deaths for every 1,000 live births. In addition to giving us key information about maternal and infant health, the infant mortality rate is an important marker of the overall health of a society. In 2017, the infant mortality rate in the United States was 5.8 deaths per 1,000 live births.

Causes of Infant Mortality

Over 22,000 infants died in the United States in 2017. The five leading causes of infant death in 2017 were:

1. Birth defects

2. Preterm birth and low birth weight

3. Maternal pregnancy complications

4. Sudden infant death syndrome

5. Injuries (e.g., suffocation)

Healthy People (www.healthypeople.gov) provides science-based, 10-year national objectives for improving the health of all Americans. One of the Healthy People 2020 objectives is to reduce the rate of all infant deaths. In 2017, 26 states met the Healthy People 2020 target of 6.0 infant deaths per 1,000 live births. Geographically, infant mortality rates in 2017 were highest among states in the south. Rates were also high in some states in the Midwest.

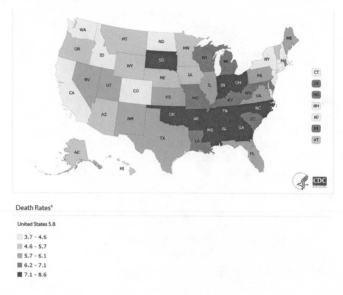

Death Rates¹

United States 5.8

| | 3.7 - 4.6
| | 4.6 - 5.7
| | 5.7 - 6.1
| | 6.2 - 7.1
| | 7.1 - 8.6

Figure 38.3. *Infant Mortality Rates by State, 2017.*

¹The number of infant deaths per 1,000 live births.

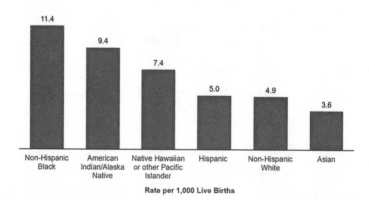

Rate per 1,000 Live Births

Figure 38.4. *Infant Mortality Rates by Race and Ethnicity, 2016.*

In 2016, infant mortality rates by race and ethnicity were as follows:

- Non-Hispanic Black: 11.4
- American Indian/Alaska Native: 9.4
- Native Hawaiian or other Pacific Islander: 7.4
- Hispanic: 5.0

- Non-Hispanic White: 4.9

- Asian: 3.6

Prevention of Infant Mortality

Often, there are no definite ways to prevent many of the leading causes of infant mortality. However, there are ways to reduce a baby's risk. Researchers continue to study the best ways to prevent and treat the causes of infant mortality and affect the contributors to infant mortality. Consider some ways to help reduce the risk.

Preventing Birth Defects

Birth defects are currently the leading cause of infant mortality in the United States. There are many different kinds of birth defects, and they can happen in any pregnancy.

There are several things pregnant women can do to help reduce the risk of certain birth defects, such as getting enough folic acid before and during pregnancy to prevent neural tube defects.

Addressing Preterm Birth, Low Birth Weight, and Their Outcomes

There is currently no definitive way to prevent preterm birth, the second-most-common cause of infant mortality in the United States. However, researchers and healthcare providers are working to address the issue on multiple fronts, including finding ways to stop preterm labor from progressing to a preterm delivery and identifying ways to improve health outcomes for infants who are born preterm. Preterm infants commonly have a low birth weight, but sometimes full-term infants are also born underweight. Causes can include a mother's chronic health condition or poor nutrition. Adequate prenatal care is essential to ensuring that full-term infants are born at a healthy weight.

There are some known risk factors for preterm birth—including having had a preterm birth with a previous pregnancy—and women with known risk factors may receive treatments to help reduce those risks. But in most cases, the cause for preterm birth is not known, so there are not always effective treatments or actions that can prevent preterm delivery.

Researchers and healthcare providers are also working to understand the health challenges faced by infants born preterm or at a low birth weight as a way to develop treatments for these challenges. For instance, preterm infants are at high risk for serious breathing problems as a result of their underdeveloped lungs. Treatments such as ventilators and steroids can help stabilize breathing to allow the lungs to develop more fully. In addition, studies suggest that infants born at low birth weight are at increased risk of certain adult health problems, such as diabetes, high blood pressure, and heart disease.

Getting Care before Conception and Delivery

During pregnancy, the mother's health, environment, and experiences affect how her fetus develops and the course of the pregnancy. By taking good care of her own health before and during pregnancy, a mother can reduce her baby's risk of many of the leading causes of infant mortality in the United States, including birth defects, preterm birth, low birth weight, sudden infant death syndrome (SIDS), and certain pregnancy complications.

Women do not need to wait until they are pregnant to take steps to improve their health. Reaching a healthy weight, getting proper nutrition, managing chronic health conditions, and seeking help for substance use and abuse, for example, can help a woman achieve better health before she is pregnant. Her improved health, in turn, can help to reduce infant mortality risks for any babies she has in the future.

Once she becomes pregnant, a mother should receive early and regular prenatal care. This type of care helps promote the best outcomes for mother and baby.

Creating a Safe Infant Sleep Environment

Sudden infant death syndrome is defined as the sudden, unexplained death of an infant younger than 1 year of age that remains unexplained even after a thorough investigation. SIDS is the third-leading cause of infant mortality in the United States.

Sudden infant death syndrome is one type of death within a broader category of causes of death called "sudden unexpected infant death" (SUID). The SUID category includes other sleep-related causes of infant death—such as accidental suffocation—as well as infections, vehicle collisions, and other causes.

As SIDS rates have been declining in the last few decades, the rates of other sleep-related causes of infant death have been increasing. Accidental injury is the fifth-leading cause of infant mortality in the United States.

Although there is no definite way to prevent SIDS, there are ways to reduce the risk of SIDS and other sleep-related causes of infant death. For example, always placing a baby on her or his back to sleep and keeping baby's sleep area free of soft objects, toys, crib bumpers, and loose bedding are important ways to reduce a baby's risk. The NICHD-led Safe to Sleep® campaign (formerly the Back to Sleep campaign) describes many ways that parents and caregivers can reduce the risk of SIDS and other sleep-related causes of infant death.

Using Newborn Screening to Detect Hidden Conditions

Newborn screening can detect certain conditions that are not noticeable at the time of birth, but that can cause serious disability or even death if not treated quickly. Infants with these conditions may seem perfectly healthy and frequently come from families with no previous history of a condition.

To perform this screening, healthcare providers take a few drops of blood from an infant's heel and apply them to special paper. The blood spots are then analyzed. If any conditions are detected, treatment can begin immediately.

Most states screen for at least 29 conditions, but some test for 50 or more conditions. Infants who are at increased or high risk for a condition because of their family history can undergo additional screening—beyond what states offer automatically—through a healthcare specialist.

Since this public health program was initiated 50 years ago, it has saved countless lives by providing early detection and intervention and by improving the quality of life for children and their families.

Chapter 39

Helping Children Cope with Death

Chapter Contents

Section 39.1—Grief and Developmental Stages...................... 356

Section 39.2—Guiding Children through Grief....................... 361

Section 39.1

Grief and Developmental Stages

This section includes text excerpted from "Grief, Bereavement, and Coping with Loss (PDQ®)—Health Professional Version," National Cancer Institute (NCI), April 20, 2017.

At one time, children were considered miniature adults, and their behaviors were expected to be modeled as such. There is a greater awareness of developmental differences between childhood and other developmental stages in the human life cycle. Differences between the grieving process for children and the grieving process for adults are recognized. It is now believed that the real issue for grieving children is not whether they grieve, but how they exhibit their grief and mourning.

The primary difference between bereaved adults and bereaved children is that intense emotional and behavioral expressions are not continuous in children. A child's grief may appear more intermittent and briefer than that of an adult, but in fact, a child's grief usually lasts longer.

The work of mourning in childhood needs to be addressed repeatedly at different developmental and chronological milestones. Because bereavement is a process that continues over time, children will revisit the loss repeatedly, especially during significant life events (e.g., going to camp, graduating from school, marrying, and experiencing the births of their own children). Children must complete the grieving process, eventually achieving resolution of grief.

Although the experience of loss is unique and highly individualized, several factors can influence a child's grief:

- Age
- Personality
- Stage of development
- Previous experiences with death
- Previous relationship with the deceased
- Environment
- Cause of death
- Patterns of interaction and communication within the family

- Stability of family life after the loss

- How the child's needs for sustained care are met

- Availability of opportunities to share and express feelings and memories

- Parental styles of coping with stress

- Availability of consistent relationships with other adults

Children do not react to loss in the same ways as adults and may not display their feelings as openly as adults do. In addition to verbal communication, grieving children may employ play, drama, art, school work, and stories. Bereaved children may not withdraw into a preoccupation with thoughts of the deceased person; they often immerse themselves in activities (e.g., they may be sad one minute and then playing outside with friends the next). Families often incorrectly interpret this behavior to mean the child does not really understand or has already gotten over death. Neither assumption may be true; children's minds protect them from thoughts and feelings that are too powerful for them to handle.

Grief reactions are intermittent because children cannot explore all their thoughts and feelings as rationally as adults can. Additionally, children often have difficulty articulating their feelings about grief. A grieving child's behavior may speak louder than any words she or he could speak. Strong feelings of anger and fear of abandonment or death may be evident in the behaviors of grieving children. Children often play death games as a way of working out their feelings and anxieties in a relatively safe setting. These games are familiar to the children and provide safe opportunities to express their feelings.

Grief and Children's Age

Death and the events surrounding it are understood differently depending on a child's age and developmental stage.

Infants

Although infants do not recognize death, feelings of loss and separation are part of developing death awareness. Children who have been separated from their mothers and deprived of nurturing can exhibit changes, such as listlessness, quietness, unresponsiveness to a smile or a coo, physical changes (including weight loss), and a decrease in activity and lack of sleep.

Ages 2 to 3 Years

In this age range, children often confuse death with sleep and can experience anxiety. In the early phases of grief, bereaved children can exhibit loss of speech and generalized distress.

Ages 3 to 6 Years

In this age range, children view death as a kind of sleep: the person is alive but in some limited way. They do not fully separate death from life and may believe that the deceased continues to live (for instance, in the ground where she or he was buried) and often ask questions about the activities of the deceased person (e.g., how is the deceased eating, going to the toilet, breathing, or playing?). Young children can acknowledge physical death but consider it a temporary or gradual event, reversible and not final (such as leaving and returning, or a game of peek-a-boo). A child's concept of death may involve magical thinking, i.e., the idea that her or his thoughts can cause actions. Children may feel that they must have done or thought something bad to become ill or that a loved one's death occurred because of some personal thought or wish. In response to death, children younger than 5 years will often exhibit disturbances in eating, sleeping, and bladder or bowel control.

Ages 6 to 9 Years

It is not unusual for children in this age range to become very curious about death, asking very concrete questions about what happens to one's body when it stops working. Death is personified as a separate person or spirit: a skeleton, ghost, angel of death, or bogeyman. Although death is perceived as final and frightening, it is not universal. Children in this age range begin to compromise, recognizing that death is final and real but mostly happens to older people (not to themselves). Grieving children can develop school phobias, learning problems, and antisocial or aggressive behaviors; they can exhibit hypochondriacal concerns or can withdraw from others. Conversely, children in this age range can become overly attentive and clinging. Boys may show an increase in aggressive and destructive behavior (e.g., acting out in school), expressing their feelings in this way rather than by openly displaying sadness. When a parent dies, children may feel abandoned by both their deceased parent and their surviving parent, since the surviving parent is frequently preoccupied with her or his own grief and is less able to emotionally support the child.

Ages 9 Years and Older

By the time a child is nine years old, death is understood as inevitable and is no longer viewed as a punishment. By the time the child is 12 years old, death is viewed as final and universal.

Table 39.1. Grief and Developmental Stages

Age	Understanding of Death	Expressions of Grief
Infancy to 2 years	Is not yet able to understand death	Quietness, crankiness, decreased activity, poor sleep, and weight loss
	Separation from mother causes changes.	
2–6 years		Asks many questions (How does she go to the bathroom? How does she eat?)
		Problems in eating, sleeping, and bladder and bowel control
		Fear of abandonment
	Death is like sleeping.	Tantrums
	Dead person continues to live and function in some ways.	Magical thinking (Did I think something or do something that caused the death? Like when I said I hate you and I wish you would die?)
	Death is temporary, not final.	
	Dead person can come back to life.	
6–9 years		Curious about death
	Death is thought of as a person or spirit (skeleton, ghost, bogeyman).	Asks specific questions
		May have exaggerated fears about school.
		May have aggressive behaviors (especially boys).
	Death is final and frightening.	Some concerns about imaginary illnesses
	Death happens to others; it will not happen to ME.	May feel abandoned

Table 39.1. Continued

Age	Understanding of Death	Expressions of Grief
		Heightened emotions, guilt, anger, shame
		Increased anxiety over own death
	Everyone will die.	Mood swings
	Death is final and cannot be changed.	Fear of rejection; not wanting to be different from peers
		Changes in eating habits
		Sleeping problems
		Regressive behaviors (loss of interest in outside activities)
		Impulsive behaviors
9 and older	Even I will die.	Feels guilty about being alive (especially related to death of a sibling or peer)

In American society, many grieving adults withdraw into themselves and limit communication. In contrast, children often talk to those around them (even strangers) as a way of watching for reactions and seeking clues to help guide their own responses. It is not uncommon for children to repeatedly ask baffling questions. For example, a child may ask, "I know Grandpa died, but when will he come home?" This is thought to be a way of testing reality for the child and confirming the story of death.

Section 39.2

Guiding Children through Grief

This section contains text excerpted from the following sources: Text beginning with the heading "Grief Expressions of Bereaved Children," is excerpted from "Grief, Bereavement, and Coping with Loss (PDQ®)—Health Professional Version," National Cancer Institute (NCI), April 20, 2017; Text beginning with the heading "Elements Related to Bereavement to Include in Emergency Management Plans" is excerpted from "Coping with the Death of a Student or Staff Member," Readiness and Emergency Management for Schools (REMS) Technical Assistance (TA) Center, U.S. Department of Education (ED), 2007. Reviewed September 2019.

Grief Expressions of Bereaved Children

There are three prominent themes in the grief expressions of bereaved children:

- Did I cause the death to happen?
- Is it going to happen to me?
- Who is going to take care of me?

Did I Cause the Death to Happen?

Children often engage in magical thinking, believing they have magical powers. If a mother says in exasperation, "You'll be the death of me," and later dies, her child may wonder whether she or he actually caused the death. Likewise, when two siblings argue, it is not unusual for one to say (or think), "I wish you were dead." If that sibling were to die, the surviving sibling might think that her or his thoughts or statements actually caused the death.

Is It Going to Happen to Me?

The death of a sibling or other child may be especially difficult because it strikes so close to the child's own peer group. If the child also perceives that the death could have been prevented (by either a parent or doctor), the child may think that she or he could also die.

Who Is Going to Take Care of Me?

Because children depend on parents and other adults for their safety and welfare, a child who is grieving the death of an important person in her or his life might begin to wonder who will provide the care that she or he needs now that the person is gone.

Interventions for Grieving Children

There are interventions that may help to facilitate and support the grieving process in children.

Explanation of Death

Silence about death (which indicates that the subject is taboo) does not help children deal with loss. When death is discussed with a child, explanations should be kept as simple and direct as possible. Each child needs to be told the truth with as much detail as can be comprehended at her or his age and stage of development. Questions should be addressed honestly and directly. Children need to be reassured about their own security (they frequently worry that they will also die or that their surviving parent will go away). A child's questions should be answered, and the child's processing of the information should be confirmed.

Correct Language

Although it is a difficult conversation to initiate with children, any discussion about death must include proper words (e.g., cancer, died, or death). Euphemisms (e.g., "he passed away," "he is sleeping," or "we lost him") should never be used because they can confuse children and lead to misinterpretations.

Planning Rituals

After a death occurs, children can and should be included in the planning of and participation in mourning rituals. As with bereaved adults, these rituals help children memorialize loved ones. Although children should never be forced to attend or participate in mourning rituals, their participation should be encouraged. Children can be encouraged to participate in the aspects of funeral or memorial services with which they feel comfortable. If the child wants to attend the funeral (or wake or memorial service), it is important that a full explanation of what to expect is given in advance. This preparation should include the layout of the room, who might be present (e.g., friends and family members), what the child will see (e.g., a casket and people crying), and what will happen. Surviving parents may be too involved in their own grief to give their children the attention they need. Therefore, it is often helpful to identify a familiar adult friend or family member who will be assigned to care for a grieving child during a funeral.

Elements Related to Bereavement to Include in Emergency Management Plans

Schools should develop emergency management plans that foster an open and supportive school climate and active parent involvement, and demonstrate a strategy, including clear staff roles and responsibilities, for responding proactively to losses that impact students and staff. Losses range from the death of a preschool classroom pet to a high school student suicide to a weather-related disaster that takes the lives of several school members. Plans should include policies for managing and screening community volunteers who may show up at school to lend support. The protocol for memorials should be defined in a school's emergency management plan.

School plans should also include policies and protocols for handling the media. If the death is likely to result in attention from the media such as might be expected in a murder, suicide, or other sudden and dramatic loss, school policies and procedures should limit direct access of the media to solely the media spokesperson for the district and the school. Students should be advised to speak with school staff and their parents or guardians if they receive inquiries from the media such as phone calls, e-mails, contacts through their personal Web pages, or in person, while staff and parents should direct all media to the spokesperson. The goal is to protect the students and the school from any unwanted media attention while facilitating accurate and appropriate information regarding the incident.

Partnering with Community Mental-Health Providers

Schools can prepare for responding to and recovering from the death of a student, staff, or faculty member by actively partnering with their community mental-health providers prior to an incident and establishing a crisis response team that includes school social workers, psychologists, and guidance counselors. All districts and schools should create an emergency management plan in collaboration with community partners, including mental-health professionals. Developing a Memorandum of Understanding (MOU) with area mental-health organizations that includes activities such as providing ongoing training of school personnel in bereavement and crisis response, supplying professional counseling services, when necessary and appropriate, to students or staff in need of assistance, and offering relief to school-based guidance counselors, social workers, and psychologists when needed could all minimize some potential barriers to recovery. Training for teachers and staff might include: an appreciation of the impact bereavement can have on learning, behavior, and development; developmental understanding of death; and age-appropriate responses to support grieving students.

Chapter 40

Collaborative Pediatric Critical Care Research Network

Pediatric critical care, or the effective and efficient care of children with critical or unstable conditions, is an important and growing sub-specialty in pediatrics. The number of pediatric intensivists, pediatric intensive care units (PICUs), and PICU beds in the United States has increased dramatically. Mortality in U.S. PICUs has fallen precipi-tously, yet survivors of childhood critical illness and injury remain at risk for morbidity and disability.

Much of the technology and many therapies in pediatric critical care have evolved without adequate study or have been adopted uncritically from adult, neonatal, or anesthetic practice. As a result, the risks and ben-efits of much intensive care practice remain largely unknown. Research is needed to make optimal decisions regarding effective critical care prac-tices. Rigorous use of appropriate scientific methodology, deployed across a network structure, achieves the numbers of patients required to provide answers more rapidly than individual sites acting alone.

In April 2004, *Eunice Kennedy Shriver* National Institute of Child Health and Human Development (NICHD) published a request for

This chapter includes text excerpted from "Collaborative Pediatric Critical Care Research Network (CPCCRN)," *Eunice Kennedy Shriver* National Institute of Child Health and Human Development (NICHD), June 17, 2019.

applications to establish CPCCRN. Clinical sites and a data coordinating center (DCC) were identified through a competitive application process. The network was renewed by the same process in 2009 and 2014.

The network is a major priority of NICHD's Pediatric Trauma and Critical Illness Branch and is supported through the cooperative agreement mechanism (UG1 for clinical sites, and U01 for the DCC) in 5-year competitive cycles. The cycle includes seven clinical sites with large PICUs and a DCC.

The network's goal is to develop an infrastructure to pursue well-designed collaborative clinical trials and meaningful descriptive studies in pediatric critical care medicine. The network seeks to reduce morbidity and mortality in pediatric critical illness and injury and to provide a framework for the development of the scientific basis of pediatric critical care practice.

Topic Areas

Collaborative Pediatric Critical Care Research Network (CPCCRN) conducts controlled observations and objective evaluations of pediatric critical care practices, including management and technology methodologies, in children with complex critical illnesses and injuries. The resulting data will help to balance the prompt implementation of technologies and treatments with effective evaluation of their safety, efficacy, cost/risk/benefit ratios, and effects on long-term outcomes for children and their families.

Research Priorities

Collaborative Pediatric Critical Care Research Network research priorities reflect the following topic areas.

Bereavement and Grief

Following the death of a child in the PICU, all parents grieve. Guidance for communicating about and considering the family's grief, emotional burden, and difficult decision-making remains largely anecdotal. Some bereaved parents are incapacitated for a prolonged period, a situation known as "complicated grief." CPCCRN investigators explore whether a follow-up meeting with the child's PICU physician after a child's death helps decrease complicated grief in these bereaved parents. Completed projects in this area include:

- **Bereavement I: Parents' Perspective.** The objective of the first phase of the CPCCRN bereavement studies was to investigate parents' perspectives on the desirability, content, and conditions of a physician-parent conference after their child's death in the PICU. This study has been completed and the results have been published.

- **Bereavement II: PICU Study.** This study was designed to investigate the extent of complicated grief symptoms and associated risk factors among parents whose child died in a PICU. This study has been completed and the results have been published.

- **Bereavement III: Physicians' Perspective.** The objective of this study was to describe physicians' experiences with and attitudes toward follow-up meetings after a child's death. This study has been completed and the results have been published.

- **Bereavement IV: Pilot Study of a Framework for Physician-Parent Follow-Up Meetings.** This study was a multicenter pilot study of video-recorded physician-parent follow-up meetings using the framework developed from the previous CPCCRN bereavement studies. This study has been completed and the results have been published.

Functional Outcomes

Two continuing priorities of the CPCCRN Advisory Committee, especially the parents who serve on the committee, are to improve processes of care and concentrate on functional outcomes of children requiring critical care. To provide a mechanism for measuring the functional outcome, CPCCRN has undertaken the following studies:

- In the Development of a Quantitative Functional Status Scale (FSS) for Pediatric Patients study, CPCCRN investigators tested a functional status scoring system that had been developed with 500 initial patients and validated with a test set of 250 additional patients. The FSS resulted in a functional status outcome measure for large outcome studies that is well-defined, quantitative, rapid, reliable, minimally dependent on subjective assessments, and applicable to hospitalized pediatric patients across a wide range of ages and inpatient environments, making it well suited for large outcome studies (Pollack, et al.; 2009; PMC3191069).

- The Trichotomous Outcome Prediction in Critical Care study has enrolled more than 10,000 PICU patients and aims to predict the outcome of PICU admissions in a trichotomous manner, using the three outcomes of good survival, poor survival, and death.

Intensive Care Clinical Processes and Protocols

To improve the evidence base for pediatric critical care practices, CPCCRN investigators selected clinical processes that are either frequently used or high-risk and implemented the following studies.

- The Pediatric Intensive Care Quality of CPR (PICqCPR) study is studying whether American Heart Association (AHA) guidelines for the proper performance of cardiopulmonary resuscitation (CPR) are utilized in the hospital setting, particularly within the PICU. The goal is to identify areas for improving CPR performance in the PICU setting to improve diastolic coronary perfusion and enhance the return of spontaneous circulation.

- The Bleeding and Thrombosis During ECMO study aimed to quantify the incidence of bleeding and thrombosis adverse events in pediatric patients requiring extracorporeal membrane oxygenation (ECMO) and to explore potential associations of complications with variations in anticoagulation protocols at different hospitals. The goal of this research is to eliminate bleeding and thrombotic complications during ECMO and to improve outcomes for these patients. Study recruitment is complete, and data analyses have begun.

- The Pediatric ECMO and Cefepime (PEACE) study enhanced the knowledge base regarding the impact of ECMO on cefepime pharmacokinetics to help improve accurate dosing. This study has been completed and the results are being published.

- The Therapeutic Hypothermia After Pediatric Cardiac Arrest (THAPCA) Trials aim to determine whether therapeutic hypothermia is as successful at treating children who experience cardiac arrest as it has been in treating adults. The trials were developed in concert with the Pediatric Emergency Care Applied Research Network, funded by the Emergency Medical Services in Children program in the Maternal and Child Health Bureau at the Health Resources Services Administration. THAPCA Trials are funded by the National Heart, Lung, and Blood Institute with CPCCRN sites serving as vanguard sites for the initial phase of the trial. The trials evaluate therapeutic hypothermia's efficacy at increasing survival rates and reducing the risk of brain injury in infants and children who experience a cardiac arrest while out of the hospital (THAPCA-OH, ClinicalTrials.gov NCT00878644) or in the hospital (THAPCA-IH, ClinicalTrials.gov NCT00880087). Subject accrual is complete for THAPCA-OH, but continues for the in-hospital trial.

- The Measuring Opioid Tolerance Induced by Fentanyl (MOTIF) study to examine the clinical factors associated with increased opioid analgesia dose among mechanically ventilated children in the PICU.

- The Variations in Pediatric Severe Asthma Care study gathered information from the Pediatric Hospital Information System (PHIS) database for hospitals that participate in CPCCRN and analyzed the data to evaluate the variation of management of critical asthma. Large variations were found between sites within the network, as well as between overall CPCCRN sites and the nation.

- Critical Care for Pediatric Asthma: Wide Care Variability and Challenges for Study

- In the Critical Asthma Mortality and Morbidity Planning study, CPCCRN investigators followed up on the PHIS analysis and conducted a retrospective medical record review of all patients admitted to CPCCRN PICUs during a 5-year period. The results confirmed significant variability of asthma management between individual sites participating in CPCCRN. The results from this and the Variations in Pediatric Severe Asthma Care study indicate areas for further research concerning drug therapy and mechanical ventilation strategies for children with critical, near-fatal asthma.

- In the R21-funded Translating an Adult Ventilator Computer Protocol to Pediatric Critical Care study, CPCCRN investigators evaluated the acceptability of computer support decisions to PICU physicians and nurses.

- The CPCCRN Core Data Project obtains descriptive information about all PICU discharges from the network clinical sites, based primarily on clinical site hospital administrative databases. The data provides a valuable resource to CPCCRN by helping to stimulate research protocols, identify the potential need for non-network partners to access additional patient populations, and provide a descriptive understanding of the critically ill infants and children cared for within the network.

Infection and Sepsis

The network concentrates on several major critical illness burdens through the following studies:

- **GM-CSF for Immunomodulation Following Trauma (GIFT-1 Study).** This is being conducted as a dose-finding study to determine the lowest tolerable dose of GM-CSF that will reverse trauma-induced immune suppression in high-risk, critically injured children. The study uses highly standardized, generalizable, rapid functional immune monitoring in a CPCCRN laboratory to determine those children at the highest risk for the development of nosocomial infection. This study is currently enrolling patients.

- **GM-CSF for Reversal of immmunopAralysis in pediatriC sEpsis-induced MODS (GRACE).** This open-label interventional trial seeks to identify the optimal dose and route of delivery (intravenous or subcutaneous) for GM-CSF in children with sepsis-induced MODS, with reversal of immunoparalysis as the primary outcome variable. The study hopes to demonstrate the role of patient-specific immunomodulation in promoting resolution of organ failure and reducing mortality from pediatric sepsis-induced MODS.

- **Microbiome, Virome, and Host Responses Preceding Ventilator-Associated Pneumonia (VAP).** This is a prospective longitudinal observational study of high-risk mechanically ventilated children with systematic bacterial and viral analyses of the respiratory tract, along with a proteomic evaluation of the host response. VAP seeks to determine whether specific taxa and patterns of bacterial microbiota contribute to VAP risk and whether bacterial communities are modulated by viral infection and host immune responses to increasing the risk of VAP in critically ill children. Enrollment in this study is complete and data are being analyzed.

- **Sepsis Induced Red Cell Dysfunction (SiRD).** This study is built on the infrastructure from the PHENOMS study (discussed in the next bullet point) and is aimed at characterizing red cell dysfunction that impairs oxygen delivery in septic children.

- **Biomarker Phenotyping of Pediatric Sepsis and Multiple Organ Failure (PHENOMS) study.** This prospective observational cohort study enrolled more than 400 children with severe sepsis and tested the hypothesis that children with inflammation pathobiology phenotypes have increased mortality, predisposing genotype and environmental risk factors, and increased C-reactive protein and ferritin levels that correlate with clinical outcomes. This study has been completed and the results have been published.

- **Life After Pediatric Sepsis Evaluation (LAPSE) study.** This prospective observational study aims to describe the postsepsis illness trajectory through serial measurements of Health-Related Quality of Life, subject functional status, and examination of organ dysfunction, as well as individual and environmental characteristics that may influence these outcomes measures. Enrollment in this study is complete and the data are being analyzed.

- **The Critical Pertussis study.** The largest prospective cohort ever assembled for a scientific study of critical pertussis, aims to characterize the acute course of critical pertussis in children. The project established trans-federal partnerships as well as partnerships with non-CPCCRN sites to conduct enhanced passive and active surveillance of 33,000 PICU admissions annually. This study has been completed and the results have been published.

- **Critical Illness Stress-induced Immune Suppression (CRISIS) Prevention trial.** It evaluated "prophylaxis" strategies used to prevent stress-induced nosocomial infection and sepsis. The study was terminated for futility after enrolling 293 subjects. Despite the early termination of this study, important information was gleaned, and the results have been published.

- **Cortisol Quantification Investigation study.** It studied adrenocortical function in children with sepsis and septic shock, commonly difficult to study because total cortisol measurements include protein-bound cortisol, which is not active. This study has been completed and the results have been published.

371

Part Seven

Legal and Economic Issues at the End of Life

Chapter 41

Getting Your Affairs in Order

Preparing and Organizing Legal Documents for the Future

No one ever plans to be sick or disabled. Yet, it is this kind of planning that can make all the difference in an emergency.

What Exactly Is an "Important Paper"?

The answer to this question may be different for every family. Remember, this is a starting place. You may have other information to add. For example, if you have a pet, you will want to include the name and address of your veterinarian. Include complete information about:

Personal Records

- Full legal name
- Social Security number (SSN)
- Legal residence
- Date and place of birth
- Names and addresses of spouse and children

This chapter includes text excerpted from "Getting Your Affairs in Order," National Institute on Aging (NIA), National Institutes of Health (NIH), June 1, 2018.

- Location of birth and death certificates and certificates of marriage, divorce, citizenship, and adoption
- Employers and dates of employment
- Education and military records
- Names and phone numbers of religious contacts
- Memberships in groups and awards received
- Names and phone numbers of close friends, relatives, doctors, lawyers, and financial advisors
- Medications are taken regularly (be sure to update this regularly)
- Location of living will and other legal documents

Financial Records

- Sources of income and assets (pension from your employer, individual retirement accounts (IRAs), 401(k)s, interest, etc.)
- Social Security and Medicare/Medicaid information
- Insurance information (life, health, long-term care, home, car) with policy numbers and agents' names and phone numbers
- Names of your banks and account numbers (checking, savings, credit union)
- Investment income (stocks, bonds, property) and stockbrokers' names and phone numbers
- Copy of most recent income tax return
- Location of most up-to-date will with an original signature
- Liabilities, including property tax—what is owed, to whom, and when payments are due
- Mortgages and debts—how and when they are paid
- Location of the original deed of trust for home
- Car title and registration
- Credit and debit card names and numbers
- Location of a safe deposit box and key

Steps for Getting Your Affairs in Order

- **Put your important papers and copies of legal documents in one place.** You can set up a file, put everything in a desk or dresser drawer, or list the information and location of papers in a notebook. If your papers are in a bank safe deposit box, keep copies in a file at home. Check each year to see if there is anything new to add.

- **Tell a trusted family member or friend where you put all your important papers.** You do not need to tell this friend or family member about your personal affairs, but someone should know where you keep your papers in case of an emergency. If you do not have a relative or friend you trust, ask a lawyer to help.

- **Discuss your end-of-life preferences with your doctor.** She or he can explain what health decisions you may have to make in the future and what treatment options are available. Talking with your doctor can help ensure your wishes are honored. Discussing advance care planning decisions with your doctor is free through Medicare during your annual wellness visit. Private health insurance may also cover these discussions.

- **Give permission in advance for your doctor or lawyer to talk with your caregiver as needed.** There may be questions about your care, a bill, or a health insurance claim. Without your consent, your caregiver may not be able to get the needed information. You can give your okay in advance to Medicare, a credit card company, your bank, or your doctor. You may need to sign and return a form.

Important Legal Documents You May Need as You Age

There are many different types of legal documents that can help you plan how your affairs will be handled in the future. Many of these documents have names that sound alike, so make sure you are getting the documents you want. Also, state laws vary, so find out about the rules, requirements, and forms used in your state.

Wills and *trusts* let you name the person you want your money and property to go to after you die.

Advance directives let you make arrangements for your care if you become sick. Two common types of advance directives are:

377

- A **living will** give you a say in your healthcare if you become too sick to make your wishes known. In a living will, you can state what kind of care you do or do not want. This can make it easier for family members to make tough healthcare decisions for you.

- A **durable power of attorney** for healthcare lets you name the person you want to make medical decisions for you if you cannot make them yourself. Make sure the person you name is willing to make those decisions for you.

For legal matters, there are ways to give someone you trust the power to act in your place.

- A **general power of attorney** lets you give someone else the authority to act on your behalf, but this power will end if you are unable to make your own decisions.

- A **durable power of attorney** allows you to name someone to act on your behalf for any legal task, but it stays in place if you become unable to make your own decisions.

Help for Getting Your Legal and Financial Papers in Order

You may want to talk with a lawyer about setting up a general power of attorney, durable power of attorney, joint account, trust, or advance directive. Be sure to ask about the lawyer's fees before you make an appointment.

You should be able to find a directory of local lawyers on the Internet or at your local library, or you can contact your local bar association for lawyers in your area. Your local bar association can also help you find what free legal aid options your state has to offer. An informed family member may be able to help you manage some of these issues.

Frequently Asked Questions about Getting Your Affairs in Order

Getting your affairs in order can be difficult, but it is an important part of preparing for the future, for you and your loved ones. It is important to gather as much information as possible to help ease the process. Here are a few questions that you may have and some answers that can help.

Who Should You Choose to Be Your Healthcare Proxy?

If you decide to choose a proxy, think about people you know who share your views and values about life and medical decisions. Your proxy might be a family member, a friend, your lawyer, or someone with whom you worship.

My Aging Parents Can No Longer Make Their Own Healthcare Decisions. How Do I Decide What Type of Care Is Right for Them?

It can be overwhelming to be asked to make healthcare decisions for someone who is no longer able to make her or his own decisions. Get a better understanding of how to make healthcare decisions for a loved one, including approaches you can take, issues you might face, and questions you can ask to help you prepare.

How Do You Help Someone with Alzheimer Disease or Dementia Get Their Affairs in Order?

A complication of diseases such as Alzheimer disease is that the person may lack or gradually lose the ability to think clearly. This change affects her or his ability to participate meaningfully in decision making and makes early planning even more important.

I Am Considering Becoming an Organ Donor. Is the Process Different for Older Adults?

There are many resources for older organ donors and recipients available from the U.S. government. You may find information for potential donors and transplant recipients over age 50, including how to register to be a donor from this link: www.nia.nih.gov/health/organ-donation-transplantation-resources-older-donors-and-recipients.

I Want to Make Sure My Affairs Are in Order before I Die, but I Am Not Sure Where to Begin

The National Institute on Aging (NIA) has free publications that can help you and your loved ones discuss key issues at the end of life, including finding hospice care, what happens at the time of death, managing grief, preparing advance directives, and other information.

Chapter 42

Patients' Rights

Chapter Contents

Section 42.1—Informed Consent... 382

Section 42.2—Health Information Privacy Rights................... 389

Section 42.3—Informed Consent for Clinical Trials 391

Section 42.1

Informed Consent

This section contains text excerpted from the following sources: Text under the heading "What Is Informed Consent?" is excerpted from "Informed Consent," National Cancer Institute (NCI), June 22, 2016. Reviewed September 2019; Text under the heading "Basic Elements of Informed Consent" is excerpted from "Informed Consent," U.S. Food and Drug Administration (FDA), May 29, 2019.

What Is Informed Consent?

Informed consent is a process through which you learn details about the trial before deciding whether to take part. This includes learning about the trial's purpose and possible risks and benefits. This is a critical part of ensuring patient safety in research.

During the informed consent process, the research team, which is made up of doctors and nurses, first explains the trial to you. The team explains the trial's:

• Purpose

• Procedures

• Risks and benefits

They will also discuss your rights, including your right to:

• Make a decision about participating

• Leave the study at any time

Before agreeing to take part in a trial, you have the right to:

• Learn about all your treatment options

• Learn all that is involved in the trial, including all details about treatment, tests, and possible risks and benefits

• Discuss the trial with the principal investigator and other members of the research team

• Both hear and read the information in language you can understand

After discussing the study with you, the research team will give you an informed consent form to read. The form includes written details about the information that was discussed with you and describes the privacy of your medical records. If you agree to take part in the study, you sign the form. But, even after you sign the consent form, you can leave the study at any time.

Basic Elements of Informed Consent
Description of Clinical Investigation

A statement that the study involves research, an explanation of the purposes of the research and the expected duration of the subject's participation, a description of the procedures to be followed, and identification of any procedures which are experimental.

A clear statement that the clinical investigation involves research is important so prospective subjects are aware that, although preliminary data (bench, animal, pilot studies, literature) may exist, the purpose of their participation is primarily to contribute to research (for example, to evaluate the safety and effectiveness of the test article, to evaluate a different dose or route of administration of an approved drug, etc.) rather than to their own medical treatment.

The U.S. Food and Drug Administration (FDA) recommends that potential subjects first be informed of the care a patient would likely receive if not part of the research and then be provided with information about the research. This sequence allows potential subjects to understand how the research differs from the care they might otherwise receive. The description should identify tests or procedures that would be part of usual care that will not be performed as well as those required by the protocol that would not be part of their care outside of the research, for example, drawing blood samples for a pharmacokinetic study. The information provided should also inform prospective subjects about the potential consequences of these differences in care. Note that all experimental procedures must be identified as such. Procedures related solely to research (for example, protocol-driven versus individualized dosing, randomized assignment to treatment, blinding of subject and investigator, and receipt of placebo if the study is placebo-controlled) must be explained.

The description of the clinical investigation must describe the test article and the control. The description should include relevant information on what is known about both the test article and the control. For example, the description should indicate whether the test article is approved/cleared for marketing and describe that use. Clarification may be provided that a marketed product may be prescribed by a healthcare practitioner for the labeled indication as well as other conditions/diseases she or he determines are reasonable. The description should also provide relevant information about any control used in the study. For example, whether the control is a medically recognized standard of care or is a placebo (including an explanation of what a placebo is). The information provided about the test article and control should include appropriate and reliable information about the benefits and risks of each, to the extent such information is available.

The consent process should outline what the subject's participation will involve in order to comply with the protocol, for example, the number of clinic visits, maintenance of diaries, and medical or dietary restrictions (including the need to avoid specific medications or activities, such as participation in other clinical investigations). If describing every procedure would make the consent form too lengthy or detailed, the FDA recommends providing the general procedures in the consent form with an addendum describing all study procedures. It may be helpful to provide a chart outlining what happens at each visit to simplify the consent form and assist the subject in understanding what participation in the clinical investigation will involve. The FDA believes that removing procedural details from the consent form will reduce its length, enhance its readability, and allow its focus to be on more important content, such as the risks and anticipated benefits if any.

The informed consent process must clearly describe the expected duration of the subject's participation in the clinical investigation, which includes their active participation as well as the long-term follow-up, if appropriate. The subject must be informed of the procedures that will occur during such followup, which may be provided in a chart as described above.

Risks and Discomforts

The informed consent process must describe the reasonably foreseeable risks or discomforts to the subject. This includes risks or discomforts of tests, interventions, and procedures required by the protocol (including standard medical procedures, exams, and tests), especially those that carry a significant risk of morbidity or mortality. Possible risks or discomforts due to changes to a subject's medical care (e.g., by changing the subject's stable medication regimen or by randomizing to placebo) should also be addressed. The explanation of potential risks of the test article and control, if any, and an assessment of the likelihood of these risks occurring should be based on information presented in the protocol, investigator's brochure, package labeling, and previous research reports.

Reasonably foreseeable discomforts to the subject must also be described. For example, the consent form should disclose the severity and duration of pain from a surgical procedure or the discomfort of prolonged immobilization for magnetic resonance imaging (MRI).

All possible risks do not need to be described in detail in the informed consent form, especially if it could be overwhelming for subjects to read. Information on risks that are more likely to occur and those that are serious should be included. The discussion may include information on whether a risk is reversible and the probability of the risk-based on existing data. Information on what may be done to mitigate the most likely to occur and serious risks and discomforts should also be considered for inclusion.

The description should not understate the probability and magnitude of the reasonably foreseeable risks and discomforts. If applicable, the consent document should include a description of the reasonably foreseeable risks not only to the subject but also to "others" (for example, radiation therapy where close proximity to subjects postprocedure may be of some risk to others). When appropriate, a statement must be included that the clinical investigation may involve currently unforeseeable risks to the subject (or to the subject's embryo or fetus, if the subject is or may become pregnant).

Benefits

The description of potential benefits should be clear, balanced, and based on reliable information to the extent such information is available. This element requires a description of the potential benefits not only to the subject (for example, "This product is intended to decrease XXX; however, we cannot guarantee that you will benefit"), but also to "others" (for example, "your participation in this research may not benefit you but may benefit future patients with your disease or condition"). Overly optimistic representations of the clinical investigation may be misleading and may violate the FDA's regulations that prohibit the promotion of investigational drugs and devices. Because the purpose of the study is to determine the safety and/or effectiveness of the test article compared to the control, it is not yet known whether the test article may or may not provide a benefit.

The FDA considers payment to subjects for participation in clinical investigations to be compensated for expenses and inconveniences, not a benefit of participation in research. If payments are provided, the consent process should not identify them as benefits.

Alternative Procedures or Treatments

To enable an informed decision about taking part in a clinical investigation, consent forms must disclose appropriate alternatives to entering the clinical investigation, if any, that might be advantageous to the subject. Prospective subjects must be informed of the care they would likely receive if they choose not to participate in the research. This includes alternatives such as approved therapies for the patient's condition, other forms of therapy (e.g., surgical), and when appropriate, supportive care with no disease-directed therapy. This disclosure must include a description of the current medically recognized standard of care, particularly in studies of serious illness. Standard of care may include uses or treatment regimens that are not included in a product's approved labeling (or, in the case of a medical device cleared under the 510(k) process, in the product's statement of intended uses). The FDA believes that treatment options lacking evidence of therapeutic value do not need to be discussed.

When disclosing appropriate alternative procedures or courses of treatment, the FDA believes a description of any reasonably foreseeable risks or discomforts and potential benefits associated with these alternatives must be disclosed. Where such descriptions or disclosures can contain quantified comparative estimates of risks and benefits (e.g., from the clinical literature), they should do so. The agency does not believe that imposing such a strict requirement for every case would be realistic or appropriate. Where such well-defined estimates are not possible, the agency believes that a description of the risks and benefits will be sufficient.

It may be appropriate to refer the subject to a healthcare professional who can more fully discuss the alternatives, for example, when alternatives include various combinations of treatments, such as radiation, surgery, and chemotherapy for some cancers. This referral should be completed prior to the subject signing and dating the consent form.

The FDA recognizes that, while an individual subject may be eligible for more than one clinical investigation, that determination and the decision as to which trial would be most appropriate for a particular subject would need to be made on a case-by-case basis. The FDA believes that the discussion of other trials for which the subject may be eligible is best left to the informed consent discussion rather than the informed consent document and may need to include the subject's primary care provider.

As applicable, the informed consent process should advise that participation in one clinical investigation may preclude an individual's eligibility to participate in other clinical investigations for the same or other indications. When there are multiple clinical investigations for evaluating the treatment of a particular disease, the sequence in which a subject may participate in the protocols may be important and should be discussed with the subject and the subject's primary care provider, if appropriate.

Confidentiality

The consent process must describe the extent to which confidentiality of records identifying subjects will be maintained and should identify all entities, for example, the study sponsor, who may gain access to the records relating to the clinical investigation. The consent process must also note the possibility that the FDA may inspect records, and should not state or imply that the FDA needs permission from the subject for access to the records. Please note that under the Health Insurance Portability and Accountability Act (HIPAA) Privacy Rule, the FDA does not need permission to inspect records containing health information. The FDA may inspect study records, for example, to assess investigator compliance with the study protocol and the validity of the data reported by the sponsor.

Under the Federal Food, Drug, and Cosmetic Act (FD&C Act), the FDA may inspect and copy all records relating to the clinical investigation. The FDA generally will not copy records that include the subject's name unless there is a reason to believe the records do not represent the actual cases studied or results obtained. When the FDA requires subject names, the FDA will generally treat such information as confidential, but on rare occasions, the FDA may be required to disclose this information to third parties, for example, to a court of law. Therefore, the consent process should not promise or imply absolute confidentiality by the FDA.

Compensation and Medical Treatment in Event of Injury

For clinical investigations involving more than minimal risk, the informed consent process must describe any compensation and medical treatments available to subjects if an injury occurs. Because available compensation and medical treatments may vary depending on the medical circumstances of the individual subject or the policies of the institution, the consent process should include an explanation to subjects of where they may obtain further information. An example of an adequate statement is, "the sponsor has made plans to pay for medical costs related to research-related injuries" followed by an explanation of how to obtain further information. If no compensation is available, the consent process should include statements, such as:

- Because of hospital policy, the hospital is not able to offer financial compensation should you be injured as a result of participating in this research. However, you are not precluded from seeking to collect compensation for injury related to malpractice, fault, or blame on the part of those involved in the research, including the hospital.

- Because of hospital policy, the hospital makes no commitment to provide free medical care or payment for any unfavorable outcomes resulting from participation in this research. Medical services will be offered at the usual charge. However, you are not precluded from seeking to collect compensation for injury related to malpractice, fault, or blame on the part of those involved in the research, including the hospital.

Contacts

The consent process must provide information on how to contact an appropriate individual for pertinent questions about the clinical investigation and the subjects' rights, and whom to contact in the event that a research-related injury to the subject occurs. This information should include contact names (or offices) and their telephone numbers. The FDA recommends that the individual or office named for questions about subjects' rights not be part of the investigational team. Subjects may be hesitant to report specific concerns or identify possible problems to someone who is part of the investigational team. In addition, the consent process should include information on whom to contact and what to do in the event of an emergency, including 24-hour contact information, if appropriate.

If contact information changes during the clinical investigation, then the new contact information must be provided to the subject. This may be done through a variety of ways, for example, a card providing the relevant contact information for the clinical investigation.

Voluntary Participation

This element requires that subjects be informed that they may decline to take part in the clinical investigation or may stop participation at any time without penalty or loss of benefits to which subjects are entitled. The language that limits the subject's right to decline to participate or withdraw from the clinical investigation must not be used. If special procedures should be followed for the subject to withdraw from the clinical investigation, the consent process must outline and explain the procedures. Also, note that subjects may not withdraw data that was collected about them prior to their withdrawal.

Section 42.2

Health Information Privacy Rights

This section includes text excerpted from "Your Health Information," U.S. Department of Health and Human Services (HHS), March 14, 2013. Reviewed September 2019.

Most of us feel that our health information is private and should be protected. That is why there is a federal law that sets rules for healthcare providers and health insurance companies about who can look at and receive our health information. This law, called the "Health Insurance Portability and Accountability Act" of 1996 (HIPAA), gives you rights over your health information, including the right to get a copy of your information, make sure it is correct, and know who has seen it.

Get It

You can ask to see or get a copy of your medical record and other health information. If you want a copy, you may have to put your request in writing and pay for the cost of copying and mailing. In most cases, your copies must be given to you within 30 days.

Check It

You can ask to change any wrong information in your file or add information to your file if you think something is missing or incomplete. For example, if you and your hospital agree that your file has the wrong result for a test, the hospital must change it. Even if the hospital believes the test result is correct, you still have the right to have your disagreement noted in your file. In most cases, the file should be updated within 60 days.

Know Who Has Seen It

By law, your health information can be used and shared for specific reasons not directly related to your care, like making sure doctors give good care, making sure nursing homes are clean and safe, reporting when the flu is in your area, or reporting as required by state or federal law. In many of these cases, you can find out who has seen your health information. You can:

- **Learn how your health information is used and shared by your doctor or health insurer.** Generally, your health information cannot be used for purposes not directly related to your care without your permission. For example, your doctor cannot give it to your employer, or share it for things like marketing and advertising, without your written authorization. You probably received a notice telling you how your health information may be used on your first visit to a new healthcare provider or when you got new health insurance, but you can ask for another copy anytime.

- **Let your providers or health insurance companies know if there is information you do not want to share.** You can ask that your health information not be shared with certain people, groups, or companies. If you go to a clinic, for example, you can ask the doctor not to share your medical records with other doctors or nurses at the clinic. You can ask for other kinds of restrictions, but they do not always have to agree to do what you ask, particularly if it could affect your care. Finally, you can also ask your healthcare provider or pharmacy not to tell your health insurance company about the care you receive or drugs you take, if you pay for the care or drugs in full and the provider or pharmacy does not need to get paid by your insurance company.

• **Ask to be reached somewhere other than home.** You can make reasonable requests to be contacted at different places or in a different way. For example, you can ask to have a nurse call you at your office instead of your home or to send mail to you in an envelope instead of on a postcard.

If you think your rights are being denied or your health information is not being protected, you have the right to file a complaint with your provider, health insurer, or the U.S. Department of Health and Human Services (HHS).

Section 42.3

Informed Consent for Clinical Trials

This section includes text excerpted from "Informed Consent for Clinical Trials," U.S. Food and Drug Administration (FDA), January 4, 2018.

Informed consent involves providing a potential participant with:

• Adequate information to allow for an informed decision about participation in the clinical investigation

• Facilitating the potential participant's understanding of the information

• An appropriate amount of time to ask questions and to discuss with family and friends the research protocol and whether you should participate

• Obtaining the potential participant's voluntary agreement to participate

• Continuing to provide information as the clinical investigation progresses or as the subject or situation requires

To be effective, the process must provide sufficient opportunity for the participant to consider whether to participate. The U.S. Food and Drug Administration (FDA) considers this to include allowing sufficient time for participants to consider the information and providing time and opportunity for the participant to ask questions and have those questions answered. The investigator (or other study staff who are conducting the informed consent interview) and the participant should exchange information and discuss the contents of the informed consent document. This process must occur under circumstances that minimize the possibility of coercion or undue influence.

As new medical products are being developed, no one knows for sure how well they will work, or what risks they will find. Clinical trials are used to answer questions, such as:

- Are new medical products safe enough to outweigh the risks related to the underlying condition?

- How should the product be used? (for example, the best dose, frequency, or any special precautions necessary to avoid problems)

- How effective is the medical product at relieving symptoms, treating or curing a condition

The main purpose of clinical trials is to "study" new medical products in people. It is important for people who are considering participation in a clinical trial to understand their role, as a "subject of research" and not as a patient.

While research subjects may get personal treatment benefit from participating in a clinical trial, they must understand that they:

- May not benefit from the clinical trial

- May be exposed to unknown risks

- Are entering into a study that may be very different from the standard medical practices that they currently know

To make an informed decision about whether to participate or not in a clinical trial, people need to be informed about:

- What will be done to them

- How the protocol (plan of research) works

- What risks or discomforts they may experience

- Participation is a voluntary decision on their part

This information is provided to potential participants through the informed consent process. Informed consent means that the purpose of the research is explained to them, including what their role would be and how the trial will work.

A central part of the informed consent process is the informed consent document. The FDA does not dictate the specific language required for the informed consent document but does require certain basic elements of consent to be included.

Before enrolling in a clinical trial, the following information must be given to each potential research subject:

- A statement explaining that the study involves research

- An explanation of the purposes of the research

- The expected length of time for participation

- A description of all the procedures that will be completed during enrollment on the clinical trial

- Information about all experimental procedures the will be completed during the clinical trial

- A description of any predictable risks

- Any possible discomforts (e.g., injections, frequency of blood test, etc.) that could occur as a result of the research

- Any possible benefits that may be expected from the research

- Information about any alternative procedures or treatment (if any) that might benefit the research subject

- A statement describing:

  - The confidentiality of information collected during the clinical trial

  - How records that identify the subject will be kept

  - The possibility that the FDA may inspect the records

- For research involving more than minimal risk information including:

  - An explanation as to whether any compensation or medical treatments are available if an injury occurs

  - What they consist of

  - Where more information may be found

  - Questions about the research

- Research subjects' rights

- Injury-related to the clinical trial

- Research subject participation is voluntary

- Research subjects have the right to refuse treatment and will not be losing any benefits for which they are entitled

- Research subjects may choose to stop participation in the clinical trial at any time without losing benefits for which they are entitled

When Appropriate, one or more of the following elements of information must also be provided in the informed consent document:

- A statement that the research treatment or procedure may involve unexpected risks (to the subject, unborn baby, if the subject is or may become pregnant)

- Any reasons why the research subject participation may be ended by the clinical trial investigator (e.g., failing to follow the requirements of the trial or changes in lab values that fall outside of the clinical trial limits)

- Added costs to the research subject that may result from participating in the trial

- The consequence of leaving a trial before it is completed (e.g., if the research and procedures require a slow and organized end of participation)

- A statement that important findings discovered during the clinical trial will be provided to the research subject

- The approximate number of research subjects that will be enrolled in the study

A potential research subject must have an opportunity to:

- Read the consent document

- Ask questions about anything they do not understand

Usually, if one is considering participating in a clinical trial, she or he may take the consent document home to discuss with family, friend or advocate.

An investigator should only get consent from a potential research subject if:

- Enough time was given to the research subject to consider whether or not to participate

- The investigator has not persuaded or influenced the potential research subject

The information must be in the language that is understandable to the research subject.

Informed consent may not include language that:

- The research subject is made to ignore or appear to ignore any of the research subject's legal rights

- Releases or appears to release the investigator, the sponsor, the institution, or its agents from their liability for negligence

Participating in clinical trials is voluntary. You have the right not to participate, or to end your participation in the clinical trial at any time.

Chapter 43

Advance Directives

What kind of medical care would you want if you were too ill or hurt to express your wishes? Advance directives are legal documents that allow you to spell out your decisions about end-of-life care ahead of time. They give you a way to tell your wishes to family, friends, and healthcare professionals and to avoid confusion later on.

A living will tells which treatments you want if you are dying or permanently unconscious. You can accept or refuse medical care. You might want to include instructions on:

- The use of dialysis and breathing machines

- If you want to be resuscitated if your breathing or heartbeat stops

- Tube feeding

- Organ or tissue donation

A durable power of attorney for healthcare is a document that names your healthcare proxy. Your proxy is someone you trust to make health decisions for you if you are unable to do so.

This chapter contains text excerpted from the following sources: Text in this chapter begins with the excerpts from "Advance Directives," MedlinePlus, National Institutes of Health (NIH), November 14, 2016. Reviewed September 2019; Text under the heading "Advance Care Planning: Healthcare Directives" is excerpted from "Advance Care Planning: Healthcare Directives," National Institute on Aging (NIA), National Institutes of Health (NIH), January 15, 2018.

Advance Care Planning: Healthcare Directives

Advance care planning is not just about old age. At any age, a medical crisis could leave you too ill to make your own healthcare decisions. Even if you are not sick now, planning for healthcare in the future is an important step toward making sure you get the medical care you would want, if you are unable to speak for yourself and doctors and family members are making the decisions for you.

Many Americans face questions about medical treatment but may not be capable of making those decisions, for example, in an emergency or at the end of life. This article will explain the types of decisions that may need to be made in such cases and questions you can think about now so you are prepared later. It can help you think about who you would want to make decisions for you if you cannot make them yourself. It will also discuss ways you can share your wishes with others. Knowing who you want to make decisions on your behalf and how you would decide might take some of the burden off family and friends.

What Is Advance Care Planning?

Advance care planning involves learning about the types of decisions that might need to be made, considering those decisions ahead of time, and then letting others know—both your family and your healthcare providers—about your preferences. These preferences are often put into an advance directive, a legal document that goes into effect only if you are incapacitated and unable to speak for yourself. This could be the result of disease or severe injury—no matter how old you are. It helps others know what type of medical care you want.

An advance directive also allows you to express your values and desires related to end-of-life care. You might think of it as a living document—one that you can adjust as your situation changes because of new information or a change in your health.

Advance Care Planning Decisions

Sometimes decisions must be made about the use of emergency treatments to keep you alive. Doctors can use several artificial or mechanical ways to try to do this. Decisions that might come up at this time relate to:

- Cardiopulmonary resuscitation (CPR)
- Ventilator use

- Artificial nutrition (tube feeding) and artificial hydration (IV, or intravenous, fluids)

- Comfort care

What Is Cardiopulmonary Resuscitation?

Cardiopulmonary resuscitation might restore your heartbeat if your heart stops or is in a life-threatening abnormal rhythm. It involves repeatedly pushing on the chest with force while putting air into the lungs. This force has to be quite strong, and sometimes ribs are broken or a lung collapses. Electric shocks, known as "defibrillation," and medicines might also be used as part of the process. The heart of a young, otherwise healthy person might resume beating normally after CPR. Often, CPR does not succeed in older adults who have multiple chronic illnesses or who are already frail.

Using a Ventilator as Emergency Treatment

Ventilators are machines that help you breathe. A tube connected to the ventilator is put through the throat into the trachea (windpipe) so the machine can force air into the lungs. Putting the tube down the throat is called "intubation." Because the tube is uncomfortable, medicines are often used to keep you sedated while on a ventilator. If you are expected to remain on a ventilator for a long time, a doctor may perform a tracheotomy or "trach" (rhymes with "make"). During this bedside surgery, the tube is inserted directly into the trachea through a hole in the neck. For long-term help with breathing, a trach is more comfortable, and sedation is not needed. People using such a breathing tube are not able to speak without special help because exhaled air does not go past their vocal cords.

Using Artificial Nutrition and Hydration Near the End of Life

If you are not able to eat, you may be fed through a feeding tube that is threaded through the nose down to your stomach. If tube feeding is still needed for an extended period, a feeding tube may be surgically inserted directly into your stomach. Hand-feeding (sometimes called "assisted oral feeding") is an alternative to tube feeding. This approach may have fewer risks, especially for people with dementia.

If you are not able to drink, you may be provided with IV fluids. These are delivered through a thin plastic tube inserted into a vein.

Artificial nutrition and hydration can be helpful if you are recovering from an illness. However, studies have shown that artificial nutrition toward the end of life does not meaningfully prolong life. Artificial nutrition and hydration may also be harmful if the dying body cannot use nutrition properly.

What Is Comfort Care at the End of Life?

Comfort care is anything that can be done to soothe you and relieve suffering while staying in line with your wishes. Comfort care includes managing shortness of breath; limiting medical testing; providing spiritual and emotional counseling; and giving medication for pain, anxiety, nausea, or constipation.

Getting Started with Advance Care Planning

Start by thinking about what kind of treatment you do or do not want in a medical emergency. It might help to talk with your doctor about how your current health conditions might influence your health in the future. For example, what decisions would you or your family face if your high blood pressure leads to a stroke? You can ask your doctor to help you understand and think through your choices before you put them in writing. Discussing advance care planning decisions with your doctor is free through Medicare during your annual wellness visit. Private health insurance may also cover these discussions.

If you do not have any medical issues now, your family medical history might be a clue to help you think about the future. Talk with your doctor about decisions that might come up if you develop health problems similar to those of other family members.

In considering treatment decisions, your personal values are key. Is your main desire to have the most days of life? Or, would your focus be on the quality of life (QOL), as you see it? What if an illness leaves you paralyzed or in a permanent coma and you need to be on a ventilator? Would you want that?

What makes life meaningful to you? If your heart stops or you have trouble breathing, would you want to undergo life-saving measures if it meant that, in the future, you could be well enough to spend time with your family? Would you be content if the emergency leaves you simply able to spend your days listening to books on tape or gazing out the window?

But, there are many other scenarios. Here are a few. What would you decide?

- If a stroke leaves you unable to move and then your heart stops, would you want CPR? What if you were also mentally impaired by a stroke—does your decision change?

- What if you are in pain at the end of life? Do you want medication to treat the pain, even if it will make you more drowsy and lethargic?

- What if you are permanently unconscious and then develop pneumonia? Would you want antibiotics and be placed on a ventilator?

For some people, staying alive as long as medically possible, or long enough to see an important event like a grandchild's wedding, is the most important thing. An advance directive can help to make that possible. Others have a clear idea about when they would no longer want to prolong their life. An advance directive can help with that, too.

Your decisions about how to handle any of these situations could be different at age 40 than at age 85. Or, they could be different if you have an incurable condition as opposed to being generally healthy. An advance directive allows you to provide instructions for these types of situations and then to change the instructions as you get older or if your viewpoint changes.

Making Your Advance Care Wishes Known

There are two main elements in an advance directive—a living will and a durable power of attorney for healthcare. There are also other documents that can supplement your advance directive. You can choose which documents to create, depending on how you want decisions to be made.

- **Living will.** A living will is a written document that helps you tell doctors how you want to be treated if you are dying or permanently unconscious and cannot make your own decisions about emergency treatment. In a living will, you can say which of the procedures described in the decisions that could come up the section you would want, which ones you would not want, and under which conditions each of your choices applies.

- **Durable power of attorney for healthcare.** A durable power of attorney for healthcare is a legal document naming a healthcare proxy, someone to make medical decisions for you at times when you are unable to do so. Your proxy, also known as a "representative," "surrogate," or "agent," should be familiar with your values and wishes. This means that she or he will be able to decide as you would when treatment decisions need to be made. A proxy can be chosen in addition to or instead of a living will. Having a healthcare proxy helps you plan for situations that cannot be foreseen, like a serious auto accident. Some people are reluctant to put specific health decisions in writing. For them, naming a healthcare agent might be a good approach, especially if there is someone they feel comfortable talking with about their values and preferences. A named proxy can evaluate each situation or treatment option independently.

• **Other advance care planning documents.** You might also want to prepare documents to express your wishes about a single medical issue or something not already covered in your advance directive. A living will usually covers only the specific life-sustaining treatments discussed earlier. You might want to give your healthcare proxy specific instructions about other issues, such as blood transfusion or kidney dialysis. This is especially important if your doctor suggests that, given your health condition, such treatments might be needed in the future.

Medical issues that might arise at the end of life include:

• A **do not resuscitate (DNR)** order tells medical staff in a hospital or nursing facility that you do not want them to try to return your heart to a normal rhythm if it stops or is beating unsustainably using CPR or other life-support measures. Sometimes this document is referred to as a do not attempt resuscitation (DNAR) or an AND (allow natural death) order. Even though a living will might say CPR is not wanted, it is helpful to have a DNR order as part of your medical file if you go to a hospital. Posting a DNR next to your bed might avoid confusion in an emergency situation. Without a DNR order, medical staff will make every effort to restore your breathing and the normal rhythm of your heart. A similar document called a "do not intubate" (DNI) order, tells medical staff in a hospital or nursing facility that you do not want to be put on a breathing machine.

• A **nonhospital DNR** order will alert emergency medical personnel to your wishes regarding measures to restore your heartbeat or breathing if you are not in the hospital.

* **Organ and tissue donation** allow organs or body parts from a generally healthy person who has died to be transplanted into people who need them. Commonly, the heart, lungs, pancreas, kidneys, corneas, liver, and skin are donated. There is no age limit for organ and tissue donation. You can carry a donation card in your wallet. Some states allow you to add this decision to your driver's license. Some people also include organ donation in their advance care planning documents. At the time of death, family members may be asked about organ donation. If those close to you, especially your proxy, know how you feel about organ donation, they will be ready to respond. There is no cost to the donor's family for this gift of life. If the person has requested a DNR order but wants to donate organs, she or he might have to indicate that the desire to donate supersedes the DNR. That is because it might be necessary to use machines to keep the heart beating until the medical staff is ready to remove the donated organs.

* **Physician Orders for Life-Sustaining Treatment (POLST) and Medical Orders for Life-Sustaining Treatment (MOLST)** forms provide guidance about your medical care preferences in the form of a doctor's orders. Typically you create a POLST or MOLST when you are near the end of life or critically ill and know the specific decisions that might need to be made on your behalf. These forms serve as a medical order in addition to your advance directive. They make it possible for you to provide guidance that healthcare professionals can act on immediately in an emergency.

A number of states use POLST and MOLST forms, which are filled out by your doctor or sometimes by a nurse practitioner or physician's assistant. The doctor fills out a POLST or MOLST after discussing your wishes with you and your family. Once signed by your doctor, this form has the same authority as any other medical order. Check with your state department of health to find out if these forms are available where you live.

How to Choose Your Healthcare Proxy

If you decide to choose a proxy, think about people you know who share your views and values about life and medical decisions. Your proxy might be a family member, a friend, your lawyer, or someone in your social or spiritual community. It is a good idea to also name an alternate proxy. It is especially important to have a detailed living will if you choose not to name a proxy.

You can decide how much authority your proxy has over your medical care—whether she or he is entitled to make a wide range of decisions or only a few specific ones. Try not to include guidelines that make it impossible for the proxy to fulfill her or his duties. For example, it is probably not unusual for someone to say in conversation, "I do not want to go to a nursing home," but think carefully about whether you want a restriction like that in your advance directive. Sometimes, for financial or medical reasons, that may be the best choice for you.

Of course, check with those you choose as your healthcare proxy and alternate before you name them officially. Make sure they are comfortable with this responsibility.

Making Your Healthcare Directives Official

Once you have talked with your doctor and have an idea of the types of decisions that could come up in the future and whom you would like as a proxy, if you want one at all, the next step is to fill out the legal forms detailing your wishes. A lawyer can help but is not required. If you decide to use a lawyer, do not depend on her or him to help you understand different medical treatments. Start the planning process by talking with your doctor.

Many states have their own advance directive forms. Your local Area Agency on Aging (AAA) can help you locate the right forms. You can find your area agency phone number by calling the Eldercare Locator toll-free at 800-677-1116 or by visiting www.eldercare.acl.gov.

Some states require your advance directive to be witnessed; a few require your signature to be notarized. A notary is a person licensed by the state to witness signatures. You might find a notary at your bank, post office, or local library, or call your insurance agent. Some notaries charge a fee.

Some states have registries that can store your advance directive for quick access by healthcare providers, your proxy, and anyone else to whom you have given permission. Private firms also will store your advance directive. There may be a fee for storing your form in a registry. If you store your advance directive in a registry and later make changes, you must replace the original with the updated version in the registry.

Some people spend a lot of time in more than one state—for example, visiting children and grandchildren. If that is your situation,

consider preparing an advance directive using forms for each state—
and keep a copy in each place, too.

What to Do after You Set Up Your Advance Directive

Give copies of your advance directive to your healthcare proxy and
alternate proxy. Give your doctor a copy of your medical records. Tell
close family members and friends where you keep a copy. If you have to
go to the hospital, give the staff there a copy to include in your records.
Because you might change your advance directive in the future, it is
a good idea to keep track of who receives a copy.

Review your advance care planning decisions from time to time—for
example, every 10 years, if not more often. You might want to revise
your preferences for care if your situation or your health changes. Or,
you might want to make adjustments if you receive a serious diagnosis; if you get married, separated, or divorced; if your spouse dies; or
if something happens to your proxy or alternate. If your preferences
change, you will want to make sure your doctor, proxy, and family
know about them.

Be Prepared

What happens if you have no advance directive or have made no
plans and you become unable to speak for yourself? In such cases, the
state where you live will assign someone to make medical decisions
on your behalf. This will probably be your spouse, your parents if
they are available, or your children if they are adults. If you have no
family members, the state will choose someone to represent your best
interests.

Always remember: an advance directive is only used if you are
in danger of dying and need certain emergency or special measures
to keep you alive, but you are not able to make those decisions on
your own. An advance directive allows you to make your wishes about
medical treatment known.

It is difficult to predict the future with certainty. You may never
face a medical situation where you are unable to speak for yourself
and make your wishes known. But, having an advance directive may
give you and those close to you some peace of mind.

Chapter 44

Financial Assistance for Long-Term or End-of-Life Care

Many older adults and caregivers worry about the cost of medical care. These expenses can use up a significant part of monthly income, even for families who thought they had saved enough.

How people pay for long-term care—whether delivered at home or in a hospital, assisted living facility, or nursing home—depends on their financial situation and the kinds of services they use. Often, they rely on a variety of payment sources, including personal funds, government programs, and private financing options.

Personal Funds

At first, many older adults pay for care in part with their own money. They may use personal savings, a pension or other retirement fund, income from stocks and bonds, or proceeds from the sale of a home.

Much home-based care is paid for using personal funds ("out of pocket"). Initially, family and friends often provide personal care and other services, such as transportation, for free. But as a person's needs increase, paid services may be needed.

This chapter includes text excerpted from "Paying for Care," National Institute on Aging (NIA), National Institutes of Health (NIH), May 1, 2017.

Many older adults also pay out-of-pocket to participate in adult day service programs, meals, and other community-based services provided by local governments and nonprofit groups. These services help them remain in their homes.

Professional care given in assisted living facilities and continuing care retirement communities are almost always paid for out of pocket, though, in some states, Medicaid may pay some costs for people who meet financial and health requirements.

Government Programs

Older adults may be eligible for some government healthcare benefits. Caregivers can help by learning more about possible sources of financial help and assisting older adults in applying for aid as appropriate. The Internet can be a helpful tool in this search.

Several federal and state programs provide help with healthcare-related costs. The Centers for Medicare and Medicaid Services (CMS) offers several programs. Over time, the benefits and eligibility requirements of these programs can change, and some benefits differ from state to state. Check with CMS or the individual programs directly for the most recent information.

Medicare

Medicare is a federal government health insurance program that pays some medical costs for people age 65 and older, and for all people with late-stage kidney failure. It also pays some medical costs for those who have gotten Social Security Disability Income (SSDI) for 24 months. It does not cover ongoing personal care at home, assisted living, or long-term care. Here are brief descriptions of what Medicare will pay for:

Medicare Part A

- Hospital costs after you pay a certain amount called the "deductible"

- Short stay in a nursing home to get care for a hospital-related medical condition

- Hospice care in the last 6 months of life

Medicare Part B

- Part of the costs for doctor's services, outpatient care, and other medical services that Part A does not cover

- Some preventive services, such as flu shots and diabetes screening

Medicare Part D

- Some medication costs

Call Medicare at 800-633-4227, toll-free TTY: 877-486-2048 to find out what costs Medicare will cover for your situation, or visit www. medicare.gov for more information.

Medicaid

Some people may qualify for Medicaid, a combined federal and state program for low-income people and families. This program covers the costs of medical care and some types of long-term care for people who have limited income and meet other eligibility requirements. Who is eligible and what services are covered vary from state to state.

Program of All-Inclusive Care for the Elderly

Some States have PACE, Program of All-Inclusive Care for the Elderly, a Medicare program that provides care and services to people who otherwise would need care in a nursing home. PACE covers medical, social service, and long-term-care costs for frail people. It may pay for some or all of the long-term care needs of a person with Alzheimer disease (AD). PACE permits most people who qualify to continue living at home instead of moving to a long-term-care facility. You will need to find out if the person who needs care qualifies for PACE. There may be a monthly charge. PACE is available only in certain states and locations within those states.

State Health Insurance Assistance Program

The State Health Insurance Assistance Program (SHIP) is a national program offered in each state that provides counseling and assistance to people and their families on Medicare, Medicaid, and Medicare supplemental insurance (Medigap) matters.

U.S. Department of Veterans Affairs

The U.S. Department of Veterans Affairs (VA) may provide long-term care or at-home care for some veterans. If your family member or relative is eligible for veterans' benefits, check with the VA or get in touch with the VA medical center nearest you. There could be a waiting list for VA nursing homes.

Social Security Disability Income

This type of Social Security is for people younger than age 65 who are disabled according to the Social Security Administration's (SSAs) definition.

For a person to qualify for SSDI, she or he must be able to show that:

• The person is unable to work

• The condition will last at least a year

• The condition is expected to result in death

Social Security has "compassionate allowances" to help people with AD, other dementias, and certain other serious medical conditions get disability benefits more quickly.

National Council on Aging

The National Council on Aging (NCOA), a private group, has a free service called "BenefitsCheckUp®." This service can help you find federal and state benefit programs that may help your family. After providing some general information about the person who needs care, you can see a list of possible benefits programs to explore. These programs can help pay for prescription drugs, heating bills, housing, meal programs, and legal services. You do not have to give a name, address, or social security number to use this service.

Private Financing Options

In addition to personal and government funds, there are several private payment options, including long-term-care insurance, reverse mortgages, certain life insurance policies, annuities, and trusts. Which option is best for a person depends on many factors, including the person's age, health status, personal finances, and risk of needing care.

Long-Term-Care Insurance

Long-term-care insurance covers many types of long-term care and benefits, including palliative and hospice care. The exact coverage depends on the type of policy you buy and what services are covered. You can purchase nursing home-only coverage or a comprehensive policy that includes both home care and facility care.

Many companies sell long-term-care insurance. It is a good idea to shop around and compare policies. The cost of a policy is based on the type and amount of services, how old you are when you buy the policy, and any optional benefits you choose.

Buying long-term-care insurance can be a good choice for younger, relatively healthy people at low risk of needing long-term care. Costs go up for people who are older, have health problems, or want more benefits. Someone who is in poor health or already receiving end-of-life care services may not qualify for long-term-care insurance.

Reverse Mortgages

A reverse mortgage is a special type of home loan that lets a homeowner convert part of the ownership value in her or his home into cash. Unlike a traditional home loan, no repayment is required until the borrower sells the home, no longer uses it as a main residence or dies.

There are no income or medical requirements to get a reverse mortgage, but you must be age 62 or older. The loan amount is tax-free and can be used for any expense, including long-term care. However, if you have an existing mortgage or other debt against your home, you must use the funds to pay off those debts first.

Life Insurance

Some life insurance policies can help pay for long-term care. Some policies offer a combination product of both life insurance and long-term-care insurance.

Policies with an "accelerated death benefit" provide tax-free cash advances while you are still alive. The advance is subtracted from the amount your beneficiaries (the people who get the insurance proceeds) will receive when you die.

You can get an accelerated death benefit if you live permanently in a nursing home, need long-term care for an extended time, are terminally ill, or have a life-threatening diagnosis, such as acquired immunodeficiency syndrome (AIDS). Check your life insurance policy to see exactly what it covers.

You may be able to raise cash by selling your life insurance policy for its current value. This option, known as a "life settlement," is usually available only to people age 70 and older. The proceeds are taxable and can be used for any reason, including paying for long-term care.

A similar arrangement called a "viatical settlement," allows a terminally ill person to sell her or his life insurance policy to an insurance company for a percentage of the death benefit on the policy. This option is typically used by people who are expected to live two years or less. A viatical settlement provides immediate cash, but it can be hard to get.

Annuities

You may choose to enter into an annuity contract with an insurance company to help pay for long-term-care services. In exchange for a single payment or a series of payments, the insurance company will send you an annuity, which is a series of regular payments over a specified period of time. There are two types of annuities: immediate annuities and deferred long-term-care annuities.

Trusts

A trust is a legal entity that allows a person to transfer assets to another person, called the "trustee." Once the trust is established, the trustee manages and controls the assets for the person or another beneficiary. You may choose to use a trust to provide flexible control of assets for an older adult or a person with a disability, which could include yourself or your spouse. Two types of trusts can help pay for long-term-care services: charitable remainder trusts and Medicaid disability trusts.

Chapter 45

Social Security Benefits

How Social Security Can Help You When a Family Member Dies

You should let Social Security know as soon as possible when a person in your family dies. Usually, the funeral director will report the person's death to Social Security. You will need to give the deceased's Social Security number (SSN) to the funeral director so they can make the report.

Some of the deceased's family members may be able to receive Social Security benefits if the deceased person worked long enough in jobs insured under Social Security to qualify for benefits. Contact Social Security as soon as you can to make sure the family gets all the benefits they are entitled to. Please read the following information carefully to learn what benefits may be available.

- The U.S Social Security Administration (SSA) can pay a one-time payment of $255 to the surviving spouse if they were

---

This chapter contains text excerpted from the following sources: Text under the heading "How Social Security Can Help You When a Family Member Dies" is excerpted from "How Social Security Can Help You When a Family Member Dies," U.S. Social Security Administration (SSA), May, 2017; Text under the heading "Social Security Lump-Sum Death Payment" is excerpted from "Social Security Lump Sum Death Payment," Benefits.gov, USA.gov, October 9, 2014. Reviewed September 2019; Text beginning with the heading "What Is a Burial Fund?" is excerpted from "Spotlight on Burial Funds—2019 Edition," U.S. Social Security Administration (SSA), February 1, 2001. Reviewed September 2019.

living with the deceased. If living apart and eligible for certain Social Security benefits on the deceased's record, the surviving spouse may still be able to get this one-time payment. If there is no surviving spouse, a child who is eligible for benefits on the deceased's record in the month of death can get this payment.

- Certain family members may be eligible to receive monthly benefits, including:

  - A widow or widower age 60 or older (age 50 or older if disabled)

  - A widow or widower any age caring for the deceased's child who is under age 16 or disabled

  - An unmarried child of the deceased who is:

    - Younger than age 18 (or up to age 19 if they are a full-time student in an elementary or secondary school)

    - Age 18 or older with a disability that began before age 22

  - A stepchild, grandchild, stepgrandchild, or adopted child under certain circumstances

  - Parents, age 62 or older, who were dependent on the deceased for at least half of their support

  - A surviving divorced spouse, under certain circumstances

If the deceased was receiving Social Security benefits, you must return the benefit received for the month of death or any later months. For example, if the person dies in July, you must return the benefit paid in August. If received by direct deposit, contact the bank or other financial institution and ask them to return any funds received for the month of death or later. If paid by check, do not cash any checks received for the month the person dies or later. Return the checks to Social Security as soon as possible.

However, eligible family members may be able to receive death benefits for the month the beneficiary died.

Contacting Social Security

The most convenient way to contact the SSA anytime, anywhere is to visit www.socialsecurity.gov. There, you can: apply for benefits; open a my Social Security account, which you can use to review your Social Security Statement, verify your earnings, print a benefit verification letter, change your direct deposit information, request a replacement Medicare card, and get a replacement SSA-1099/1042S; obtain valuable information; find publications; get answers to frequently asked questions; and much more.

If you do not have access to the Internet, the SSA offers many automated services by telephone, 24 hours a day, 7 days a week. Call the SSA at toll-free at 800-772-1213 or at our TTY number, 800-325-0778, if you are deaf or hard of hearing.

Social Security Lump-Sum Death Payment
Program Description

The Social Security Lump-Sum Death Payment (LSDP) Benefits are a federally funded program managed by the SSA. A surviving spouse or child may receive a special lump-sum death payment of $255 if they meet certain requirements.

Program Requirements

To qualify for this benefit the surviving spouse must be living in the same household with the worker when she or he died. If they were living apart, the surviving spouse can still receive the lump-sum if, during the month the worker died, she or he:

- Was already receiving benefits on the worker's record, or
- Became eligible for benefits upon the worker's death

If there is no eligible surviving spouse, the lump-sum can be paid to the worker's child (or children) if, during the month the worker died, the child:

- Was already receiving benefits on the worker's record, or
- Became eligible for benefits upon the worker's death

What Is a Burial Fund?

A burial fund is a money set aside to pay for burial expenses. For example, this money can be in a bank account, other financial instruments, or a prepaid burial arrangement.

Some states allow an individual to prepay for their burial by contracting with a funeral home and paying in advance for their funeral. You should discuss this with your local social security office.

415

Does a Burial Fund Count as a Resource for Supplemental Security Income?

Generally, you and your spouse can set aside up to $1,500 each to pay for burial expenses. In most cases, this money will not count as a resource for Supplemental Security Income (SSI).

If you (and your spouse) own life insurance policies or have other burial arrangements in addition to your $1,500 burial funds, some of the money in the burial fund may count toward the resource limit of $2,000 for an individual or $3,000 for a couple.

Does Interest Earned on Your (And Your Spouse's) Burial Fund Count as a Resource or Income for Supplemental Security Income?

No. Interest earned on your (or your spouse's) burial fund that you leave in the fund does not count as a resource or income for SSI and does not affect your SSI benefit.

How Can You Set Up a Burial Fund?

Any account you set up must clearly show that the money is set aside to pay burial expenses. You can do this either by:

- Titling the account as a burial fund

- Signing a statement saying

  - How much has been set aside for burial expenses

  - For whose burial, the money is set aside

  - How the money has been set aside

  - The date you first considered the money set aside for burial expenses

What Happens When You Spend Money from a Burial Fund

If you spend any money from a burial fund on items unrelated to burial expenses, there may be a penalty.

Chapter 46

Duties of a Personal Representative (Executor)

Personal Representative

Generally, a Health Insurance Portability and Accountability Act (HIPAA)—covered healthcare provider or health plan must allow your personal representative to inspect and receive a copy of protected health information about you that they maintain.

Naming a Personal Representative

Your personal representative can be named several ways; state law may affect this process. If a person can make healthcare decisions for you using a healthcare power of attorney, the person is your personal representative.

This chapter contains text excerpted from the following sources: Text under the heading "Personal Representatives" is excerpted from "Personal Representatives," U.S. Department of Health and Human Services (HHS), June 16, 2017; Text under the heading "Who Must Be Recognized as the Individual's Personal Representative" is excerpted from "Guidance: Personal Representatives," U.S. Department of Health and Human Services (HHS), September 19, 2013. Reviewed September 2019; Text beginning with the heading "General Responsibilities of an Estate Administrator" is excerpted from "Deceased Taxpayers—Understanding the General Duties as an Estate Administrator," Internal Revenue Service (IRS), July 16, 2019.

Children

The personal representative of a minor child is usually the child's parent or legal guardian. State laws may affect guardianship.

In cases where a custody decree exists, the personal representative is the parent(s) who can make healthcare decisions for the child under the custody decree.

Deceased Persons

When an individual dies, the personal representative for the deceased is the executor or administrator of the deceased individual's estate or the person who is legally authorized by a court or by state law to act on the behalf of the deceased individual or her or his estate.

Exceptions

A provider or plan may choose not to treat a person as your personal representative if the provider or plan reasonably believes that the person might endanger you in situations of domestic violence, abuse, or neglect.

Who Must Be Recognized as the Individual's Personal Representative

The following chart displays who must be recognized as the personal representative for a category of individuals:

Table 46.1. Personal Representative

If the Individual Is:	The Personal Representative Is:
An Adult or An Emancipated Minor	A person with legal authority to make healthcare decisions on behalf of the individual *Examples*: Healthcare power of attorney Court-appointed legal guardian A general power of attorney or durable power of attorney that includes the power to make healthcare decisions
An Unemancipated Minor	A parent, guardian, or other person acting in loco parentis with legal authority to make healthcare decisions on behalf of the minor child

Table 46.1. Continued

If the Individual Is:	The Personal Representative Is:
Deceased	A person with legal authority to act on behalf of the decedent or the estate (not restricted to persons with authority to make healthcare decisions) *Examples*: Executor or administrator of the estate Next of kin or other family members (if relevant law provides authority)

General Responsibilities of an Estate Administrator

When a person dies a probate proceeding may be opened. Depending on state law, probate will generally open within 30 to 90 days from the date of death.

One of the probate court's first actions will be to appoint a legal representative for the decedent and her or his estate. The legal representative may be a surviving spouse, another family member, the executor named in the decedent's will or an attorney. The term "estate administrator" to is used to refer to the appointed legal representative. The probate court will issue letters testamentary authorizing the estate administrator of the decedent to act on the decedent's behalf. You will need the letters testamentary to handle the decedent's tax and other matters.

In general, the responsibilities of an estate administrator are to collect all the decedent's assets, pay creditors and distribute the remaining assets to heirs or other beneficiaries. As an estate administrator, your first responsibility is to provide the probate court with an accounting of the decedent's assets and debts. Some assets may need to be appraised to determine their value. All debts will need to be verified and creditor claims against the estate must be filed.

Tax Responsibilities of an Estate Administrator

A decedent and their estate are separate taxable entities. So, if filing requirements are satisfied, an estate administrator may have to file different types of tax returns.

First, an estate administrator may need to file income tax returns for the decedent (Form 1040 series). The decedent's Form 1040 for the year of death, and for any preceding years for which a return was not filed, is required if the decedent's income for those years was above the filing requirement.

Second, an estate administrator may need to file income tax returns for the estate (Form 1041). To file this return you will need to get a tax identification number for the estate (called an "employer identification number" or "EIN"). An estate is required to file an income tax return if assets of the estate generate more than $600 in annual income. For example, if the decedent had interest, dividend or rental income when alive, then after death that income becomes income of the estate and may trigger the requirement to file an estate income tax return.

If the estate operates a business after the owner's death, the estate administrator is required to secure a new employer identification number for the business, report wages or income under the new EIN and pay any taxes that are due.

Some or all of the information you need to file income tax returns for the decedent and their estate may be in the decedent's personal records. The Internal Revenue Service (IRS) can help by providing copies of income documents (Forms W-2 or 1099 for example) and copies of filed tax returns or transcripts of tax accounts.

Third, an estate administrator may need to file an estate tax return (Form 706). The estate tax is a tax on the transfer of assets from the decedent to their heirs and beneficiaries. In general, the estate tax only applies to large estates.

Chapter 47

Understanding the Family and Medical Leave Act (FMLA)

Family and Medical Leave Act

The Family and Medical Leave Act (FMLA) entitles eligible employees of covered employers to take unpaid, job-protected leave for specified family and medical reasons with continuation of group health insurance coverage under the same terms and conditions as if the employee had not taken leave. Eligible employees are entitled to:

- Twelve work weeks of leave in a 12-month period for:

  - The birth of a child and to care for the newborn child within one year of birth

  - The placement with the employee of a child for adoption or foster care and to care for the newly placed child within one year of placement

This chapter contains text excerpted from the following sources: Text under the heading "Family and Medical Leave Act" is excerpted from "Family and Medical Leave Act," U.S. Department of Labor (DOL), August 5, 2019; Text under the heading "Rules and General Information about the Family and Medical Leave Act" is excerpted from "Wage and Hour Division— The Family and Medical Leave Act," U.S. Department of Labor (DOL), February 5, 2013. Reviewed September 2019.

- To care for the employee's spouse, child, or parent who has a serious health condition

- A serious health condition that makes the employee unable to perform the essential functions of her or his job

- Any qualifying exigency arising out of the fact that the employee's spouse, son, daughter, or parent is a covered military member on "covered active duty"

- Twenty-six workweeks of leave during a single 12 month period to care for a covered servicemember with a serious injury or illness if the eligible employee is the service member's spouse, son, daughter, parent, or next of kin (military caregiver leave).

Rules and General Information about the Family and Medical Leave Act

The following paragraphs provide general information about which employers are covered by the FMLA, when employees are eligible and entitled to take FMLA leave, and what rules apply when employees take FMLA leave.

Covered Employers

The FMLA only applies to employers that meet certain criteria. A covered employer is a:

- Private-sector employer, with 50 or more employees in 20 or more workweeks in the current or preceding calendar year, including a joint employer or successor in interest to a covered employer

- Public agency, including a local, state, or federal government agency, regardless of the number of employees it employs

- Public or private elementary or secondary school, regardless of the number of employees it employs

Eligible Employees

Only eligible employees are entitled to take FMLA leave. An eligible employee is one who:

- Works for a covered employer

- Has worked for the employer for at least 12 months

- Has at least 1,250 hours of service for the employer during the 12 month period immediately preceding the leave*

- Works at a location where the employer has at least 50 employees within 75 miles

Special hours of service eligibility requirements apply to airline flight crew employees.

The 12-months of employment do not have to be consecutive. That means any time previously worked for the same employer (including seasonal work) could, in most cases, be used to meet the 12-month requirement. If the employee has a break in service that lasted seven years or more, the time worked prior to the break will not count unless the break is due to service covered by the Uniformed Services Employment and Reemployment Rights Act (USERRA), or there is a written agreement, including a collective bargaining agreement, outlining the employer's intention to rehire the employee after the break-in service.

Leave Entitlement

Eligible employees may take up to 12 workweeks of leave in a 12-month period for one or more of the following reasons:

- The birth of a son or daughter or placement of a son or daughter with the employee for adoption or foster care

- To care for a spouse, son, daughter, or parent who has a serious health condition

- For a serious health condition that makes the employee unable to perform the essential functions of her or his job

- For any qualifying exigency arising out of the fact that a spouse, son, daughter, or parent is a military member on covered active duty or call to covered active duty status

An eligible employee may also take up to 26 workweeks of leave during a "single 12-month period" to care for a covered servicemember with a serious injury or illness, when the employee is the spouse, son, daughter, parent, or next of kin of the servicemember. The "single 12-month period" for military caregiver leave is different from the 12-month period used for other FMLA leave reasons.

Under some circumstances, employees may take FMLA leave on an intermittent or reduced schedule basis. That means an employee may take leave in separate blocks of time or by reducing the time she or he works each day or week for a single qualifying reason. When leave is needed for planned medical treatment, the employee must make a reasonable effort to schedule treatment so as not to unduly disrupt the employer's operations. If FMLA leave is for the birth, adoption, or foster placement of a child, use of intermittent or reduced schedule leave requires the employer's approval.

Under certain conditions, employees may choose, or employers may require employees, to "substitute" (run concurrently) accrued paid leave, such as sick or vacation leave, to cover some or all of the FMLA leave period. An employee's ability to substitute accrued paid leave is determined by the terms and conditions of the employer's normal leave policy.

Notice

Employees must comply with their employer's usual and customary requirements for requesting leave and provide enough information for their employer to reasonably determine whether the FMLA may apply to the leave request. Employees generally must request leave 30 days in advance when the need for leave is foreseeable. When the need for leave is foreseeable less than 30 days in advance or is unforeseeable, employees must provide notice as soon as possible and practicable under the circumstances.

When an employee seeks leave for an FMLA-qualifying reason for the first time, the employee need not expressly assert FMLA rights or even mention the FMLA. If an employee later requests additional leave for the same qualifying condition, the employee must specifically reference either the qualifying reason for leave or the need for FMLA leave.

Covered employers must:

1. Post a notice explaining rights and responsibilities under the FMLA (and may be subject to a civil money penalty of up to $110 for willful failure to post)

2. Include information about the FMLA in their employee handbooks or provide information to new employees upon hire

3. When an employee requests FMLA leave or the employer acquires knowledge that leave may be for an FMLA-qualifying reason, provide the employee with notice concerning her or his eligibility for FMLA leave and her or his rights and responsibilities under the FMLA

4. Notify employees whether leave is designated as FMLA leave and the amount of leave that will be deducted from the employee's FMLA entitlement

Certification

When an employee requests FMLA leave due to her or his own serious health condition or a covered family member's serious health condition, the employer may require certification in support of the leave from a healthcare provider. An employer may also require second or third medical opinions (at the employer's expense) and periodic recertification of a serious health condition.

Job Restoration and Health Benefits

Upon return from FMLA leave, an employee must be restored to her or his original job or to an equivalent job with equivalent pay, benefits, and other terms and conditions of employment. An employee's use of FMLA leave cannot be counted against the employee under a "no-fault" attendance policy. Employers are also required to continue group health insurance coverage for an employee on FMLA leave under the same terms and conditions as if the employee had not taken leave.

Other Provisions

Special rules apply to employees of local education agencies. Generally, these rules apply to intermittent or reduced schedule FMLA leave or the taking of FMLA leave near the end of a school term.

Salaried executive, administrative, and professional employees of covered employers who meet the Fair Labor Standards Act (FLSA) criteria for exemption from minimum wage and overtime under the FLSA regulations, 29 CFR Part 541, do not lose their FLSA-exempt status by using any unpaid FMLA leave. This special exception to the "salary basis" requirements for FLSA's exemption extends only to an eligible employee's use of FMLA leave.

Enforcement

It is unlawful for any employer to interfere with, restrain, or deny the exercise of or the attempt to exercise any right provided by the FMLA. It is also unlawful for an employer to discharge or discriminate against any individual for opposing any practice, or because of involvement in any proceeding, related to the FMLA. The Wage and Hour Division is responsible for administering and enforcing the FMLA for most employees. Most federal and certain congressional employees are also covered by the law but are subject to the jurisdiction of the U.S. Office of Personnel Management (OPM) or Congress. If you believe that your rights under the FMLA have been violated, you may file a complaint with the Wage and Hour Division (WHD) or file a private lawsuit against your employer in court.

Part Eight

Final Arrangements

Chapter 48

Funeral Services: An Overview

When a loved one dies, grieving family members and friends often are confronted with dozens of decisions about the funeral—all of which must be made quickly and often under great emotional duress. What kind of funeral should it be? What funeral provider should you use? Should you bury or cremate the body, or donate it to science? What are you legally required to buy? What about the availability of environmentally friendly or "green" burials? What other arrangements should you plan? And, practically, how much is it all going to cost?

Funeral Planning Tips

Many funeral providers offer various "packages" of goods and services for different kinds of funerals. When you arrange for a funeral, you have the right to buy goods and services separately. That is, you do not have to accept a package that may include items you do not want. Here are some tips to help you shop for funeral services:

- **Shop around in advance.** Compare prices from at least two funeral homes. Remember that you can supply your own casket or urn.

This chapter includes text excerpted from "Shopping for Funeral Services," Federal Trade Commission (FTC), July 2012. Reviewed September 2019.

- **Ask for a price list.** The law requires funeral homes to give you written price lists for products and services.

- **Resist pressure to buy goods and services you do not really want or need.**

- **Avoid emotional overspending.** It is not necessary to have the fanciest casket or the most elaborate funeral to properly honor a loved one.

- **Recognize your rights.** Laws regarding funerals and burials vary from state to state. It is a smart move to know which goods or services the law requires you to purchase and which are optional.

- **Apply the same smart shopping techniques you use for other major purchases.** You can cut costs by limiting the viewing to one day or one hour before the funeral, and by dressing your loved one in a favorite outfit instead of costly burial clothing.

- **Shop in advance.** It allows you to comparison shop without time constraints, creates an opportunity for family discussion, and lifts some of the burden from your family.

The Federal Trade Commission Funeral Rule and Rights

The Funeral Rule, enforced by the Federal Trade Commission (FTC), makes it possible for you to choose only those goods and services you want or need and to pay only for those you select, whether you are making arrangements when a death occurs or in advance. The Rule allows you to compare prices among funeral homes, and makes it possible for you to select the funeral arrangements you want at the home you use. (The Rule does not apply to third-party sellers, such as casket and monument dealers, or cemeteries that lack an on-site funeral home.)

The FTC Funeral Rule gives you the right to:

- **Buy only the funeral arrangements you want.** You have the right to buy separate goods (such as caskets) and services (such as embalming or a memorial service). You do not have to accept a package that may include items you do not want.

- **Get price information on the telephone.** Funeral directors must give you price information on the telephone if you ask for it. You do not have to give them your name, address, or telephone number first. Although they are not required to do so, many funeral homes mail their price lists, and some post them online.

- **Get a written, itemized price list when you visit a funeral home.** The funeral home must give you a General Price List (GPL) that is yours to keep. It lists all the items and services the home offers, and the cost of each one.

- **See a written casket price list before you see the actual caskets.** Sometimes, detailed casket price information is included on the funeral home's GPL. More often, though, it is provided on a separate casket price list. Get the price information before you see the caskets, so that you can ask about lower-priced products that may not be on display.

- **See a written outer burial container price list.** Outer burial containers are not required by state law anywhere in the United States, but many cemeteries require them to prevent the grave from caving in. If the funeral home sells containers, but does not list their prices on the GPL, you have the right to look at a separate container price list before you see the containers. If you do not see the lower-priced containers listed, ask about them.

- **Receive a written statement after you decide what you want, and before you pay.** It should show exactly what you are buying and the cost of each item. The funeral home must give you a statement listing every good and service you have selected, the price of each, and the total cost immediately after you make the arrangements.

- **Get an explanation in the written statement from the funeral home that describes any legal cemetery or crematory requirement** that requires you to buy any funeral goods or services.

- **Use an "alternative container" instead of a casket for cremation.** No state or local law requires the use of a casket for cremation. A funeral home that offers cremations must tell you that alternative containers are available, and must make them available. They might be made of unfinished wood, pressed wood, fiberboard, or cardboard.

- **Provide the funeral home with a casket or urn you buy elsewhere.** The funeral provider cannot refuse to handle a

431

casket or urn you bought online, at a local casket store, or somewhere else—or charge you a fee to do it. The funeral home cannot require you to be there when the casket or urn is delivered to them.

* **Make funeral arrangements without embalming.** No state law requires routine embalming for every death. Some states require embalming or refrigeration if the body is not buried or cremated within a certain time; some states do not require it at all. In most cases, refrigeration is an acceptable alternative. In addition, you may choose services such as direct cremation and immediate burial, which do not require any form of preservation. Many funeral homes have a policy requiring embalming if the body is to be publicly viewed, but this is not required by law in most states. Ask if the funeral home offers private family viewing without embalming. If some form of preservation is a practical necessity, ask the funeral home if refrigeration is available.

Funeral Costs and Pricing Checklist

Funeral costs include basic services fee for the funeral director and staff, charges for other services and merchandise, and cash advances. Make copies of the checklist and use it when you shop with several funeral homes to compare costs.

Funeral Fees
Basic Fees

The Funeral Rule allows funeral providers to charge a basic services fee that customers have to pay. The basic services fee includes services that are common to all funerals, regardless of the specific arrangement. These include funeral planning, securing the necessary permits and copies of death certificates, preparing the notices, sheltering the remains, and coordinating the arrangements with the cemetery, crematory or other third parties. The fee does not include charges for optional services or merchandise.

Merchandise Fees

Charges for other services and merchandise, include costs for optional goods and services such as transporting the remains; embalming and other preparation; use of the funeral home for the viewing, ceremony or memorial service; use of equipment and staff for a grave-side service; use of a hearse or limousine; a casket, outer burial container or alternate container; and cremation or interment.

Cash Advances

Cash advances are fees charged by the funeral home for goods and services it buys from outside vendors on your behalf, including flowers, obituary notices, pallbearers, officiating clergy, and organists and soloists. Some funeral providers charge you their cost for the items they buy on your behalf. Others add a service fee to the cost. The Funeral Rule requires those who charge an extra fee to disclose that fact in writing, although it does not require them to specify the amount of their markup. The Rule also requires funeral providers to tell you if there are refunds, discounts, or rebates from the supplier on any cash advance item.

Calculating the Actual Cost of a Funeral

The funeral provider must give you an itemized statement of the total cost of the funeral goods and services you have selected when you are making the arrangements. If the funeral provider does not know the cost of the cash advance items at the time, she or he is required to give you a written "good faith estimate." This statement also must disclose any legal cemetery or crematory requirements that you purchase specific funeral goods or services.

The Funeral Rule does not require any specific format for this information. Funeral providers may include it in any document they give you at the end of your discussion about funeral arrangements.

Services and Products
Embalming

Many funeral homes require embalming if you are planning a viewing or visitation. But, embalming generally is not necessary or legally required if the body is buried or cremated shortly after death. Eliminating this service can save you hundreds of dollars. Under the Funeral Rule, a funeral provider:

- May not provide embalming services without permission

- May not falsely state that embalming is required by law

- Must disclose in writing that embalming is not required by law, except in certain special cases

433

- May not charge a fee for unauthorized embalming unless embalming is required by state law

- Must disclose in writing that you usually have the right to choose a disposition, such as direct cremation or immediate burial, that does not require embalming if you do not want this service

- Must disclose in writing that some funeral arrangements, such as a funeral with viewing, may make embalming a practical necessity and, if so, a required purchase

Caskets

For a "traditional" full-service funeral:
A casket often is the single most expensive item you will buy if you plan a "traditional" full-service funeral. Caskets vary widely in style and price and are sold primarily for their visual appeal. Typically, they are constructed of metal, wood, fiberboard, fiberglass or plastic. Although an average casket costs slightly more than $2,000, some mahogany, bronze or copper caskets sell for as much as $10,000.

When you visit a funeral home or showroom to shop for a casket, the Funeral Rule requires the funeral director to show you a list of caskets the company sells, with descriptions and prices, before showing you the caskets. Industry studies show that the average casket shopper buys one of the first three models shown, generally the middle-priced of the three.

So it is in the seller's best interest to start out by showing you higher-end models. If you have not seen some of the lower-priced models on the price list, ask to see them—but do not be surprised if they are not prominently displayed, or not on display at all.

Traditionally, caskets have been sold only by funeral homes. But more and more, showrooms and websites operated by "third-party" dealers are selling caskets. You can buy a casket from one of these dealers and have it shipped directly to the funeral home. The Funeral Rule requires funeral homes to agree to use a casket you bought elsewhere, and does not allow them to charge you a fee for using it.

No matter where or when you are buying a casket, it is important to remember that its purpose is to provide a dignified way to move the body before burial or cremation. No casket, regardless of its qualities or cost, will preserve a body forever. Metal caskets frequently are described as "gasketed," "protective" or "sealer" caskets. These terms mean that the casket has a rubber gasket or some other feature that is designed to delay the penetration of water into the casket and prevent rust. The Funeral Rule forbids claims that these features help preserve the remains indefinitely because they do not. They just add to the cost of the casket.

Most metal caskets are made from rolled steel of varying gauges—the lower the gauge, the thicker the steel. Some metal caskets come with a warranty for longevity. Wooden caskets generally are not gasketed and do not have a warranty for longevity. They can be hardwood, such as mahogany, walnut, cherry or oak, or softwood such as pine. Pine caskets are a less expensive option, but funeral homes rarely display them. Manufacturers of both wooden and metal caskets usually offer warranties for workmanship and materials.

For Cremation

Many families that choose to have their loved ones cremated rent a casket from the funeral home for the visitation and funeral, eliminating the cost of buying a casket. If you opt for visitation and cremation, ask about the rental option. For those who choose a direct cremation without a viewing or other ceremony where the body is present, the funeral provider must offer an inexpensive unfinished wood box or alternative container, a nonmetal enclosure—pressboard, cardboard or canvas—that is cremated with the body.

Under the Funeral Rule, funeral directors who offer direct cremations:

- May not tell you that state or local law requires a casket for direct cremations, because none do

- Must disclose in writing your right to buy an unfinished wood box or an alternative container for a direct cremation, and

- Must make an unfinished wood box or other alternative container available for direct cremations

Burial Vaults or Grave Liners

Burial vaults or grave liners, also known as "burial containers," are commonly used in "traditional" full-service funerals. The vault or liner is placed in the ground before burial, and the casket is lowered into it at the burial. The purpose is to prevent the ground from caving in as the casket deteriorates over time. A grave liner is made of reinforced concrete and will satisfy any cemetery requirement. Grave liners cover only the top and sides of the casket. A burial vault is more substantial and expensive than a grave liner. It surrounds the casket in concrete or another material and may be sold with a warranty of protective strength.

State laws do not require a vault or liner, and funeral providers may not tell you otherwise. However, keep in mind that many cemeteries require some type of outer burial container to prevent the grave from sinking in the future. Neither grave liners nor burial vaults are designed to prevent the eventual decomposition of human remains. It is illegal for funeral providers to claim that a vault will keep water, dirt, or other debris from penetrating into the casket if that is not true.

Before showing you any outer burial containers, a funeral provider is required to give you a list of prices and descriptions. It may be less expensive to buy an outer burial container from a third-party dealer than from a funeral home or cemetery. Compare prices from several sources before you select a model.

Preservation Processes and Products

As far back as the ancient Egyptians, people have used oils, herbs and special body preparations to help preserve the bodies of their dead. Yet, no process or products have been devised to preserve a body in the grave indefinitely. The Funeral Rule prohibits funeral providers from telling you that it can be done. For example, funeral providers may not claim that either embalming or a particular type of casket will preserve the body of the deceased for an unlimited time.

Funeral Pricing Checklist

Make copies of this checklist and check with several funeral homes to compare costs.

"Simple" disposition of the remains:

Immediate burial _____

Immediate cremation _____

If the cremation process is extra, how much is it? _____

Donation of the body to a medical school or hospital _____

"Traditional," full-service burial or cremation:

Basic services fee for the funeral director and staff _____

Pickup of body _____

Embalming _____

Other preparation of body _____

Least expensive casket _____

Description, including model # _____

Outer burial container (vault) _____
Description _____
Visitation/viewing—staff and facilities _____
Funeral or memorial service—staff and facilities _____
Graveside service, including staff and equipment _____
Hearse _____
Other vehicles _____
Total _____
Other services:
Forwarding body to another funeral home _____
Receiving body from another funeral home _____
Cemetery/mausoleum costs:
Cost of lot or crypt (if you do not already own one) _____
Perpetual care _____
Opening and closing the grave or crypt _____
Grave liner, if required _____
Marker/monument (including setup) _____

Types of Funerals

Every family is different, and not everyone wants the same type of funeral. Funeral practices are influenced by religious and cultural traditions, costs, and personal preferences. These factors help determine whether the funeral will be elaborate or simple, public or private, religious or secular, and where it will be held. They also influence whether the body will be present at the funeral, if there will be a viewing or visitation, and if so, whether the casket will be open or closed, and whether the remains will be buried or cremated.

"Traditional" Full-Service Funeral

This type of funeral, often referred to by funeral providers as a "traditional" funeral, usually includes a viewing or visitation and formal funeral service, use of a hearse to transport the body to the funeral site and cemetery, and burial, entombment, or cremation of the remains.

It is generally the most expensive type of funeral. In addition to the funeral home's basic services fee, costs often include embalming and dressing the body; rental of the funeral home for the viewing or service; and use of vehicles to transport the family if they do not use their own. The costs of a casket, cemetery plot or crypt and other funeral goods and services also must be factored in.

437

Direct Burial

The body is buried shortly after death, usually in a simple container. No viewing or visitation is involved, so no embalming is necessary. A memorial service may be held at the graveside or later. Direct burial usually costs less than the "traditional" full-service funeral. Costs include the funeral home's basic services fee, as well as transportation and care of the body, the purchase of a casket or burial container and a cemetery plot or crypt. If the family chooses to be at the cemetery for the burial, the funeral home often charges an additional fee for a graveside service.

Direct Cremation

The body is cremated shortly after death, without embalming. The cremated remains are placed in an urn or other container. No viewing or visitation is involved. The remains can be kept in the home, buried, or placed in a crypt or niche in a cemetery, or buried or scattered in a favorite spot. Direct cremation usually costs less than the "traditional" full-service funeral. Costs include the funeral home's basic services fee, as well as transportation and care of the body. A crematory fee may be included or, if the funeral home does not own the crematory, the fee may be added on. There also will be a charge for an urn or other container. The cost of a cemetery plot or crypt is included only if the remains are buried or entombed.

Funeral providers who offer direct cremations also must offer to provide an alternative container that can be used in place of a casket.

Choosing a Funeral Provider

Many people do not realize that in most states they are not legally required to use a funeral home to plan and conduct a funeral. However, because they have little experience with the many details and legal requirements involved and may be emotionally distraught when it is time to make the plans, they find the services of a professional funeral home to be a comfort.

People often select a funeral home or cemetery because it is close to home, has served the family in the past, or has been recommended by someone they trust. But, limiting the search to just one funeral home may risk paying more than necessary for the funeral or narrowing their choice of goods and services.

Comparison Shopping for a Funeral Home / Provider

Comparison shopping does not have to be difficult, especially if it is done before the need for a funeral arises. Thinking ahead can help you make informed and thoughtful decisions about funeral arrangements. It allows you to choose the specific items you want and need, and to compare the prices several funeral providers charge.

If you visit a funeral home in person, the funeral provider is required by law to give you a General Price List (GPL) itemizing the cost of the items and services the home offers. If the GPL does not include specific prices of caskets or outer burial containers, the law requires the funeral director to show you the price lists for those items before showing you the items.

Sometimes it is more convenient and less stressful to "price shop" funeral homes by telephone. The Funeral Rule requires funeral directors to provide price information on the phone to any caller who asks for it. In addition, many funeral homes are happy to mail you their price lists, although that is not required by law.

When comparing prices, be sure to consider the total cost of all the items together, in addition to the costs of single items. Every funeral home should have price lists that include all the items essential for the different types of arrangements it offers. Many funeral homes offer package funerals that may cost less than buying individual items or services. Offering package funerals is permitted by law, as long as an itemized price list also is provided. But, you cannot accurately compare total costs unless you use the price lists.

In addition, there is a trend toward consolidation in the funeral home industry, and many neighborhood funeral homes may appear to be locally owned when in fact, they are owned by a national corporation. If this issue is important to you, you may want to ask if the funeral home is independent and locally owned.

439

Chapter 49

Planning a Funeral

Choosing a Funeral Provider

Many people do not realize that in most states they are not legally required to use a funeral home to plan and conduct a funeral. However, because they have little experience with the many details and legal requirements involved and may be emotionally distraught when it is time to make the plans, they find the services of a professional funeral home to be a comfort.

People often select a funeral home or cemetery because it is close to home, has served the family in the past, or has been recommended by someone they trust. But, limiting the search to just one funeral home may risk paying more than necessary for the funeral or narrowing their choice of goods and services.

Comparison Shopping for a Funeral Home/Provider

Comparison shopping does not have to be difficult, especially if it is done before the need for a funeral arises. Thinking ahead can help you make informed and thoughtful decisions about funeral arrangements.

This chapter contains text excerpted from the following sources: Text under the heading "Choosing a Funeral Provider" is excerpted from "Choosing a Funeral Provider," Federal Trade Commission (FTC), July 2012. Reviewed September 2019; Text under the heading "Planning Your Own Funeral" is excerpted from "Planning Your Own Funeral," Federal Trade Commission (FTC), July 2012. Reviewed September 2019.

It allows you to choose the specific items you want and need, and to compare the prices several funeral providers charge.

If you visit a funeral home in person, the funeral provider is required by law to give you a general price list (GPL) itemizing the cost of the items and services the home offers. If the GPL does not include specific prices of caskets or outer burial containers, the law requires the funeral director to show you the price lists for those items before showing you the items.

Sometimes it is more convenient and less stressful to "price shop" funeral homes by telephone. The Funeral Rule requires funeral directors to provide price information on the phone to any caller who asks for it. In addition, many funeral homes are happy to mail you their price lists, although that is not required by law.

When comparing prices, be sure to consider the total cost of all the items together, in addition to the costs of single items. Every funeral home should have price lists that include all the items essential for the different types of arrangements it offers. Many funeral homes offer package funerals that may cost less than buying individual items or services. Offering package funerals is permitted by law, as long as an itemized price list also is provided. But, you cannot accurately compare total costs unless you use the price lists.

In addition, there is a trend toward consolidation in the funeral home industry, and many neighborhood funeral homes may appear to be locally owned when in fact, they are owned by a national corporation. If this issue is important to you, you may want to ask if the funeral home is independent and locally owned.

Planning Your Own Funeral

To help relieve their families, an increasing number of people are planning their own funerals, designating their funeral preferences, and sometimes paying for them in advance. They see funeral planning as an extension of will and estate planning.

Funeral Planning Tips

Thinking ahead can help you make informed and thoughtful decisions about funeral arrangements. It allows you to choose the specific items you want and need, and compare the prices offered by several funeral providers. It also spares your survivors the stress of making these decisions under the pressure of time and strong emotions. You can make arrangements directly with a funeral establishment.

An important consideration when planning a funeral preneed is where the remains will be buried, entombed, or scattered. In the short time between the death and burial of a loved one, many family members find themselves rushing to buy a cemetery plot or grave—often without careful thought or a personal visit to the site. That is why it is in the family's best interest to buy cemetery plots before you need them.

You may wish to make decisions about your arrangements in advance, but not pay for them in advance. Keep in mind that over time, prices may go up and businesses may close or change ownership. However, in some areas with increased competition, prices may go down over time. It is a good idea to review and revise your decisions every few years, and to make sure your family is aware of your wishes.

Put your preferences in writing, give copies to family members and your attorney, and keep a copy in a handy place. Do not designate your preferences in your will, because a will often is not found or read until after the funeral. And avoid putting the only copy of your preferences in a safe deposit box. That is because your family may have to make arrangements on a weekend or holiday, before the box can be opened.

Prepaying

Millions of Americans have entered into contracts to arrange their funerals and prepay some or all of the expenses involved. Laws of individual states govern the prepayment of funeral goods and services; various states have laws to help ensure that these advance payments are available to pay for the funeral products and services when they are needed. But, protections vary widely from state to state, and some state laws offer little or no effective protection. Some state laws require the funeral home or cemetery to place a percentage of the prepayment in a state-regulated trust or to purchase a life insurance policy with death benefits assigned to the funeral home or cemetery.

If you are thinking about prepaying for funeral goods and services, it is important to consider these issues before putting down any money:

- What are you are paying for? Are you buying only merchandise, such as a casket and vault, or are you purchasing funeral services as well?

- What happens to the money you have prepaid? States have different requirements for handling funds paid for prearranged funeral services.

- What happens to the interest income on money that is prepaid and put into a trust account?

- Are you protected if the firm you dealt with goes out of business?

- Can you cancel the contract and get a full refund if you change your mind?

- What happens if you move to a different area or die while away from home? Some prepaid funeral plans can be transferred, but often at an added cost.

Be sure to tell your family about the plans you have made; let them know where the documents are filed. If your family is not aware that you have made plans, your wishes may not be carried out. And if family members do not know that you have prepaid the funeral costs, they could end up paying for the same arrangements. You may wish to consult an attorney on the best way to ensure that your wishes are followed.

Chapter 50

Military Funeral Planning

How Do I Plan a Burial for a Veteran or Other Family Member?

If you have a preneed decision letter confirming that the veteran, spouse, or dependent family members can be buried in a Veterans Affairs (VA) national cemetery:

- To start, you may want to choose a funeral director to help you plan the burial. Then either you or the funeral director can call the National Cemetery Scheduling Office at 800-535-1117 to request a burial.

- You need not do anything else except prepare yourself and your family for the funeral.

- Find out what to expect at a military funeral or memorial service.

If you do not have a preneed decision letter:

- To start, you may want to choose a funeral director to help you plan the burial. Then either you or the funeral director will need to take these 3 steps to apply for a burial.

This chapter includes text excerpted from "Plan a Burial for a Veteran, Spouse, or Dependent Family Member," U.S. Department of Veterans Affairs (VA), November 7, 2018.

Gather Documents to Identify the Veteran, Spouse, or Dependent Family Member

- You will need:

    - The Certificate of Release or Discharge from Active Duty (DD214) or other discharge documents of the veteran or service member whose military service will be used to determine eligibility for burial in a VA national cemetery. If you cannot find these documents, please ask for our help to get them.

- Find out which discharge documents we accept along with your application.

- You will also need the information listed below about the veteran, service member, or dependent family member:

    - Name

    - Gender

    - Social Security number or military service number (veteran ID)

    - Date of birth

    - Relationship to the service member or veteran whose military service will be used to decide the eligibility

    - Marital status

    - Date of death (and zip code and county at the time of death)

- You will need information about the next-of-kin (the closest living relative of the veteran, service member, or dependent family member), including the person's:

    - Name

    - Relationship to the veteran, service member, or dependent family member

    - Social Security number

    - Phone number

    - Address

- You may also need more information in certain cases:

    - If the person was married, you will also need the surviving spouse's status as a veteran, service member, or family member.

446

- If the person has any children with disabilities, you will need the status and detailed information for any disabled children who may be buried in the future in a national cemetery.

- If the person's spouse passed away previously and was buried in a VA national cemetery, you will need the full name of the spouse as well as the cemetery section and site number where they are buried.

Decide on the Burial Details and Gather All Related Information

- You will need to provide the following information:
  - The cemetery where you would prefer the veteran, spouse, dependent family member be buried
    - Find a VA national cemetery.
    - Find a state veterans cemetery.
  - The type of burial you would like for the person (casket or cremation) and the size of the casket or cremation urn
  - The type of gravesite memorial you would like. This may be a headstone, grave marker, niche cover, or medallion.

- If the person is a veteran or reservist, you will also need to confirm whether you would like burial honors or memorial items, such as:
  - A burial flag
  - A Presidential Memorial Certificate (PMC)
  - Other possible military honors beyond the playing of "taps" and flag folding and presentation
  - Gravesite memorials and burial honors

Contact the National Cemetery Scheduling Office

The funeral director you have chosen can help you with these steps too:

- For burial in a national cemetery, fax any discharge papers to the National Cemetery Scheduling Office at 866-900-6417. Or scan and e-mail the papers to NCA.Scheduling@va.gov with the person's name you are requesting burial benefits for in the subject line.

- Then call 800-535-1117 to confirm the burial application.

447

Can I Get Information about the Burial at Sea Program?

- If you have questions about the Burial at Sea (BAS) program, please contact the United States Navy Mortuary Affairs office toll-free at 866-787-0081, Monday through Friday, 8:30 a.m. to 5:00 p.m. (ET).

Can I Get Help Paying for Burial Costs?

- If you are the spouse of record (the legally recognized spouse) or a designated (legally chosen) family member of a veteran, you may be able to get financial help for burial and funeral costs.

Chapter 51

Cremation Explained

Cremation is the second most common method of disposition in the United States and gains in popularity every year. It is the most common option in Japan, India, England, and other countries. For most individuals, the selection of cremation is motivated by religious practice and cultural preference. Additional reasons for choosing cremation over traditional burial are lower cost, ease, more options for memorialization, and environmental considerations.

Cremation is generally less expensive than a traditional burial. The National Funeral Directors Association (NFDA) estimates the average cost of a traditional funeral to be $4,782. This price does not include cemetery charges, such as grave space, burial fees, monuments, or markers, which generally add thousands to the final cost. Cremations, on the other hand, the average $1,200. Although cremation is typically perceived to be a wholly different form of service, most firms provide elements from the traditional burial service. For example, memorial services, where the body is viewed in a rented casket, are becoming more common. Based on information from the Cremation Association of North America, the actual cremation service itself costs approximately $110 to $150. Also, many people who preplan and prepay for their funeral services select cremation.

Some consumers perceive cremation to be simpler than traditional burial, and this simplicity appeals to a growing share of the market.

This chapter includes text excerpted from "Economic Impact Analysis of Proposed Other Solid Waste Incinerator Regulation," U.S. Environmental Protection Agency (EPA), September 1999. Reviewed October 2019.

There are fewer transactions in the cremation process; a consumer may only have to interact with a funeral director rather than with cemeteries and other agencies. Funeral directors provide most legal services as part of the cremation fee, reducing the burden on families.

Cremation also provides more options for memorialization. Remains can be stored in an urn at someone's home, a cemetery, or mausoleum. The remains can also be scattered at sea, in a park, or at other locations (where permitted by law) per the deceased's request. Finally, cremated remains do not require the relatively large burial plots needed for traditional burial, reducing the cemeteries' pressure on the environment. When cremains are buried, the individual plot is significantly smaller than the plot used in traditional burial.

Cremation Process

There are many different classes of crematories; however, the technology employed by each unit-type is essentially the same. The technology has changed little in the latter half of the twentieth century. Crematories vary according to size and capacity. They are typically large, front-loaded units that weigh between 20,000 and 30,000 pounds. Combustion takes place in two chambers at an average rate of 100 to 150 pounds per hour. Crematories use natural gas, electricity, and propane to power the unit and facilitate the combustion process.

The primary chamber is preheated to about 1292°F. The body is enclosed in a combustible container, such as a wooden coffin, cardboard box, or plastic bag. The operator increases the temperature to between 1652 and 2012°F. The body stays in the primary chamber between 1 and 2 hours, depending on body size. After the remains have cooled, the bones are crushed to the consistency of coarse sand. Finally, all the remains are placed in either an urn or a plastic bag for transport.

Chapter 52

Medical
Certification of Death

Death Certification

A death certificate is a permanent record of an individual's death. One purpose of the death certificate is to obtain a simple description of the sequence or process leading to death rather than a record describing all medical conditions present at death.

Causes of death on the death certificate represent a medical opinion that might vary among individual physicians. In signing the death certificate, the physician, medical examiner, or coroner certifies that, in her or his medical opinion, the individual died from the reported causes of death. The certifier's opinion and confidence in that opinion are based upon her or his training, knowledge of medicine, available medical history, symptoms, diagnostic tests, and available autopsy results for the decedent. Even if extensive information is available to the certifier, causes of death may be difficult to determine, so the certifier may indicate uncertainty by qualifying the causes on the death certificate.

Cause-of-death data are important for surveillance, research, design of public health and medical interventions, and funding decisions for

This chapter includes text excerpted from "Possible Solutions to Common Problems in Death Certification," Centers for Disease Control and Prevention (CDC), November 6, 2015. Reviewed September 2019.

research and development. While the death certificate is a legal document used for legal, family, and insurance purposes, it may not be the only record used, because, in some cases, the death certificate may only be admissible as proof of death.

Difficulties in Death Certification
Uncertainty

Often several acceptable ways of writing a cause-of-death statement exist. Optimally, a certifier will be able to provide a simple description of the process leading to death that is etiologically clear and to be confident that this is the correct sequence of causes. However, realistically, description of the process is sometimes difficult because the certifier is not certain.

In this case, the certifier should think through the causes about which he/she is confident and what possible etiologies could have resulted in these conditions. The certifier should select the causes that are suspected to have been involved and use words such as "probable" or "presumed" to indicate that the description provided is not completely certain. If the initiating condition reported on the death certificate could have arisen from a preexisting condition but the certifier cannot determine the etiology, he/she should state that the etiology is unknown, undetermined, or unspecified, so it is clear that the certifier did not have enough information to provide even a qualified etiology.

The Elderly

When preparing a cause-of-death statement for an elderly decedent, the causes should present a clear and distinct etiological sequence, if possible. Causes of death on the death certificate should not include terms, such as "senescence," "old age," "infirmity," and "advanced age" because they have little value for public health or medical research. Age is recorded elsewhere on the death certificate. When malnutrition is involved, the certifier should consider if other medical conditions could have led to malnutrition.

When a number of conditions or multiple organs/system failure resulted in death, the physician, medical examiner, or coroner should choose a single sequence to describe the process leading to death and list the other conditions in Part II of the certification section. "Multiple system failure" could be included as an "other significant condition" but also specify the systems involved. In other instances, conditions listed in Part II of the death certificate may include causes that resulted

452

from the underlying cause but did not fit into the sequence resulting in death.

If the certifier cannot determine a descriptive sequence of causes of death despite carefully considering all the information available and circumstances of death did not warrant investigation by the medical examiner or coroner, death may be reported as "unspecified natural causes." If any potentially lethal medical conditions are known but cannot be cited as part of the sequence leading to death, they should be listed as other significant conditions.

Infant Deaths

Maternal conditions may have initiated or affected the sequence that resulted in infant death. These maternal conditions should be reported in the cause-of-death statement in addition to the infant causes.

When sudden infant death syndrome (SIDS) is suspected, a complete investigation should be conducted, typically by a medical examiner. If the infant is under one year of age, no cause of death is determined after scene investigation, clinical history is reviewed, and a complete autopsy is performed, then the death can be reported as SIDS. If the investigation is not complete, the death may be reported as presumed to be SIDS.

Avoid Ambiguity

Most certifiers will find themselves, at some point, in the circumstance in which they are unable to provide a simple description of the process of death. In this situation, the certifier should try to provide a clear sequence, qualify the causes about which he/she is uncertain, and be able to explain the certification chosen.

When processes such as the following are reported, additional information about the etiology should be reported if possible:

Table 52.1. Death Certification

Cardiovascular		
Acute myocardial infarction	Congestive heart failure	Myocardial infarction
Arrhythmia	Cardiomyopathy	Shock
Atrial fibrillation	Dysrhythmia	Ventricular fibrillation
Cardiac arrest	Heart failure	Ventricular tachycardia

Table 52.1. Continued

Cardiovascular		
Cardiac dysrhythmia	Hypotension	
Central Nervous System		
Altered mental status	Cerebral edema	Open (or closed) head injury
Anoxic encephalopathy	Dementia (when not otherwise specified)	Seizures
Brain injury	Epidural hematoma	Subdural hematoma
Brain stem herniation	Increased intracranial pressure	Subarachnoid hemorrhage
Cerebrovascular accident	Intracranial Hemorrhage	Uncal herniation
Cerebellar tonsillar herniation	Metabolic encephalopathy	
Respiratory		
Aspiration	Pneumonia	Pulmonary insufficiency
Pleural effusions	Pulmonary embolism	Pulmonary edema
Gastrointestinal		
Biliary obstruction	Diarrhea	Hepatic failure
Bowel obstruction	End-stage liver disease	Hepatorenal syndrome
Cirrhosis	Gastrointestinal hemorrhage	Perforated gallbladder
Blood, Renal, Immune		
Coagulopathy	Hepatorenal syndrome	Renal failure
Disseminated intravascular coagulopathy	Immunosuppression	Thrombocytopenia
End-stage renal disease	Pancytopenia	Urinary tract infection
Not System-Oriented		
Abdominal hemorrhage	Decubiti	Hyponatremia
Ascites	Dehydration	Multi-organ failure
Anoxia	Exsanguination	Necrotizing soft-tissue infection
Bacteremia	Failure to thrive	Peritonitis
Bedridden	Gangrene	Sepsis
Carcinogenesis	Hemothorax	Septic shock
Carcinomatosis	Hyperglycemia	Shock
Chronic bedridden state	Hyperkalemia	Volume depletion

If the certifier is unable to determine the etiology of a process such as those shown above, the process must be qualified as being of an unknown, undetermined, probable, presumed, or unspecified etiology so it is clear that a distinct etiology was not inadvertently or carelessly omitted.

The following conditions and types of death might seem to be specific but when the medical history is examined further may be found to be complications of an injury or poisoning (possibly occurring long ago):

- Subdural hematoma

- Epidural hematoma

- Subarachnoid hemorrhage

- Fracture

- Pulmonary embolism

- Thermal burns/chemical burns

- Sepsis

- Hyperthermia

- Hypothermia

- Hip fracture

- Seizure disorder

- Drug or alcohol overdose/drug or alcohol abuse

Is it possible that the underlying cause of death was the result of an injury or poisoning? If it might be, check with the medical examiner/coroner to find out if the death should be reported to her or him.

When indicating neoplasms as a cause of death indicate the following:

1. Primary site or that the primary site is unknown

2. Benign or malignant

3. Cell type or that the cell type is unknown

4. Grade of a neoplasm

5. Part or lobe of an organ affected (e.g., a well-differentiated squamous cell carcinoma, lung, left upper lobe)

Medical Examiner or Coroner

The medical examiner/coroner investigates deaths that are unexpected, unexplained, or if an injury or poisoning was involved. State laws often provide guidelines for when a medical examiner/coroner must be notified. In the case of deaths known or suspected to have resulted from injury or poisoning, report the death to the medical examiner/coroner as required by state law. The medical examiner/ coroner will either complete the cause-of-death section of the death certificate or waive that responsibility. If the medical examiner/coroner does not accept the case, then the certifier will need to complete the cause-of-death section.

Chapter 53

If Death Occurs While
Traveling

Death of a friend, relative, or coworker can be immensely distressing. The situation is aggravated when death occurs abroad, where grieving people may be unfamiliar with local processes, language, and culture. Whether dealing with the death locally or from their home country, next of kin could face large, unanticipated costs, and labor-intensive administrative steps. Depending on the circumstances surrounding the dead, some countries may require an autopsy. Besides relatives, sources of support include the local consulate or embassy, travel insurance provider, tour operator, faith-based and aid organizations, and the deceased's employer. There likely will need to be an official identification of the body. A body can be identified by witness statements of those who knew the person well, analyzing deoxyribonucleic acid (DNA) samples, checking fingerprints, reviewing dental radiographs, or inspecting surgical implants.

Death Onboard a Conveyance

The Federal Aviation Administration (FAA) requires that flight attendants receive training in cardiopulmonary resuscitation (CPR) and in the proper use of an automated external defibrillator (AED) at

This chapter includes text excerpted from "Travelers' Health—Death during Travel," Centers for Disease Control and Prevention (CDC), June 24, 2019.

least once every 2 years. Under federal law, there are Good Samaritan laws for actions brought in a federal or state court resulting out of acts or omissions when people assist in a medical emergency during flight unless there is gross negligence or willful misconduct. If CPR is performed in the aircraft cabin, once it has been continued for 30 minutes or longer with no signs of life within this period, and no shocks advised by an AED, the person may be presumed dead and resuscitation efforts halted. Airlines may choose to specify additional criteria, depending upon the availability of a ground-to-air medical consultation service or a physician aboard.

Cruise ships are usually better equipped than aircraft and carry medical professionals to provide clinical care. If the death occurs on a cruise ship despite medical interventions, the crew is usually able to provide logistic support to repatriate the body. Cruise ships are equipped with morgues and carry body bags.

The U.S. regulations require that all deaths aboard commercial flights and ships destined for the United States be reported to the Centers for Disease Control and Prevention (CDC).

Obtaining Department of State Assistance

When a U.S. citizen dies outside the United States, the deceased person's next of kin or legal representative should notify U.S. consular officials at the Department of State (DOS). Consular personnel is available 24 hours a day, 7 days a week, to provide assistance to U.S. citizens for overseas emergencies.

If the next of kin or legal representative is in a foreign country with the deceased U.S. citizen, she or he should contact the nearest U.S. embassy or consulate for assistance. Contact information for U.S. embassies, consulates, and consular agencies overseas may be found at the DOS website (www.usembassy.gov).

If a family member, domestic partner, or legal representative is in a different country from the deceased person, she or he should call the DOS's Office of Overseas Citizens Services in Washington, DC, from 8 a.m. to 5 p.m. Eastern time, Monday through Friday, at 888-407-4747 (toll-free) or 202-501-4444. For emergency assistance after working hours or on weekends and holidays, call the DOS switchboard at 202-647-4000 and ask to speak with the Overseas Citizens Services duty officer. In addition, the U.S. embassy closest to or in the country where the U.S. citizen died can provide assistance (www.usembassy.gov).

The DOS has no funds to assist in the return of remains of U.S. citizens who die abroad. U.S. consular officers assist the next of kin by conveying instructions to the appropriate offices within the foreign country and providing information to the family on how to transmit the necessary private funds to cover the costs of preparing and repatriating human remains. The process can be expensive and lengthy. Upon issuance of a local (foreign) death certificate, the nearest U.S. embassy or consulate may prepare a consular report of the death of an American abroad. Copies of that report are provided to the next of kin or legal representative and may be used in U.S. courts to settle estate matters. If there is no next of kin or legal representative in-country, a consular officer will act as a provisional conservator of the deceased's personal effects.

Importation of Human Remains for Interment or Cremation
General Guidance

Except for cremated remains, human remains intended for interment (placement in a grave or tomb) or cremation after entry into the United States must be accompanied by a death certificate stating the cause of death. A death certificate is an official document signed by a coroner, healthcare provider, or other official authorized to make a declaration of the cause of death. Death certificates written in a language other than English must be accompanied by an English translation. If a death certificate is not available in time for returning the remains, the U.S. embassy or consulate should provide a consular mortuary certificate stating whether the person died from a disease classified as quarantinable in the United States. Any requirements of the country of origin, air carrier, U.S. Customs and Border Protection (CBP), and the Transportation Security Administration (TSA) must also be met. The CDC regulates the importation of human remains and provides guidance for their importation. The requirements are more stringent if the person died from a disease classified as quarantinable in the United States.

Exportation of Human Remains

The Centers for Disease Control and Prevention (CDC) does not regulate the exportation of human remains outside the United States, although other state and local regulations may apply. The U.S. Postal Service (UPS) is the only courier authorized to ship cremated remains. Exporters of human remains and travelers taking human remains out of the United States should be aware that the importation requirements of the destination country and the air carrier must be met. Information regarding these requirements may be obtained from the foreign embassy or consulate (www.state.gov/s/cpr/rls) and the air carrier.

Chapter 54

Grief, Bereavement, and Coping with Loss

People cope with the loss of a loved one in different ways. Most people who experience grief will cope well. Others will have severe grief and may need treatment. There are many things that can affect the grief process of someone who has lost a loved one to cancer. They include:

- The personality of the person who is grieving

- The relationship with the person who died

- The loved one's cancer experience and the way the disease progressed

- The grieving person's coping skills and mental health history

- The amount of support the grieving person has

- The grieving person's cultural and religious background

- The grieving person's social and financial position

This chapter includes text excerpted from "Grief, Bereavement, and Coping with Loss (PDQ®)—Patient Version," National Cancer Institute (NCI), March 6, 2013. Reviewed September 2019.

This chapter describes the different types of grief reactions and treatments for grief. It is intended as a resource to help caregivers.

Bereavement and Grief

Bereavement is the period of sadness after losing a loved one through death.

Grief and mourning occur during the period of bereavement. Grief and mourning are closely related. Mourning is the way we show grief in public. The way people mourn is affected by beliefs, religious practices, and cultural customs. People who are grieving are sometimes described as bereaved.

Grief is the normal process of reacting to the loss.

Grief is an emotional response to the loss of a loved one. Common grief reactions include the following:

- Feeling emotionally numb

- Feeling unable to believe the loss occurred

- Feeling anxiety from the distress of being separated from the loved one

- Mourning along with depression

- A feeling of acceptance

Types of Grief Reactions
Anticipatory Grief

Anticipatory grief may occur when a death is expected.

Anticipatory grief occurs when a death is expected, but before it happens. It may be felt by the families of people who are dying and by the person dying. Anticipatory grief helps family members get ready emotionally for the loss. It can be a time to take care of unfinished business with the dying person, such as saying "I love you" or "I forgive you."

Like grief that occurs after the death of a loved one, anticipatory grief involves mental, emotional, cultural, and social responses. However, anticipatory grief is different from grief that occurs after death. Symptoms of anticipatory grief include the following:

- Depression

- Feeling a greater than usual concern for the dying person

- Imagining what the loved one's death will be like

- Getting ready emotionally for what will happen after the death

Anticipatory grief may help the family but not the dying person. Anticipatory grief helps family members cope with what is to come. For the patient who is dying, anticipatory grief may be too much to handle and may cause her or him to withdraw from others.

Anticipatory grief does not always occur.

Some researchers report that anticipatory grief is rare. Studies showed that periods of acceptance and recovery usually seen during grief are not common before the patient's actual death. The bereaved may feel that trying to accept the loss of a loved one before death occurs may make it seem that the dying patient has been abandoned.

Also, grief felt before the death will not decrease the grief felt afterward or make it last a shorter time.

Normal Grief

Normal or common grief begins soon after a loss and symptoms go away over time.

During normal grief, the bereaved person moves toward accepting the loss and is able to continue normal day-to-day life even though it is hard to do. Common grief reactions include:

- Emotional numbness, shock, disbelief, or denial. These often occur right after the death, especially if the death was not expected.

- Anxiety over being separated from the loved one. The bereaved may wish to bring the person back and become lost in thoughts of the deceased. Images of death may occur often in the person's everyday thoughts.

- Distress that leads to crying; sighing; having dreams, illusions, and hallucinations of the deceased; and looking for places or things that were shared with the deceased

- Anger

- Periods of sadness, loss of sleep, loss of appetite, extreme tiredness, guilt, and loss of interest in life. Day-to-day living may be affected

In normal grief, symptoms will occur less often and will feel less severe as time passes. Recovery does not happen in a set period of time. For most bereaved people having normal grief, symptoms lessen between six months and two years after the loss.

Many bereaved people will have grief bursts or pangs.

Grief bursts or pangs are short periods (20 to 30 minutes) of very intense distress. Sometimes these bursts are caused by reminders of the deceased person. At other times they seem to happen for no reason.

Grief is sometimes described as a process that has stages.

There are several theories about how the normal grief process works. Experts have described different types and numbers of stages that people go through as they cope with loss. At this time, there is not enough information to prove that one of these theories is more correct than the others.

Although many bereaved people have similar responses as they cope with their losses, there is no typical grief response. The grief process is personal.

Complicated Grief

There is no right or wrong way to grieve, but studies have shown that there are patterns of grief that are different from the most common. This has been called "complicated grief."

Complicated grief reactions that have been seen in studies include:

- **Minimal grief reaction:** A grief pattern in which the person has no, or only a few, signs of distress or problems that occur with other types of grief.

- **Chronic grief:** A grief pattern in which the symptoms of common grief last for a much longer time than usual. These symptoms are a lot like the ones that occur with major depression, anxiety, or posttraumatic stress.

Factors that Affect Complicated Grief

Researchers study grief reactions to try to find out what might increase the chance that complicated grief will occur.

Studies have looked at how the following factors affect the grief response:

Whether the Death Is Expected or Unexpected

It may seem that any sudden, unexpected loss might lead to more difficult grief. However, studies have found that bereaved people with high self-esteem and/or a feeling that they have control over life are likely to have a normal grief reaction even after an unexpected loss. Bereaved people with low self-esteem and/or a sense that life cannot be controlled are more likely to have complicated grief after an unexpected loss. This includes more depression and physical problems.

The Personality of the Bereaved

Studies have found that people with certain personality traits are more likely to have long-lasting depression after a loss. These include people who are very dependent on the loved one (such as a spouse) and people who deal with distress by thinking about it all the time.

The Religious Beliefs of the Bereaved

Some studies have shown that religion helps people cope better with grief. Other studies have shown it does not help or causes more distress. Religion seems to help people who go to church often. The positive effect on grief may be because church-goers have more social support.

Whether the Bereaved Is Male or Female

In general, men have more problems than women do after a spouse's death. Men tend to have worse depression and more health problems than women do after the loss. Some researchers think this may be because men have less social support after a loss.

The Age of the Bereaved

In general, younger bereaved people have more problems after a loss than older bereaved people do. They have more severe health problems, grief symptoms, and other mental and physical symptoms. Younger bereaved people, however, may recover more quickly than older bereaved people do, because they have more resources and social support.

The Amount of Social Support the Bereaved Has

Lack of social support increases the chance of having problems coping with a loss. Social support includes the person's family, friends, neighbors, and community members who can give psychological, physical, and financial help. After the death of a close family member, many people have a number of related losses. The death of a spouse, for

465

example, may cause a loss of income, changes in lifestyle, and day-to-day living. These are all related to social support.

Treatment of Grief

Normal grief may not need to be treated.

Most bereaved people work through grief and recover within the first six months to two years. Researchers are studying whether bereaved people experiencing normal grief would be helped by formal treatment. They are also studying whether treatment might prevent complicated grief in people who are likely to have it.

For people who have serious grief reactions or symptoms of distress, treatment may be helpful.

Complicated grief may be treated with different types of psychotherapy (talk therapy).

Researchers are studying the treatment of mental, emotional, social, and behavioral symptoms of grief. Treatment methods include discussion, listening, and counseling.

Complicated grief treatment (CGT) is a type of grief therapy that was helpful in a clinical trial.

Complicated grief treatment has three phases:

- The first phase includes talking about the loss and setting goals toward recovery. The bereaved are taught to work on these two things.

- The second phase includes coping with the loss by retelling the story of death. This helps bereaved people who try not to think about their loss.

- The last phase looks at the progress that has been made toward recovery and helps the bereaved make future plans. The bereaved feelings about ending the sessions are also discussed.

In a clinical trial of patients with complicated grief, CGT was compared to interpersonal psychotherapy (IPT). IPT is a type of psychotherapy that focuses on a person's relationships with others and is helpful in treating depression. In patients with complicated grief, CGT was more helpful than IPT.

Cognitive-behavioral therapy (CBT) for complicated grief was helpful in a clinical trial.

Cognitive-behavioral therapy works with the way a person's thoughts and behaviors are connected. CBT helps the patient learn skills that change attitudes and behaviors by replacing negative thoughts and changing the rewards of certain behaviors.

A clinical trial compared CBT to counseling for complicated grief. Results showed that patients treated with CBT had more improvement in symptoms and general mental distress than those in the counseling group.

Depression related to grief is sometimes treated with drugs.

There is no standard drug therapy for depression that occurs with grief. Some healthcare professionals think depression is a normal part of grief and does not need to be treated. Whether to treat grief-related depression with drugs is up to the patient and the healthcare professional to decide.

Clinical trials of antidepressants for depression related to grief have found that the drugs can help relieve depression. However, they give less relief and take longer to work than they do when used for depression that is not related to grief.

Chapter 55

Mourning the Death of a Spouse

When your spouse dies, your world changes. You are in mourning—feeling grief and sorrow at the loss. You may feel numb, shocked, and fearful. You may feel guilty for being the one who is still alive. At some point, you may even feel angry at your spouse for leaving you. All of these feelings are normal. There are no rules about how you should feel. There is no right or wrong way to mourn.

When you grieve, you can feel both physical and emotional pain. People who are grieving often cry easily and can have:

- Trouble sleeping

- Little interest in food

- Problems with concentration

- A hard time making decisions

- In addition to dealing with feelings of loss, you may also need to put your own life back together. This can be hard work. Some people feel better sooner than they expect. Others may take longer.

This chapter includes text excerpted from "Mourning the Death of a Spouse," National Institute on Aging (NIA), National Institutes of Health (NIH), June 3, 2017.

As time passes, you may still miss your spouse. But for most people, the intense pain will lessen. There will be good and bad days. You will know you are feeling better when there are more good days than bad. Do not feel guilty if you laugh at a joke or enjoy a visit with a friend.

There are many ways to grieve and to learn to accept the loss. Try not to ignore your grief. Support may be available until you can manage your grief on your own. It is especially important to get help with your loss if you feel overwhelmed or very depressed by it.

Family and compassionate friends can be a great support. They are grieving, too, and some people find that sharing memories is one way to help each other. Feel free to share stories about the one who is gone. Sometimes, people hesitate to bring up the loss or mention the dead person's name because they worry this can be hurtful. But, people may find it helpful to talk directly about their loss. You are all coping with the death of someone you cared for.

For some people, mourning can go on so long that it becomes unhealthy. This can be a sign of serious depression and anxiety. Talk with your doctor if sadness keeps you from carrying on with your day-to-day life. Support may be available until you can manage the grief on your own.

How Grief Counseling Can Help

Sometimes people find grief counseling makes it easier to work through their sorrow. Regular talk therapy with a grief counselor or therapist can help people learn to accept death and, in time, start a new life.

There are also support groups where grieving people help each other. These groups can be specialized—parents who have lost children or people who have lost spouses, for example—or they can be for anyone learning to manage grief. Check with religious groups, local hospitals, nursing homes, funeral homes, or your doctor to find support groups in your area.

An essential part of hospice is providing grief counseling to the family of someone who was under their care. You can also ask hospice workers for bereavement support at this time, even if hospice was not used before the death.

Remember to take good care of yourself. You might know that grief affects how you feel emotionally, but you may not realize that it can also have physical effects. The stress of death and your grief could even make you sick. Eat well, exercise, get enough sleep, and get back to doing things you used to enjoy, such as going to the movies, walking, or reading. Accept offers of help or companionship from friends and family. It is good for you and for them.

Remember that your children are grieving, too. It will take time for the whole family to adjust to life without your spouse. You may find that your relationship with your children and their relationships with each other have changed. Open, honest communication is important.

Mourning takes time. It is common to have rollercoaster emotions for a while.

Taking Care of Yourself while Grieving

In the beginning, you may find that taking care of details and keeping busy, helps. For a while, family and friends may be around to assist you. But, there comes a time when you will have to face the change in your life.

Here are some ideas to keep in mind:

- **Take care of yourself.** Grief can be hard on your health. Exercise regularly, eat healthy food and get enough sleep. Bad habits, such as drinking too much alcohol or smoking, can put your health at risk.

- **Try to eat right.** Some widowed people lose interest in cooking and eating. It may help to have lunch with friends. Sometimes, eating at home alone feels too quiet. Turning on the radio or TV during meals can help. For information on nutrition and cooking for one, look for helpful books at your local library or bookstore or online (www.nia.nih.gov/health/ smart-food-choices-healthy-aging).

- **Talk with caring friends.** Let family and friends know when you want to talk about your spouse. They may be grieving too and may welcome the chance to share memories. Accept their offers of help and company, when possible.

- **Visit with members of your religious community.** Many people who are grieving find comfort in their faith. Praying, talking with others of your faith, reading religious or spiritual texts, or listening to uplifting music also may bring comfort.

- **See your doctor.** Keep up with visits to your healthcare provider. If it has been a while, schedule a physical and bring your doctor up to date on any preexisting medical conditions and any new health issues that may be of concern. Let your

471

healthcare provider know if you are having trouble taking care of your everyday activities, such as getting dressed or fixing meals.

Does Everyone Feel the Same Way after a Death?

Men and women share many of the same feelings when a spouse dies. Both may deal with the pain of loss, and both may worry about the future. But, there also can be differences.

Many married couples divide up their household tasks. One person may pay bills and handle car repairs. The other person may cook meals and mow the lawn. Splitting up jobs often works well until there is only one person who has to do it all. Learning to manage new tasks—from chores to household repairs to finances—takes time, but it can be done.

Being alone can increase concerns about safety. It is a good idea to make sure there are working locks on the doors and windows. If you need help, ask your family or friends.

Facing the future without a husband or wife can be scary. Many people have never lived alone. Those who are both widowed and retired may feel very lonely and become depressed. Talk to your doctor about how you are feeling.

Make Plans and Be Active

After years of being part of a couple, it can be upsetting to be alone. Many people find it helps to have things to do every day. Whether you are still working or are retired, write down your weekly plans. You might:

- Take a walk with a friend
- Visit the library
- Volunteer
- Try an exercise class
- Join a singing group
- Join a bowling league
- Offer to watch your grandchildren
- Consider adopting a pet
- Take a class at a nearby senior center, college, or recreation center
- Stay in touch with family and friends, either in person or online

Getting Your Legal and Financial Paperwork in Order

When you feel stronger, you should think about getting your legal and financial affairs in order. For example, you might need to:

- Write a new will and advance directive.

- Look into a durable power of attorney for legal matters and healthcare, in case you are unable to make your own medical decisions in the future.

- Put joint property (such as a house or car) in your name.

- Check on changes you might need to make to your health insurance as well as your life, car, and homeowner's insurance.

- Sign up for Medicare by your 65th birthday.

- Make a list of bills you will need to pay in the next few months: for instance, state and federal taxes and your rent or mortgage.

When you are ready, go through your husband's or wife's clothes and other personal items. It may be hard to give away these belongings. Instead of parting with everything at once, you might make three piles: one to keep, one to give away, and one "not sure." Ask your children or others to help. Think about setting aside items such as a special piece of clothing, watch, favorite book, or picture to give to your children or grandchildren as personal reminders of your spouse.

Going Out after the Death of a Spouse

Having a social life on your own can be tough. It may be hard to think about going to parties or other social events by yourself. It can be hard to think about coming home alone. You may be anxious about dating. Many people miss the feeling of closeness that marriage brings. After a time, some are ready to have a social life again.

Here are some things to remember:

- Go at a comfortable pace. There is no rush.

- It is okay to make the first move when it comes to planning things to do.

- Try group activities. Invite friends over for a potluck dinner or go to a senior center.

- With married friends, think about informal outings such as walks, picnics, or movies rather than couple's events that remind you of the past.

- Find an activity you like. You may have fun and meet people who like to do the same thing.

- You can develop meaningful relationships with friends and family members of all ages.

- Many people find that pets provide important companionship.

Part Nine

Mortality Statistics

Chapter 56

Life Expectancy: Global Trends

The world is on the brink of a demographic milestone. Since the beginning of recorded history, young children have outnumbered their elders. In about five years' time, however, the number of people aged 65 or older will outnumber children under age 5. Driven by falling fertility rates and remarkable increases in life expectancy, population aging will continue, even accelerate. The number of people aged 65 or older is projected to grow from an estimated 524 million in 2010 to nearly 1.5 billion in 2050, with most of the increase in developing countries.

The remarkable improvements in life expectancy over the past century were part of a shift in the leading causes of disease and death. At the dawn of the 20th century, the major health threats were infectious and parasitic diseases that most often claimed the lives of infants and children. Currently, noncommunicable diseases that more commonly affect adults and older people impose the greatest burden on global health.

In developing countries, the rise of chronic noncommunicable diseases, such as heart disease, cancer, and diabetes reflects changes in lifestyle and diet, as well as aging. The potential economic and societal costs of noncommunicable diseases of this type rise sharply with

This chapter includes text excerpted from "Global Health and Aging," National Institute on Aging (NIA), National Institutes of Health (NIH), October 2011. Reviewed September 2019.

age and have the ability to affect economic growth. A World Health Organization (WHO) analysis in 23 low- and middle-income countries estimated the economic losses from three noncommunicable diseases (heart disease, stroke, and diabetes) in these countries would total US$83 billion between 2006 and 2015.

Reducing severe disability from disease and health conditions is one key to holding down health and social costs. The health and economic burden of disability also can be reinforced or alleviated by environmental characteristics that can determine whether an older person can remain independent despite physical limitations. The longer people can remain mobile and care for themselves, the lower are the costs for long-term care to families and society.

Because many adult and older-age health problems were rooted in early life experiences and living conditions, ensuring good child health can yield benefits for older people. In the meantime, generations of children and young adults who grew up in poverty and ill health in developing countries will be entering old age in the coming decades, potentially increasing the health burden of older populations in those countries.

With continuing declines in death rates among older people, the proportion aged 80 or older is rising quickly, and more people are living past 100. The limits to life expectancy and lifespan are not as obvious as once thought. And there is mounting evidence from cross-national data that—with appropriate policies and programs—people can remain healthy and independent well into old age and can continue to contribute to their communities and families.

The potential for an active, healthy old age is tempered by one of the most daunting and potentially costly consequences of ever-longer life expectancies: the increase in people with dementia, especially Alzheimer disease (AD). Most dementia patients eventually need constant care and help with the most basic activities of daily living, creating a heavy economic and social burden. The prevalence of dementia rises sharply with age. An estimated 25–30 percent of people aged 85 or older have dementia. Unless new and more effective interventions are found to treat or prevent AD, prevalence is expected to rise dramatically with the aging of the population in the United States and worldwide.

Aging is taking place alongside other broad social trends that will affect the lives of older people. Economies are globalizing, people are more likely to live in cities, and technology is evolving rapidly. Demographic and family changes mean there will be fewer older people with families to care for them. People now have fewer children, are less likely to be married, and are less likely to live with older generations.

With declining support from families, society will need better information and tools to ensure the well-being of the world's growing number of older citizens.

Humanity's Aging

In 2010, an estimated 524 million people were aged 65 or older—8 percent of the world's population. By 2050, this number is expected to nearly triple to about 1.5 billion, representing 16 percent of the world's population. Although more developed countries have the oldest population profiles, the vast majority of older people—and the most rapidly aging populations—are in less developed countries. Between 2010 and 2050, the number of older people in less developed countries is projected to increase more than 250 percent, compared with a 71 percent increase in developed countries.

This remarkable phenomenon is being driven by declines in fertility and improvements in longevity. With fewer children entering the population and people living longer, older people are making up an increasing share of the total population. In more developed countries, fertility fell below the replacement rate of two live births per woman by the 1970s, down from nearly three children per woman around 1950. Even more crucial for population aging, fertility fell with surprising speed in many less developed countries from an average of six children in 1950 to an average of two or three children in 2005. In 2006, fertility was at or below the two-child replacement level in 44 less developed countries.

Most developed nations have had decades to adjust to their changing age structures. It took more than 100 years for the share of France's population aged 65 or older to rise from 7 percent to 14 percent. In contrast, many less developed countries are experiencing a rapid increase in the number and percentage of older people, often within a single generation. For example, the same demographic aging that unfolded over more than a century in France will occur in just two decades in Brazil. Developing countries will need to adapt quickly to this reality. Many less-developed nations will need policies that ensure the financial security of older people, and that provide the health and social care they need, without the same extended period of economic growth experienced by aging societies in the West. In other words, some countries may grow old before they grow rich. In some countries, the sheer number of people entering older ages will challenge national infrastructures, particularly health systems. This numeric surge in older people is dramatically illustrated in the world's two most populous countries: China and India. China's older population—those over age 65—will likely swell to 330 million by 2050 from 110 million. India's current older population of 60 million is projected to exceed 227 million in 2050, an increase of nearly 280 percent. By the middle of this century, there could be 100 million Chinese over the age of 80. This is an amazing achievement considering that there were fewer than 14 million people this age on the entire planet just a century ago.

Living Longer

The dramatic increase in average life expectancy during the 20th century ranks as one of society's greatest achievements. Although most babies born in 1900 did not live past age 50, life expectancy at birth now exceeds 83 years in Japan—the current leader—and is at least 81 years in several other countries. Less developed regions of the world have experienced a steady increase in life expectancy since World War II, although not all regions have shared in these improvements. (One notable exception is the fall in life expectancy in many parts of Africa because of deaths caused by the human immunodeficiency virus(HIV)/acquired immunodeficiency syndrome (AIDS) epidemic.) The most dramatic and rapid gains have occurred in East Asia, where life expectancy at birth increased from less than 45 years in 1950 to more than 74 years.

These improvements are part of a major transition in human health spreading around the globe at different rates and along different pathways. This transition encompasses a broad set of changes that include a decline from high to low fertility; a steady increase in life expectancy at birth and at older ages; and a shift in the leading causes of death and illness from infectious and parasitic diseases to noncommunicable diseases and chronic conditions. In early nonindustrial societies, the risk of death was high at every age, and only a small proportion of people reached old age. In modern societies, most people live past middle age, and deaths are highly concentrated at older ages.

The victories against infectious and parasitic diseases are a triumph for public health projects of the 20th century, which immunized millions of people against smallpox, polio, and major childhood killers such as measles. Even earlier, better living standards, especially more nutritious diets, and cleaner drinking water began to reduce serious infections and prevent deaths among children. More children were surviving their vulnerable early years and reaching adulthood. In fact, more than 60 percent of the improvement in female life expectancy at birth in developed countries between 1850 and 1900 occurred because more children

480

were living to age 15, not because more adults were reaching old age. It was not until the 20th century that mortality rates began to decline within the older ages. Research shows a surprising and continuing improvement in life expectancy among those aged 80 or above.

The progressive increase in survival in these oldest age groups was not anticipated by demographers, and it raises questions about how high the average life expectancy can realistically rise and about the potential length of the human lifespan. While some experts assume that life expectancy must be approaching an upper limit, data on life expectancies between 1840 and 2007 show a steady increase averaging about three months of life per year. The country with the highest average life expectancy has varied over time. In 1840 it was Sweden and now it is Japan—but the pattern is strikingly similar. So far there is little evidence that life expectancy has stopped rising even in Japan.

The rising life expectancy within the older population itself is increasing the number and proportion of people at very old ages. The "oldest old" (people aged 85 or older) constitute 8 percent of the world's 65-and-over population: 12 percent in more developed countries and 6 percent in less developed countries. In many countries, the oldest old are now the fastest-growing part of the total population. On a global level, the 85-and-over population is projected to increase 351 percent between 2010 and 2050, compared to a 188 percent increase for the population aged 65 or older and a 22 percent increase for the population under age 65.

The global number of centenarians is projected to increase 10-fold between 2010 and 2050. In the mid-1990s, some researchers estimated that, over the course of human history, the odds of living from birth to age 100 may have risen from 1 in 20,000,000 to 1 in 50 for females in low mortality nations, such as Japan and Sweden. This group's longevity may increase even faster than current projections assume— previous population projections often underestimated decreases in mortality rates among the oldest old.

New Disease Patterns

The transition from high to low mortality and fertility that accompanied socioeconomic development has also meant a shift in the leading causes of disease and death. Demographers and epidemiologists describe this shift as part of an "epidemiologic transition" characterized by the waning of infectious and acute diseases and the emerging importance of chronic and degenerative diseases. High death rates from infectious diseases are commonly associated with poverty, poor diets,

481

and limited infrastructure found in developing countries. Although many developing countries still experience high child mortality from infectious and parasitic diseases, one of the major epidemiologic trends of the current century is the rise of chronic and degenerative diseases in countries throughout the world—regardless of income level.

Evidence from the multicountry Global Burden of Disease project and other international epidemiologic research shows that health problems associated with wealthy and aged populations affect a wide and expanding swath of the world population. Over the next 10 to 15 years, people in every world region will suffer more death and disability from such noncommunicable diseases as heart disease, cancer, and diabetes than from infectious and parasitic diseases. The myth that noncommunicable diseases affect mainly affluent and aged populations were dispelled by the project, which combines information about mortality and morbidity from every world region to assess the total health burden from specific diseases. The burden is measured by estimating the loss of healthy years of life due to a specific cause based on detailed epidemiological information. In 2008, noncommunicable diseases accounted for an estimated 86 percent of the burden of disease in high-income countries, 65 percent in middle-income countries, and a surprising 37 percent in low-income countries.

By 2030, noncommunicable diseases are projected to account for more than one-half of the disease burden in low-income countries and more than three-fourths in middle-income countries. Infectious and parasitic diseases will account for 30 percent and 10 percent, respectively, in low- and middle-income countries. Among the 60-and-over population, noncommunicable diseases already account for more than 87 percent of the burden in low-, middle-, and high-income countries.

But, the continuing health threats from communicable diseases for older people cannot be dismissed, either. Older people account for a growing share of the infectious disease burden in low-income countries. Infectious disease programs, including those for HIV/AIDS, often neglect older people and ignore the potential effects of population aging. Yet, antiretroviral therapy is enabling more people with HIV/AIDS to survive to older ages. And, there is growing evidence that older people are particularly susceptible to infectious diseases for a variety of reasons, including immunosenescence (the progressive deterioration of immune function with age) and frailty. Older people already suffering from one chronic or infectious disease are especially vulnerable to additional infectious diseases. For example, type 2 diabetes and tuberculosis are well known "comorbid risk factors" that have serious health consequences for older people.

482

Chapter 57

Mortality Trends in the United States

This chapter discusses the final 2017 U.S. mortality data on deaths and death rates by demographic and medical characteristics. These data provide information on mortality patterns among U.S. residents by variables, such as sex, race and ethnicity, and cause of death. Life expectancy estimates, age-specific death rates, age-adjusted death rates by race and ethnicity and sex, 10 leading causes of death, and 10 leading causes of infant death were analyzed by comparing 2017 and 2016 final data.

How Long Can We Expect to Live?

In 2017, life expectancy at birth was 78.6 years for the total U.S. population—a decrease from 78.7 years in 2016. For males, life expectancy changed from 76.2 in 2016 to 76.1 in 2017. For females, life expectancy remained the same at 81.1.

The life expectancy for females was consistently higher than it was for males. In 2017, the difference in life expectancy between females and males increased 0.1 years from 4.9 years in 2016 to 5.0 years in 2017.

In 2017, life expectancy at age 65 for the total population was 19.5 years, an increase of 0.1 years from 2016. Life expectancy at age 65 was 20.6 years for females and 18.1 years for males, both unchanged

This chapter includes text excerpted from "Mortality in the United States, 2017," Centers for Disease Control and Prevention (CDC), November 29, 2018.

from 2016. The difference in life expectancy at age 65 between females and males was 2.5 years, unchanged from 2016.

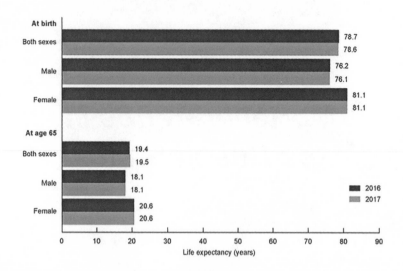

Figure 57.1. *Life Expectancy at Selected Ages, by Sex: The United States, 2016 and 2017.* (Source: National Center for Health Statistics (NCHS), National Vital Statistics System (NVSS), Mortality.)

Note: Life expectancies for 2016 were revised using updated Medicare data; therefore, figures may differ from those previously published.

What Are the Age-Adjusted Death Rates for Race–Ethnicity–Sex Groups?

The age-adjusted death rate for the total population increased by 0.4 percent from 728.8 per 100,000 standard population in 2016 to 731.9 in 2017. Age-adjusted death rates increased in 2017 from 2016 for non-Hispanic White males (0.6%) and non-Hispanic White females (0.9%). The age-adjusted death rate decreased for non-Hispanic Black females (0.8%). Rates did not change significantly for non-Hispanic Black males, Hispanic males, and Hispanic females from 2016 to 2017.

Did Age-Specific Death Rates Change among Those Aged 15 Years and Over?

Death rates increased significantly between 2016 and 2017 for age groups 25 to 34 (2.9%), 35 to 44 (1.6%), and 85 and over (1.4%).

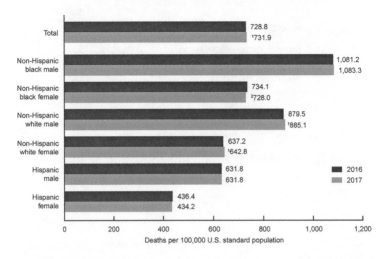

Figure 57.2. *Age-Adjusted Death Rates, by Race and Ethnicity and Sex: The United States, 2016 and 2017.* (Source: National Center for Health Statistics (NCHS), National Vital Statistics System (NVSS), Mortality.)

[1]*Statistically significant increase in age-adjusted death rate from 2016 to 2017 (p < 0.05).* [2]*Statistically significant decrease in age-adjusted death rate from 2016 to 2017 (p < 0.05).*

The death rate decreased significantly for the age group 45 to 54 (1.0%).

Rates for other age groups did not change significantly between 2016 and 2017.

What Are the Leading Causes of Death?

In 2017, the 10 leading causes of death (heart disease, cancer, unintentional injuries, chronic lower respiratory diseases, stroke, Alzheimer disease (AD), diabetes, influenza and pneumonia, kidney disease, and suicide) remained the same as in 2016. Causes of death are ranked according to the number of deaths. The 10 leading causes accounted for 74 percent of all deaths in the United States in 2017.

From 2016 to 2017, age-adjusted death rates increased for 7 of 10 leading causes of death and decreased by 1. The rate increased 4.2 percent for unintentional injuries, 0.7 percent for chronic lower respiratory diseases, 0.8 percent for stroke, 2.3 percent for AD, 2.4 percent for diabetes, 5.9 percent for influenza and pneumonia, and 3.7 percent for suicide. The rate decreased by 2.1 percent for cancer. Rates for heart disease and kidney disease did not change significantly.

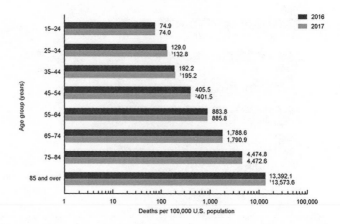

Figure 57.3. *Death Rates for Ages 15 Years and Over: The United States, 2016 and 2017.* (Source: National Center for Health Statistics (NCHS), National Vital Statistics System (NVSS), Mortality.)

[1]*Statistically significant increase in age-specific death rate from 2016 to 2017 (p < 0.05).*
[2]*Statistically significant decrease in age-specific death rate from 2016 to 2017 (p < 0.05).*
Note: Rates are plotted on a logarithmic scale.

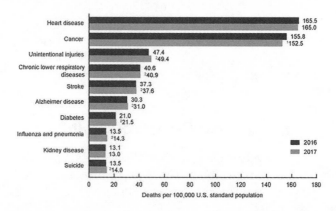

Figure 57.4. *Age-Adjusted Death Rates for the 10 Leading Causes of Death: The United States, 2016 and 2017.* (Source: National Center for Health Statistics (NCHS), National Vital Statistics System (NVSS), Mortality.)
[1]*Statistically significant decrease in age-adjusted death rate from 2016 to 2017 (p < 0.05). [2]Statistically significant increase in the age-adjusted death rate from 2016 to 2017 (p < 0.05).*
Note: A total of 2,813,503 resident deaths were registered in the United States in 2017. The 10 leading causes accounted for 74.0 percent of all deaths in the United States in 2017. Causes of death are ranked according to the number of deaths. Rankings for 2016 data are not shown. Data table for Figure 57.4 includes the number of deaths for leading causes.

What Are the Leading Causes of Infant Death?

The infant mortality rate (IMR)—the ratio of infant deaths to live births in a given year—is generally regarded as a good indicator of the overall health of a population. IMR changed from 587.0 infant deaths per 100,000 live births in 2016 to 579.3 in 2017, but this change was not statistically significant.

The 10 leading causes of infant death in 2017 accounted for 67.8 percent of all infant deaths in the United States. The leading causes remained the same as in 2016 although maternal complications became the third leading cause while sudden infant death syndrome became the fourth, and diseases of the circulatory system became the eighth leading cause while respiratory distress of newborn became the ninth. Causes of infant death are ranked according to the number of infant deaths. IMR for unintentional injuries increased by 10.7 percent from 30.9 infant deaths per 100,000 live births in 2016 to 34.2 in 2017. Mortality rates for other leading causes of infant death did not change significantly.

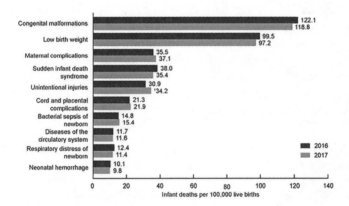

Figure 57.5. *Infant Mortality Rates for the 10 Leading Causes of Infant Death in 2017: The United States, 2016 and 2017.* (Source: National Center for Health Statistics (NCHS), National Vital Statistics System (NVSS), Mortality.)

[1]*Statistically significant increase in mortality rate from 2016 to 2017 ($p < 0.05$). Note: A total of 22,335 deaths occurred in children under age 1 year in the United States in 2017, with an infant mortality rate of 579.3 infant deaths per 100,000 live births. The 10 leading causes of infant death in 2017 accounted for 67.8 percent of all infant deaths in the United States. A total of 23,161 infant deaths occurred in 2016, with an infant mortality rate of 587.0 infant deaths per 100,000 live births. Causes of death are ranked according to the number of deaths. Rankings for 2016 data are not shown. Data table for Figure 57.5 includes the number of deaths under age 1 year for the leading causes of infant death.*

Summary

In 2017, a total of 2,813,503 resident deaths were registered in the United States—69,255 more deaths than in 2016. From 2016 to 2017, the age-adjusted death rate for the total population increased by 0.4 percent, and life expectancy at birth decreased by 0.1 years. Age-specific death rates between 2016 and 2017 increased for age groups 25 to 34, 35 to 44, and 85 and over, and decreased for age group 45 to 54. Age-adjusted death rates increased for non-Hispanic White males and non-Hispanic White females and decreased for non-Hispanic Black females.

The 10 leading causes of death in 2017 remained the same as in 2016. Age-adjusted death rates increased for seven leading causes and decreased for one. Life expectancy at birth decreased 0.1 years from 78.7 years in 2016 to 78.6 in 2017, largely because of increases in mortality from unintentional injuries, suicide, diabetes, and influenza and pneumonia, with unintentional injuries making the largest contribution.

In 2017, a total of 22,335 deaths occurred among children under age 1 year, which was 826 fewer infant deaths than in 2016. The leading causes of infant death were the same in 2017 and 2016 although maternal complications became the third leading cause while sudden infant death syndrome became the fourth, and diseases of the circulatory system became the eighth leading cause while respiratory distress of newborn became the ninth. The only significant change among the 10 leading causes of infant death was a 10.7 percent increase in infant mortality rate (IMR) for unintentional injuries.

Definitions
Cause of Death

Based on medical information—including injury diagnoses and external causes of injury—entered on death certificates filed in the United States. This information is classified and coded in accordance with the International Statistical Classification of Diseases (ICD) and Related Health Problems, Tenth Revision.

Death Rates

For 2017, based on population estimates for July 1, 2017, that is consistent with the April 1, 2010, census. These population estimates (as well as population figures for the 2010 census) are available on the National Center for Health Statistics' (NCHS) website. Age-adjusted death rates are useful when comparing different populations because they remove the potential bias that can occur when the populations being compared have different age structures. NCHS uses the direct method of standardization.

Infant Mortality Rate

Computed by dividing the number of infant deaths in a calendar year by the number of live births registered for that same time period. Infant mortality rate (IMR) is the most widely used index for measuring the risk of dying during the first year of life.

Leading Causes of Death

Ranked according to the number of deaths assigned to rankable causes.

Life Expectancy

The expected average number of years of life remaining at a given age. It is denoted by ex, which means the average number of subsequent years of life for someone now aged x. Life expectancy estimates for 2017 are based on a methodology first implemented with the 2008 final mortality data. Life expectancies for 2016 were revised using updated Medicare data; therefore, figures may differ from those previously published. Life expectancies for 2017 may change slightly when updated Medicare data become available.

Data Source and Methods

The data shown in this report reflect information collected by NCHS for 2016 and 2017 from death certificates filed in all 50 states and the District of Columbia (DC) and compiled into national data known as the "National Vital Statistics System" (NVSS). The standard presentation of life expectancy estimates is rounded to one decimal place. Changes in life expectancy, computed using figures rounded to one decimal, may slightly overestimate or underestimate the actual change. Changes in life expectancy from 2016 to 2017 using unrounded estimates were less than 0.1 years. Death rates shown in this report are calculated based on postcensal population estimates as of July 1, 2016, and July 1, 2017, which are consistent with the April 1, 2010, census. Differences between death rates were evaluated using a two-tailed z test.

Chapter 58

Leading Causes of Death in the United States

The 15 leading causes of death in 2017 accounted for 80 percent of all deaths in the United States. The leading causes of death in 2017 remained the same as in 2016, although chronic liver disease and cirrhosis, the 12th leading cause of death in 2016, became the 11th leading cause in 2017, and septicemia, the 11th leading cause of death in 2016, became the 12th leading cause in 2017. By rank, the 15 leading causes of death in 2017 were:

1. Diseases of heart (heart disease)

2. Malignant neoplasms (cancer)

3. Accidents (unintentional injuries)

4. Chronic lower respiratory diseases

5. Cerebrovascular diseases (stroke)

6. Alzheimer disease (AD)

7. Diabetes mellitus (diabetes)

8. Influenza and pneumonia

9. Nephritis, nephrotic syndrome and nephrosis (kidney disease)

This chapter includes text excerpted from "National Vital Statistics Reports," Centers for Disease Control and Prevention (CDC), June 24, 2019.

10. Intentional self-harm (suicide)

11. Chronic liver disease and cirrhosis

12. Septicemia

13. Essential hypertension and hypertensive renal disease (hypertension)

14. Parkinson disease (PD)

15. Pneumonitis due to solids and liquids

Death rates vary greatly by age. As a result, the shifting age distribution of a population can significantly influence changes in crude death rates over time. Age-adjusted death rates, in contrast, eliminate the influence of such differences in the population age structure. Therefore, whereas causes of death are ranked according to the number of deaths, age-adjusted death rates are used to depict trends for leading causes of death in this report because they are better than crude rates for showing changes in mortality over time and among causes of death.

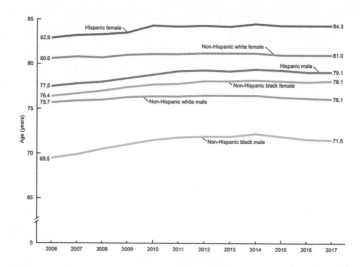

Figure 58.1. *Life Expectancy, by Race and Hispanic Origin and Sex: The United States, 2006–2017.* (Source: National Center for Health Statistics (NCHS), National Vital Statistics System, Mortality.)

From 2016 to 2017, age-adjusted death rates increased significantly for 10 of the 15 leading causes of death and decreased to 1 of the 15 leading causes. The rate for the top leading cause of death, heart disease, decreased 0.3 percent in 2017 from 2016, but this change was not significant. The rate for the second leading cause of death, cancer, decreased 2.1 percent, continuing a gradual but consistent downward trend since 1993. Deaths from these two diseases combined accounted for 44.3 percent of deaths in the United States in 2017.

Leading causes of death that showed significant increases in 2017 from 2016 were unintentional injuries (4.2%), chronic lower respiratory diseases (0.7%), stroke (0.8%), AD (2.3%), diabetes (2.4%), influenza and pneumonia (5.9%), suicide (3.7%), chronic liver disease and cirrhosis (1.9%), hypertension (4.7%), and PD (5.0%).

The observed changes from 2016 to 2017 in the age-adjusted death rates for heart disease, kidney disease, septicemia, and pneumonitis due to solids and liquids were not significant.

Assault (homicide), the 16th leading cause of death in 2017, dropped from among the 15 leading causes of death in 2010 but is still a major issue for some age groups. In 2017, the age-adjusted rate for homicide did not change. Homicide was among the 15 leading causes of death in 2017 for age groups under 1 year (13th), 1 to 4 (4th), 5 to 14 (5th), 15 to 24 (3rd), 25 to 34 (3rd), 35 to 44 (5th), and 45 to 54 (10th) (19).

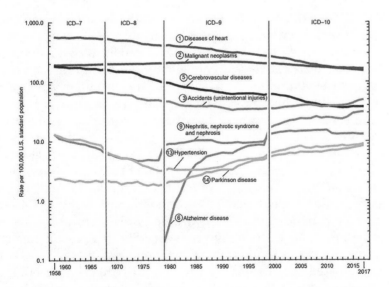

Figure 58.2. *Age-Adjusted Death Rates for Selected Leading Causes of Death: The United States, 1958–2017.* (Source: National Center for Health Statistics (NCHS), National Vital Statistics System (NVSS), Mortality.)

Notes: ICD is the International Classification of Diseases. Circled numbers indicate the ranking of conditions as the leading causes of death in 2017.

Although the human immunodeficiency virus (HIV) disease has not been among the 15 leading causes of death since 1997 (26), it is still considered a major public health problem for some age groups. Historically, for all ages combined, HIV disease mortality reached its highest level in 1995 after a period of increase from 1987 through 1994. Subsequently, the rate for this disease decreased an average of 33.0 percent per year from 1995 through 1998, and 6.4 percent per year from 1999 through 2017 (19,27). In 2017, HIV disease was among the 15 leading causes of death for age groups 15 to 24 (15th), 25 to 34 (9th), 35 to 44 (10th), 45 to 54 (14th), and 55 to 64 (14th).

Enterocolitis due to *Clostridium difficile* (*C. difficile*)—a predominantly antibiotic-associated inflammation of the intestines caused by *C. difficile*, a gram-positive, anaerobic, spore-forming bacillus—is of growing concern. The disease is often acquired in hospitals or other healthcare facilities with long-term patients or residents. The number of deaths from *C. difficile* climbed from 793 deaths in 1999 to a high of 8,085 deaths in 2011.

In 2017, the number of deaths from *C. difficile* was 6,118. In 2017, the age-adjusted death rate for this cause was 1.6 deaths per 100,000 U.S. standard population, a decrease of 11.1 percent from the rate in 2016 (1.8). In 2017, *C. difficile* ranked as the 19th leading cause of death for the population aged 65 and over. Approximately 87 percent of deaths from *C. difficile* occurred among people aged 65 and over.

The relative risk of death in one population group compared with another can be expressed as a ratio. Ratios based on age-adjusted death rates show that males have higher rates than females for 13 of the 15 leading causes of death, with rates for males being at least twice as great as those for females for 3 of these leading causes. The largest ratio was for suicide (3.7). Other large ratios were evident for PD (2.3), unintentional injuries (2.1), chronic liver disease and cirrhosis and pneumonitis due to solids and liquids (1.9 each), heart disease and diabetes (1.6 each), cancer and kidney disease (1.4 each), influenza and pneumonia (1.3), chronic lower respiratory diseases and septicemia (1.2 each), and hypertension (1.1). Age-adjusted rates were lower for males than for females for one leading cause, AD (0.7).

Age-adjusted death rates for the non-Hispanic Black population were higher than for the non-Hispanic White population for 8 of the 15 leading causes of death. The largest ratios were for kidney disease (2.2) and hypertension and diabetes (2.1 each). Other causes for which the ratio was high include septicemia (1.7), stroke (1.4), heart disease (1.2), and cancer and influenza and pneumonia (1.1 each). For six of the leading causes, age-adjusted rates were lower for the non-Hispanic

494

Black population than for the non-Hispanic White population. The smallest non-Hispanic Black-to-non-Hispanic White ratio was for suicide (0.4); that is, the risk of dying from suicide was more than two times greater for the non-Hispanic White population than for the non-Hispanic Black population.

Other conditions with a low non-Hispanic Black-to-non-Hispanic White ratio were PD (0.5), chronic lower respiratory diseases and chronic liver disease and cirrhosis (0.7 each), unintentional injuries (0.8), and AD (0.9).

Leading causes of death in 2017 for the total population and for specific subpopulations are further detailed in a companion National Vital Statistics Report (NVSR) on leading causes by age, race, Hispanic origin, and sex.

Age-adjusted death rates for the non-Hispanic White population were higher than for the Hispanic population for 11 of the 15 leading causes of death. The largest ratios were for chronic lower respiratory diseases (2.7) and suicide (2.6). Other causes for which the ratio was high include unintentional injuries and pneumonitis due to solids and liquids (1.7 each); heart disease, cancer, and PD (1.5 each); AD, influenza and pneumonia, and septicemia (1.3 each); and stroke (1.1). Age-adjusted rates were lower for the non-Hispanic White population than for the Hispanic population for diabetes (0.7) and chronic liver disease and cirrhosis (0.8).

Other Select Causes
Drug-Induced Mortality

In 2017, a total of 73,990 persons died of drug-induced causes in the United States. This category includes deaths from poisoning and medical conditions caused by the use of legal or illegal drugs, as well as deaths from poisoning due to medically prescribed and other drugs. It excludes deaths indirectly related to drug use, as well as newborn deaths due to the mother's drug use.

In 2017, the age-adjusted death rate for drug-induced causes for the total population increased significantly, by 9.6 percent from 20.8 in 2016 to 22.8 in 2017. For males in 2017, the age-adjusted death rate for drug-induced causes was 2.0 times the rate for females. The rate for drug-induced causes increased by 10.5 percent for males and 7.0 percent for females in 2017 from 2016. The age-adjusted death rate for non-Hispanic White males was 14.4 percent higher than for non-Hispanic Black males and 122.6 percent higher than for Hispanic males. The rate for non-Hispanic White females was 60.8 percent

495

higher than for non-Hispanic Black females and 265.5 percent higher than for Hispanic females.

Among the major race–ethnicity–sex groups, the age-adjusted death rates for drug-induced causes increased significantly in 2017 from 2016 for non-Hispanic White males (9.0%), non-Hispanic White females (7.5%), non-Hispanic Black males (22.9%), non-Hispanic Black females (14.7%), and Hispanic males (13.5%). The rate for Hispanic females did not change significantly.

Alcohol-Induced Mortality

In 2017, a total of 35,823 persons died of alcohol-induced causes in the United States. This category includes deaths from dependent and nondependent use of alcohol, as well as deaths from accidental poisoning by alcohol. It excludes unintentional injuries, homicides, and other causes indirectly related to alcohol use, as well as deaths due to fetal alcohol syndrome.

The age-adjusted death rate for alcohol-induced causes for the total, male, and female populations did not change significantly from 2016 to 2017. For males, the age-adjusted death rate for alcohol-induced causes in 2017 was 2.7 times the rate for females. The age-adjusted death rate for non-Hispanic White males was 35.8 percent higher than for non-Hispanic Black males and 12.4 percent lower than for Hispanic males. The rate for non-Hispanic White females was 69.4 percent higher than for non-Hispanic Black females and 74.3 percent higher than for Hispanic females.

Among the major race–ethnicity–sex groups, the age-adjusted rate for alcohol-induced death increased significantly in 2017 from 2016 for non-Hispanic White males (2.8%). The rates for non-Hispanic White females, non-Hispanic Black males, non-Hispanic Black females, Hispanic males, and Hispanic females did not change significantly.

Firearm-Related Mortality

In 2017, 39,773 persons died from firearm-related injuries in the United States. In 2017, the age-adjusted death rate for firearm-related injuries for the total population increased significantly, by 1.7 percent from 11.8 in 2016 to 12.0 in 2017. For males in 2017, the age-adjusted death rate for firearm-related injuries was 6.1 times the rate for females. The rate of firearm-related mortality increased by 2.0 percent for males from 2016 to 2017. The rate for females in 2017 was unchanged from 2016. The age-adjusted death rate for non-Hispanic White males was

54.9 percent lower than for non-Hispanic Black males and 73.9 percent higher than for Hispanic males. The rate for non-Hispanic White females was 15.6 percent lower than for non-Hispanic Black females and 111.1 percent higher than for Hispanic females.

Among the major race–ethnicity–sex groups, the age-adjusted death rates for firearm-related injuries increased significantly in 2017 from 2016 for non-Hispanic White males (3.2%). The rates for non-Hispanic White females, non-Hispanic Black males, non-Hispanic Black females, Hispanic males, and Hispanic females did not change significantly.

Chapter 59

Life Expectancy at Birth

Expectation of Life at Birth and at Specific Ages

Life expectancy at birth represents the average number of years that a group of infants would live if the group was to experience throughout life the age-specific death rates present in the year of birth.

The life table data are shown in this report for 2001 to 2017 are based on a revised methodology first presented with final data reported for 2008. The life table methodology was revised by changing the smoothing technique used to estimate the life table functions at the oldest ages.

The methods used to produce life expectancies by Hispanic origin are based on death rates adjusted for misclassification. In contrast, the age-specific and age-adjusted death rates shown in this report for the Hispanic population are not adjusted for misclassification of Hispanic origin. Thus, it shows Hispanic deaths and death rates as collected by the registration areas, and these match the deaths and death rates produced using the mortality data file.

Life tables were generated for both sexes and by each sex for the following populations:

- Total U.S. population

- Non-Hispanic White population

This chapter includes text excerpted from "National Vital Statistics Reports," Centers for Disease Control and Prevention (CDC), June 24, 2019.

• Non-Hispanic Black population

• Hispanic population

In 2017, life expectancy at birth for the U.S. population was 78.6 years, 0.1 years lower than in 2016. The general trend in U.S. life expectancy since 1900 has been one of improvement. However, decreases in life expectancy occurred in 2015 and 2017, and these were the only decreases in the last 20 years. In 2017, life expectancy for males (76.1 years) was 0.1 years lower than in 2016. Life expectancy for females (81.1 years) was the same as in 2016. From 1900 through the late 1970s, the gap in life expectancy between the sexes widened from 2.0 to 7.8 years. The gap between sexes has narrowed since its peak in the 1970s. In 2017, the difference in life expectancy between the sexes increased for the second consecutive year to 5.0 years, a 0.1-year increase from 4.9 years in 2016.

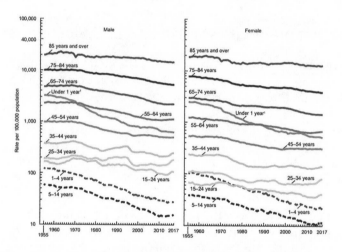

Figure 59.1. *Death Rates, by Age and Sex: The United States, 1955–2017.* (Source: National Center for Health Statistics (NCHS), National Vital Statistics System (NVSS), Mortality.)
[1]Rates are based on population estimates which differ from infant mortality rates (based on live births).

Life expectancy figures by Hispanic origin have been available starting with data for 2006. Life expectancy decreased by 0.1 years for the non-Hispanic White population (from 78.6 years in 2016 to 78.5 in 2017). Life expectancy for the non-Hispanic Black population in 2017 (74.9) was the same as in 2016. The difference in life expectancy between the non-Hispanic White and non-Hispanic Black populations decreased by 0.1 years, from 3.7 years in 2016 to 3.6 years in 2017. The non-Hispanic White–non-Hispanic Black gap generally narrowed from 2006 to 2014 but widened in 2015 and 2016 before decreasing in 2017. Life expectancy for the Hispanic population (81.8) was the same as in 2016. Life expectancy was 1.5 years higher in 2017 compared with 2006. The difference in life expectancy between the Hispanic and non-Hispanic White populations was 3.3 years in 2017, an increase of 0.1 years from 2016, but the same as in 2014 and 2015. Prior to 2014, the non-Hispanic White–Hispanic gap was widening gradually.

Among the six Hispanic origin–race–sex groups in 2017, Hispanic females had the highest life expectancy at birth (84.3 years), followed by non-Hispanic White females (81.0), Hispanic males (79.1), non-Hispanic Black females (78.1), non-Hispanic White males (76.1), and non-Hispanic Black males (71.5).

Life expectancy for two of the six Hispanic-origin–race–sex groups decreased in 2017 from 2016. Life expectancy decreased to 0.1 years for both non-Hispanic White males and non-Hispanic Black males. Life expectancy for non-Hispanic Black females increased by 0.1 years. Life expectancy for non-Hispanic White females and Hispanic males and females was unchanged.

Life expectancy for both males and females was higher by three years or more for the Hispanic population than for the nonHispanic White and non-Hispanic Black populations. Various hypotheses have been proposed to explain favorable mortality outcomes among Hispanic persons. The most prevalent hypotheses are the healthy migrant effect, which argues that Hispanic immigrants are selected for their good health and robustness; the "salmon bias" effect, which posits that U.S. residents of Hispanic origin may return to their country of origin to die or when ill; and the "cultural effect," which argues that culturally influenced family structure, lifestyle behaviors, and social networks may confer a protective barrier against the negative effects of low socioeconomic and minority status.

Life tables shown in this report may be used to compare life expectancies at selected ages from birth to 100 years. For example, on the basis of mortality experienced in 2017, a person aged 50 could expect to live an average of 31.6 more years, for a total of 81.6 years. A person aged 65 could expect to live an average of 19.4 more years, for a total of 84.4 years, and a person aged 85 could expect to live an average of 6.6 more years, for a total of 91.6 years. While life expectancy at some ages decreased from 2016 to 2017 (at ages 90 and 95), life expectancy increased at ages 55 and 75.

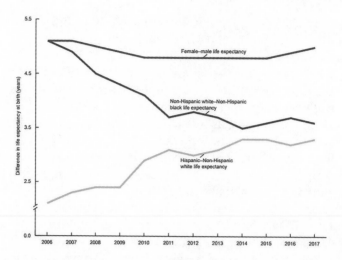

Figure 59.2. *Differences in Female-Male, Non-Hispanic White–Non-Hispanic Black, and Hispanic–Non-Hispanic White Life Expectancy: The United States, 2006–2017.* (Source: National Center for Health Statistics (NCHS), National Vital Statistics System (NVSS), Mortality.)

Chapter 60

Infant and Maternal Mortality Trends and Disparities

Trends in Infant Mortality and Infant Age at Death

- In 2017, there were 22,341 infant deaths reported in the United States; the U.S. infant mortality rate was 5.79 deaths per 1,000 live births, not statistically different from the rate of 5.87 in 2016.

- The U.S. infant mortality rate has generally trended downward since 1995 (the first year the linked birth/infant death file has been available) and has declined 16 percent since 2005, the most recent high (6.86).

- The 2017 neonatal mortality rate (infant deaths at less than 28 days) was 3.85, not significantly different from the rate in 2016 (3.88); the neonatal mortality rate has generally declined since 1995 and is down 15 percent since 2005 (4.54).

- The 2017 postneonatal mortality rate (infant deaths at 28 days or greater) was 1.94, not statistically different from the postneonatal mortality rate in 2016 (1.99); the postneonatal mortality rate has also generally declined since 1995 and is down 16 percent since 2005 (2.32).

This chapter includes text excerpted from "National Vital Statistics Reports," Centers for Disease Control and Prevention (CDC), August 1, 2019.

Race and Hispanic Origin

• In 2017, infant mortality continues to vary by race; infants of non-Hispanic Black women had the highest mortality rate (10.97 infant deaths per 1,000 births), followed by infants of non-Hispanic AIAN (9.21), non-Hispanic NHOPI (7.64), Hispanic (5.10), non-Hispanic White (4.67), and nonHispanic Asian (3.78) women).

• Infants of non-Hispanic Black women also had the highest neonatal mortality rate in 2017 (7.16) compared with infants of the other race and Hispanic-origin groups; the lowest neonatal mortality rate was for infants of non-Hispanic Asian women (2.71).

• In 2017, postneonatal mortality rates were higher for infants of non-Hispanic Black (3.82), non-Hispanic NHOPI (3.82), and non-Hispanic AIAN (4.41) women than for infants of Hispanic (1.54), non-Hispanic White (1.63), and nonHispanic Asian (1.08) women; infants of non-Hispanic Asian women had the lowest postneonatal mortality rate.

• Among Hispanic-origin subgroups in 2017, infants of Puerto Rican women had the highest infant mortality rate (6.48), followed by infants of Mexican (5.05), Central and South American (4.48), and Cuban (3.98) women.

Maternal Age

• Mortality rates were highest for infants of women under age 20 (9.01 infant deaths per 1,000 births), decreased through infants of women aged 30 to 34 (4.76), and then increased among infants born to older mothers (5.35 and 6.97 for women aged 35 to 39 and 40 and over, respectively).

• Mortality rates for infants of women under age 20 were 89 percent higher than those for infants of women aged 30 to 34, the group with the lowest rates.

State

• By state, infant mortality ranged from a low of 3.66 infant deaths per 1,000 births in Massachusetts to a high of 8.73 in Mississippi.

• Eleven states had infant mortality rates significantly lower than the national infant mortality rate of 5.79: California,

Colorado, Connecticut, Idaho, Massachusetts, Minnesota, New Hampshire, New Jersey, New York, North Dakota, and Washington.

- Fifteen states and the District of Columbia had infant mortality rates significantly higher than the U.S. infant mortality rate: Alabama, Arkansas, Georgia, Indiana, Kentucky, Louisiana, Maryland, Michigan, Mississippi, North Carolina, Ohio, Oklahoma, South Carolina, South Dakota, and Tennessee.

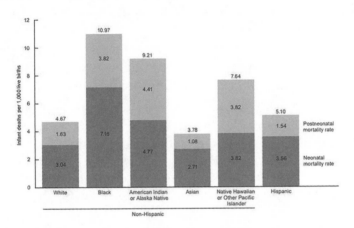

Figure 60.1. *Infant, Neonatal, and Postneonatal Mortality Rates, by Race and Hispanic Origin: The United States, 2017* (Source: National Center for Health Statistics (NCHS), National Vital Statistics System (NVSS), Linked Birth/Infant Death File.)
Note: Neonatal and postneonatal rates may not add to the total infant mortality rate due to rounding.

Gestational Age

- In 2017, 67 percent of infant deaths were to infants born preterm (less than 37 weeks of gestation).

- Infant mortality rates were highest for infants born before 28 weeks of gestation (384.39 infant deaths per 1,000 births), rates declined through 41 weeks (1.51), and then increased at 42 weeks or more (3.98).

- In 2017, the mortality rate for infants born before 28 weeks of gestation was 183 times the rate for term infants (37–41 weeks of gestation) (2.10).

Leading Causes of Infant Death

• In 2017, the five leading causes of all infant deaths were congenital malformations (21% of infant deaths), disorders related to short gestation and low birth weight (17%), maternal complications (6%), sudden infant death syndrome (SIDS) (6%), and unintentional injuries (6%).

• In 2017, mortality rates for the five leading causes of infant death were 119.2 infant deaths per 100,000 births for congenital malformations, 97.4 for disorders related to short gestation and low birthweight, 37.2 for maternal complications, 35.3 for SIDS, and 34.1 for unintentional injuries.

• From 2016 through 2017, infant mortality rates for SIDS declined (38.0 infant deaths per 100,000 live births to 35.3), whereas rates for unintentional injuries increased (30.8 to 34.1).

• The five leading causes of death by race and Hispanic origin and Hispanic subgroup were the same as for all infants except for non-Hispanic Asian and Central and South American infants. Infants of non-Hispanic Black women had the highest mortality rates for disorders related to short gestation and low birth weight (241.5) and maternal complications (83.3).

• Infants of non-Hispanic Asian women had the lowest mortality rates of all race and Hispanic-origin groups for congenital malformations (84.7) and unintentional injuries (10.0). Infants of non-Hispanic White women had the lowest mortality rates for maternal complications (23.6); infants of non-Hispanic White and non-Hispanic Asian women had the lowest mortality rates for low birth weight (63.2 and 65.0, respectively).

Table 60.1. Infant Mortality Rate, by Gestational Age: The United States, 2015–2017.

Year	Less than 32 Weeks	32 to 33 Weeks	34 to 36 Weeks	37 to 41 Weeks	42 Weeks or More
Deaths per 1,000 Live Births					
2017	187.56	20.5	8.5	2.1	3.98
2016	190.15	20.12	8.65	2.19	4.31
2015	193.54	20.79	8.76	2.17	4.2

(Source: National Center for Health Statistics (NCHS), National Vital Statistics System (NVSS), Linked Birth/Infant Death File.)

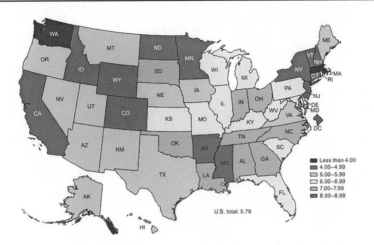

Figure 60.2. *Infant Mortality Rates, by State: The United States, 2017.*
(Source: National Center for Health Statistics (NCHS), National Vital
Statistics System (NVSS), Linked Birth/Infant Death File.)

Preterm-Related Causes of Death

- In 2017, 7,675 out of 22,341 infant deaths (34%) in the United
  States were preterm-related, unchanged from 2016 (34%).

- The total preterm-related infant mortality rate was 199.1
  infant deaths per 100,000 live births in 2017, which was
  not statistically different from the 2016 rate (201.6); the
  preterm-related infant mortality rate declined 8 percent from
  2010 (216.3) through 2017.

- In 2017, 41 percent of deaths for infants of non-Hispanic Black
  women and 44 percent of deaths for infants of Cuban women
  were due to preterm-related causes; the percentage of infant
  deaths due to preterm-related causes was lowest for infants of
  non-Hispanic AIAN (26%), non-Hispanic NHOPI (28%), and
  non-Hispanic White (29%) women.

- The preterm-related infant mortality rate for non-Hispanic
  Black women (454.1) was more than three times as high as that
  for non-Hispanic White women (135.1).

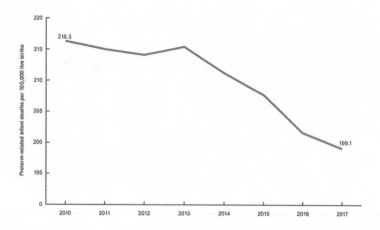

Figure 60.3. *Preterm-Related Cause of Death Infant Mortality Rate: The United States, 2010–2017.* (Source: National Center for Health Statistics (NCHS), National Vital Statistics System (NVSS), Linked Birth/Infant Death File)

Note: A cause of death was considered preterm-related if 75 percent or more of infants whose deaths were attributed to that cause were born at under 37 weeks of gestation, and the cause of death was a direct consequence of preterm birth.

Table 60.2. Percentages and Rates for Preterm-Related Infant Deaths: United States, 2010–2017 Percentages and Rates for Preterm-Related Infant Deaths: United States, 2010–2017.

Year	Percent	Deaths per 100,000 live births
2017	34.4	199.1
2016	34.4	201.6
2015	35.2	207.7
2014	36.3	211.2
2013	36.1	215.4
2012	35.8	214.1
2011	35.4	215
2010	35.2	216.3

Source: National Center for Health Statistics (NCHS), National Vital Statistics System (NVSS), Linked Birth/Infant Death File.)

Chapter 61

Work-Related Fatalities

There were a total of 5,147 fatal work injuries recorded in the United States in 2017, down slightly from the 5,190 fatal injuries reported in 2016, as reported by the U.S. Bureau of Labor Statistics. The fatal injury rate decreased to 3.5 per 100,000 full-time equivalents (FTE) workers from 3.6 in 2016.

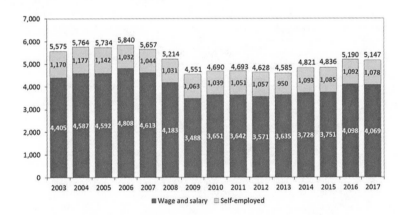

Figure 61.1. *Number of Fatal Work Injuries by Employee Status, 2013–2017.*

This chapter includes text excerpted from "National Census of Fatal Occupational Injuries in 2017," U.S. Bureau of Labor Statistics (BLS), U.S. Department of Labor (DOL), December 18, 2018.

Type of Incident

Fatal falls were at their highest level in the 26-year history of the Census of Fatal Occupational Injuries (CFOI) accounting for 887 (17%) worker deaths. Transportation incidents remained the most frequent fatal event in 2017 with 2,077 (40%) occupational fatalities. Violence and other injuries by persons or animals decreased 7 percent in 2017 with homicides and suicides decreasing by 8 percent and 5 percent, respectively.

- Unintentional overdoses due to nonmedical use of drugs or alcohol while at work increased 25 percent from 217 in 2016 to 272 in 2017. This was the fifth consecutive year in which unintentional workplace overdose deaths have increased by at least 25 percent.

- Contact with objects and equipment incidents were down 9 percent (695 in 2017 from 761 in 2016) with caught in running equipment or machinery deaths down 26 percent (76 in 2017 from 103 in 2016).

- Fatal occupational injuries involving confined spaces rose 15 percent to 166 in 2017 from 144 in 2016.

- Crane-related workplace fatalities fell to their lowest level ever recorded in CFOI, 33 deaths in 2017.

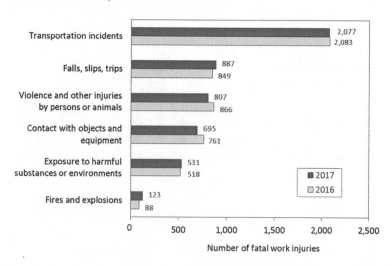

Figure 61.2. *Number of Fatal Work Injuries by Major Event, 2016–2017.*

Occupation

The transportation and material moving the occupational group and the construction and extraction occupational group accounted for 47 percent of worker deaths in 2017. Within the occupational subgroup driver/sales workers and truck drivers, heavy and tractor-trailer truck drivers had the largest number of fatal occupational injuries with 840. This represented the highest value for heavy and tractor-trailer truck drivers since the occupational series began in 2003. Fishers and related fishing workers and logging workers had the highest published rates of fatal injury in 2017.

* Grounds maintenance workers (including first-line supervisors) incurred 244 fatalities in 2017. This was a small decrease from the 2016 figure but was still the second-highest total since 2003. A total of 36 deaths were due to falls from trees, and another 35 were due to being struck by a falling tree or branch.

* There were 258 fatalities among farmers, ranchers, and other agricultural managers in 2017. Approximately 63 percent of these farmers were age 65 and over with 48 being age 80 or over. Of the 258 deaths, 103 involved a farm tractor.

* Police and sheriff's patrol officers incurred 95 fatal occupational injuries in 2017, fewer than the 108 fatalities in 2016.

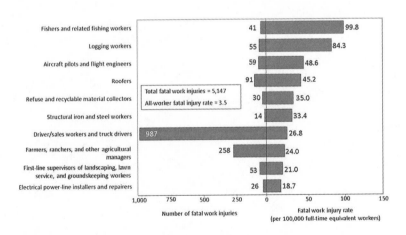

Figure 61.3. *Civilian Occupation with High Fatal Work Injury Rates, 2017*

Other Key Findings of the 2017 Census of Fatal Occupational Injuries

- 15 percent of the fatally-injured workers in 2017 were age 65 or over—a series high. In 1992, the first year CFOI published national data, that figure was 8 percent. These workers also had a higher fatality rate than other age groups in 2017.

- Fatalities incurred by non-Hispanic Black or African American workers and non-Hispanic Asian workers each decreased 10 percent from 2016 to 2017.

- Fatal occupational injuries in the private manufacturing industry and wholesale trade industry were the lowest since this series began in 2003.

- Workplace fatalities in the private mining, quarrying, and oil and gas extraction industry increased 26 percent to 112 in 2017 from a series low of 89 in 2016. Over 70 percent of these fatalities were incurred by workers in the oil and gas extraction industries.

- A total of 27 states had fewer fatal workplace injuries in 2017 than 2016, while 21 states and the District of Columbia (DC) had more; California and Maine had the same number as 2016. A total of 192 metropolitan statistical areas (MSAs) had five or more fatal work injuries in 2017.

Chapter 62

Childhood Risk of Injury-Related Death

Unintentional injuries—such as those caused by burns, drowning, falls, poisoning, and road traffic—are the leading cause of morbidity and mortality among children in the United States. Each year, among those 0 to 19 years of age, more than 12,000 people die from unintentional injuries and more than 9.2 million are treated in emergency departments (EDs) for nonfatal injuries.

The Centers for Disease Control and Prevention (CDC) Childhood Injury Report: Patterns of Unintentional Injuries among 0 to 19-Year-Olds in the United States, uses data from the National Vital Statistics Systems (NVSS) and the National Electronic Injury Surveillance System (NEISS)—All Injury Program to provide an overview of unintentional injuries related to drowning, falls, fires or burns, poisoning, suffocation, and transportation-related injuries among others. Results are presented by age group and sex, as well as the geographic distribution of injury death rates by state.

Key findings from the report include the following:

Injury Deaths

- On average, 12,175 children 0 to 19 years of age died each year in the United States from an unintentional injury.

This chapter includes text excerpted from "CDC Childhood Injury Report," Centers for Disease Control and Prevention (CDC), February 6, 2019.

- Males had higher injury death rates than females.

  - The death rate for males was almost two times the rate for females, and males had a higher injury death rate compared to females in all childhood age groups.

- Injuries due to transportation were the leading cause of death for children.

  - The highest death rates were among occupants of motor vehicles in traffic.

  - There were also a substantial number of pedestrian and pedal cyclist deaths among children.

- Combining all unintentional injury deaths among those between 0 and 19 years, motor vehicle traffic-related deaths were the leading cause.

- The leading causes of injury death differed by age group.

  - For children less than 1 year of age, two-thirds of injury deaths were due to suffocation.

  - Drowning was the leading cause of injury death for those 1 to 4 years of age.

  - For children 5 to 19 years of age, the most injury deaths were due to being an occupant in a motor vehicle traffic crash.

- The risk of injury death varied by race.

  - Injury death rates were highest for American Indian and Alaska Natives and were lowest for Asian or Pacific Islanders.

  - Overall death rates for Whites and African Americans were approximately the same.

- Injury death rates varied by state depending upon the cause of death.

  - Overall, states with the lowest injury death rates were in the northeast. Fire and burn death rates were highest in some of the southern states.

  - Death rates from transportation-related injuries were highest in some southern states and some states of the upper plains, while lowest rates occurred in states in the northeast region.

- For injury causes with an overall low burden, death rates greatly varied by age.

  - The poisoning death rate for those older than 15 years of age was at least five times the rates of the younger age groups, and the suffocation death rate for infants was over 16 times the rates for all older age groups.

Nonfatal Injuries

- An estimated 9.2 million children annually had an initial emergency department visit for an unintentional injury.

- Males generally had higher nonfatal injury rates than females.

  - For children 1 to 19 years of age, nonfatal injury rates were higher among males than females, while the rates were approximately the same for those under one year.

- Injuries due to falls were the leading cause of nonfatal injury.

  - Each year, approximately 2.8 million children had an initial emergency department visit for injuries from a fall.

  - For children, less than one year of age falls accounted for over 50 percent of nonfatal injuries.

- The majority of nonfatal injuries are from five causes.

  - Falls were the leading cause of nonfatal injury for all age groups of less than 15.

  - For children ages 0 to 9, the next two leading causes were being struck by or against an object and animal bites or insect stings.

  - For children 10 to 14 years of age, the next leading causes were being struck by or against an object and overexertion.

  - For children 15 to 19 years of age, the three leading causes of nonfatal injuries were being struck by or against an object, falls, and motor vehicle occupant injuries.

- Nonfatal injury rates varied by age group.

  - Nonfatal suffocation rates were highest for those less than 1 year of age.

  - Rates for fires or burns and drowning were highest for children 4 years and younger.

- Children 1 to 4 years of age had the highest rates of nonfatal falls and poisoning.

- Injury rates related to motor vehicles was highest in children 15 to 19 years of age.

Chapter 63

Suicide Facts and Statistics

Suicide

- Suicide was the tenth leading cause of death for all ages in 2013.

- There were 41,149 suicides in 2013 in the United States—a rate of 12.6 per 100,000 is equal to 113 suicides each day or one every 13 minutes.

- Based on data about suicides in 16 National Violent Death Reporting System (NVDRS) states in 2010, 33.4 percent of suicide decedents tested positive for alcohol, 23.8 percent for antidepressants, and 20 percent for opiates, including heroin and prescription pain killers.

- Suicide results in an estimated $51 billion in combined medical and work loss costs.

Nonfatal Suicidal Thoughts and Behavior

- Among adults aged ≥18 years in the United States during 2013:

  - An estimated 9.3 million adults (3.9% of the adult U.S. population) reported having suicidal thoughts in the past year.

This chapter includes text excerpted from "Suicide—Facts at a Glance," Centers for Disease Control and Prevention (CDC), 2015. Reviewed September 2019.

- The percentage of adults having serious thoughts about suicide was highest among adults aged 18 to 25 (7.4%), followed by adults aged 26 to 49 (4%), then by adults aged 50 or older (2.7%).

- An estimated 2.7 million people (1.1%) made a plan about how they would attempt suicide in the past year.

- The percentage of adults who made a suicide plan in the past year was higher among adults aged 18 to 25 (2.5%) than among adults aged 26 to 49 (1.35%) and those aged 50 or older (0.6%).

- An estimated 1.3 million adults aged 18 or older (0.6%) attempted suicide in the past year. Among these adults who attempted suicide, 1.1 million also reported making suicide plans (0.2 million did not make suicide plans).

- Among students in grades 9 to 12 in the United States during 2013:

  - 17 percent of students seriously considered attempting suicide in the previous 12 months (22.4% of females and 11.6% of males).

  - 13.6 percent of students made a plan about how they would attempt suicide in the previous 12 months (16.9% of females and 10.3% of males).

  - 8 percent of the students attempted suicide one or more times in the previous 12 months (10.6% of females and 5.4% of males).

  - 2.7 percent of students made a suicide attempt that resulted in an injury, poisoning, or an overdose that required medical attention (3.6% of females and 1.8% of males).

Gender Disparities

- Males take their own lives at nearly four times the rate of females and represent 77.9 percent of all suicides.

- Females are more likely than males to have suicidal thoughts.

- Suicide is the seventh leading cause of death for males and the fourteenth leading cause for females.

- Firearms are the most commonly used method of suicide among males (56.9%).

• Poisoning is the most common method of suicide for females (34.8%).

Racial and Ethnic Disparities

• Suicide is the eighth leading cause of death among American Indians/Alaska Natives across all ages.

• Among American Indians/Alaska Natives aged 10 to 34 years, suicide is the second leading cause of death.

• The suicide rate among American Indian/Alaska Native adolescents and young adults ages 15 to 34 (19.5 per 100,000) is 1.5 times higher than the national average for that age group (12.9 per 100,000).

• The percentages of adults aged 18 or older having suicidal thoughts in the previous 12 months were 2.9 percent among Blacks, 3.3 percent among Asians, 3.6 percent among Hispanics, 4.1 percent among Whites, 4.6 percent among Native Hawaiians /Other Pacific Islanders, 4.8 percent among American Indians/ Alaska Natives, and 7.9 percent among adults reporting two or more races.

• Among Hispanic students in grades 9-12, the prevalence of having seriously considered attempting suicide (18.9%), having made a plan about how they would attempt suicide (15.7%), having attempted suicide (11.3%), and having made a suicide attempt that resulted in an injury, poisoning, or overdose that required medical attention (4.1%) was consistently higher than White and Black students.

Age Group Differences

• Suicide is the third leading cause of death among persons aged 10 to 14, the second among persons aged 15 to 34 years, the fourth among persons aged 35 to 44 years, the fifth among persons aged 45 to 54 years, the eighth among persons 55 to 64 years, and the seventeenth among persons 65 years and older.

• In 2011, middle-aged adults accounted for the largest proportion of suicides (56%), and from 1999 to 2010, the suicide rate among this group increased by nearly 30 percent.

519

- Among adults aged 18 to 22 years, similar percentages of full-time college students and other adults in this age group had suicidal thoughts (8 and 8.7%, respectively) or made suicide plans (2.4 and 3.1%).

- Full-time college students aged 18 to 22 years were less likely to attempt suicide (0.9 versus 1.9%) or receive medical attention as a result of a suicide attempt in the previous 12 months (0.3 versus 0.7%).

Nonfatal, Self-Inflicted Injuries

- In 2013, 494,169 people were treated in emergency departments for self-inflicted injuries.

- Nonfatal, self-inflicted injuries (including hospitalized and emergency department treated and released) resulted in an estimated $10.4 billion in combined medical and work loss costs.

Chapter 64

Alcohol-Attributable Deaths

Alcohol Use in the United States

* Prevalence of drinking

  * According to the 2015 National Survey on Drug Use and Health (NSDUH), 86.4 percent of people ages 18 or older reported that they drank alcohol at some point in their lifetime; 70.1 percent reported that they drank in the past year; 56 percent reported that they drank in the past month.

* Prevalence of binge drinking and heavy alcohol use

  * In 2015, 26.9 percent of people ages 18 or older reported that they engaged in binge drinking in the past month; 7 percent reported that they engaged in heavy alcohol use in the past month.

Alcohol-Use Disorder in the United States

* Adults (ages 18+)

* According to the 2015 NSDUH, 15.1 million adults ages 18 and older (6.2% of this age group) had alcohol-use disorder (AUD). This includes 9.8 million men (8.4% of men in this age group) and 5.3 million women (4.2% of women in this age group)

This chapter includes text excerpted from "Alcohol Facts and Statistics," National Institute on Alcohol Abuse and Alcoholism (NIAAA), August 2018.

- About 6.7 percent of adults who had AUD in the past year received treatment. This includes 7.4 percent of males and 5.4 percent of females with AUD in this age group.

- Youth (ages 12 to 17)

- According to the 2015 NSDUH, an estimated 623,000 adolescents ages 12 to 17 (2.5% of this age group) had AUD. This number includes 298,000 males (2.3% of males in this age group) and 325,000 females (2.7% of females in this age group). About 5.2 percent of youth who had AUD in the past year received treatment. This includes 5.1 percent of males and 5.3 percent of females with AUD in this age group.

Alcohol-Related Deaths

- An estimated 88,0008 people (approximately 62,000 men and 26,000 women) die from alcohol-related causes annually, making alcohol the third leading preventable cause of death in the United States. The first is tobacco, and the second is poor diet and physical inactivity.

- In 2014, alcohol-impaired driving fatalities accounted for 9,967 deaths (31% of overall driving fatalities).

Economic Burden

- In 2010, alcohol misuse cost the United States $249 billion.

- Three-quarters of the total cost of alcohol misuse is related to binge drinking.

Global Burden

- In 2012, 3.3 million deaths, or 5.9 percent of all global deaths (7.6% for men and 4.1% for women), were attributable to alcohol consumption.

- In 2014, the World Health Organization (WHO) reported that alcohol contributed to more than 200 diseases and injury-related health conditions, most notably DSM-full time alcohol dependence, liver cirrhosis, cancers, and injuries. In 2012, 5.1 percent of the burden of disease and injury worldwide (139 million disability-adjusted life-years) was attributable to alcohol consumption.

- Globally, alcohol misuse was the fifth leading risk factor for premature death and disability in 2010. Among people between the ages of 15 and 49, it is the first. In the age group 20 to 39 years, approximately 25 percent of the total deaths are alcohol-attributable.

Family Consequences

- More than 10 percent of U.S. children live with a parent with alcohol problems, according to a 2012 study.

Underage Drinking

- Prevalence of underage alcohol use

  - **Prevalence of drinking:** According to the 2015 NSDUH, 33.1 percent of 15-year-olds report that they have had at least 1 drink in their lives. About 7.7 million people ages 12 to 20 (20.3% of this age group) reported drinking alcohol in the past month (19.8% of males and 20.8% of females).

  - **Prevalence of binge drinking:** According to the 2015 NSDUH, approximately 5.1 million people (about 13.4%) ages 12 to 20 (13.4% of males and 13.3% of females) reported binge drinking in the past month.

  - **Prevalence of heavy alcohol use:** According to the 2015 NSDUH, approximately 1.3 million people (about 3.3%) ages 12 to 20 (3.6% of males and 3% of females) reported heavy alcohol use in the past month.

- Consequences of underage alcohol use

  - Research indicates that alcohol use during the teenage years could interfere with normal adolescent brain development and increase the risk of developing AUD. In addition, underage drinking contributes to a range of acute consequences, including injuries, sexual assaults, and even deaths— including those from car crashes.

Alcohol and College Student

- Prevalence of alcohol use

  - **Prevalence of drinking:** According to the 2015 NSDUH, 58 percent of full-time college students ages 18 to 22 drank alcohol in the past month compared with 48.2 percent of other persons of the same age.

- **Prevalence of binge drinking:** According to the 2015 NSDUH, 37.9 percent of college students ages 18 to 22 reported binge drinking in the past month compared with 32.6 percent of other persons of the same age.

- **Prevalence of heavy alcohol use:** According to the 2015 NSDUH, 12.5 percent of college students ages 18 to 22 reported heavy alcohol use in the past month compared with 8.5 percent of other persons of the same age.

- Consequences—researchers estimate that each year:
  - 1,825 college students between the ages of 18 and 24 die from alcohol-related unintentional injuries, including motor-vehicle crashes.
  - 696,000 students between the ages of 18 and 24 are assaulted by another student who has been drinking.
  - 97,000 students between the ages of 18 and 24 report experiencing alcohol-related sexual assault or date rape.
  - Roughly 20 percent of college students meet the criteria for AUD.
  - About 1 in 4 college students report academic consequences from drinking, including missing class, falling behind in class, doing poorly on exams or papers, and receiving lower grades overall.

Alcohol and Pregnancy

- The prevalence of fetal alcohol syndrome (FAS) in the United States was estimated by the Institute of Medicine (IOM) in 1996 to be between 0.5 and 3 cases per 1,000.

- More reports from specific U.S. sites report the prevalence of FAS to be 2 to 7 cases per 1,000, and the prevalence of fetal alcohol spectrum disorders (FASD) to be as high as 20 to 50 cases per 1,000.

Alcohol and the Human Body

- In 2015, of the 78,529 liver disease deaths among individuals ages 12 and older, 47 percent involved alcohol. Among males,

49,695 liver disease deaths occurred and 49.5 percent involved alcohol. Among females, 28,834 liver disease deaths occurred and 43.5 percent involved alcohol.

- Among all cirrhosis deaths in 2013, 47.9 percent were alcohol-related. The proportion of alcohol-related cirrhosis was highest (76.5%) among deaths of a person aged 25 to 34, followed by deaths of a person aged 35 to 44, at 70 percent.

- In 2009, alcohol-related liver disease was the primary cause of almost 1 in 3 liver transplants in the United States.

- Drinking alcohol increases the risk of cancers of the mouth, esophagus, pharynx, larynx, liver, and breast.

Chapter 65

Deaths from Stroke

Stroke Statistics

- Stroke kills about 140,000 Americans each year—that's 1 out of every 20 deaths.

- Someone in the United States has a stroke every 40 seconds. Every 4 minutes, someone dies of a stroke.

- Every year, more than 795,000 people in the United States have a stroke. About 610,000 of these are first or new strokes.

- About 185,000 strokes—nearly 1 of 4—are in people who have had a previous stroke.

- About 87 percent of all strokes are ischemic strokes, in which blood flow to the brain is blocked.

- Stroke costs the United States an estimated $34 billion each year. This total includes the cost of healthcare services, medicines to treat stroke, and missed days of work.

- Stroke is a leading cause of serious long-term disability. Stroke reduces mobility in more than half of stroke survivors age 65 and over.

This chapter includes text excerpted from "Stroke Facts," Centers for Disease Control and Prevention (CDC), September 6, 2017.

Stroke Statistics by Race and Ethnicity

- Stroke is the fifth leading cause of death for Americans, but the risk of having a stroke varies with race and ethnicity.

- The risk of having a first stroke is nearly twice as high for blacks as for Whites and Blacks have the highest rate of death due to stroke.

- Though stroke death rates have declined for decades among all races/ethnicities, Hispanics have seen an increase in death rates since 2013.

Stroke Risk Varies by Age

- Stroke risk increases with age, but strokes can—and do—occur at any age.

- In 2009, 34 percent of people hospitalized for stroke were less than 65 years old.

Early Action Is Important for Stroke

Know the warning signs and symptoms of stroke so that you can act fast if you or someone you know might be having a stroke. The chances of survival are greater when emergency treatment begins quickly.

- In one survey, most respondents—93 percent—recognized sudden numbness on one side as a symptom of stroke. Only 38 percent were aware of all major symptoms and knew to call 9-1-1 when someone was having a stroke.

- Patients who arrive at the emergency room within 3 hours of their first symptoms often have less disability three months after a stroke than those who received delayed care.

Americans at Risk for Stroke

High blood pressure, high cholesterol, smoking, obesity, and diabetes are leading causes of stroke. One in three U.S. adults has at least one of these conditions or habits.

Part Ten

Additional Help and Information

Chapter 66

Glossary of End-of-Life Terms

accelerated death benefit (ADB): A life insurance policy feature that lets you use some of the policy's death benefit prior to death.

activities of daily living (ADLs): Basic actions that independently functioning individuals perform on a daily basis.

acute care: Recovery is the primary goal of acute care. Physician, nurse, or other skilled professional services are typically required and usually provided in a doctor's office or hospital. Acute care is usually short term.

adult day services (ADS): Services provided during the day at a community-based center. Programs address the individual needs of functionally or cognitively impaired adults. These structured, comprehensive programs provide social and support services in a protective setting during any part of a day, but not 24-hour care. Many adult day service programs include health-related services.

advanced directive: Legal document that specifies whether you would like to be kept on artificial life support if you become permanently unconscious or are otherwise dying and unable to speak for yourself. It also specifies other aspects of healthcare you would like under those circumstances.

This glossary contains terms excerpted from documents produced by several sources deemed reliable.

Alzheimer disease (AD): Progressive, degenerative form of dementia that causes severe intellectual deterioration. First symptoms are impaired memory, followed by impaired thought and speech, and finally complete helplessness.

amino acid: One of several molecules that join together to form proteins. There are 20 common amino acids found in proteins.

anemia: A condition in which the number of red blood cells is below normal.

anesthetic: A drug that causes insensitivity to pain and is used for surgeries and other medical procedures.

annuity: A contract in which an individual gives an insurance company money that is later distributed back to the person over time. Annuity contracts traditionally provide a guaranteed distribution of income over time, until the death of the person or persons named in the contract or until a final date, whichever comes first.

antibiotic: A drug used to treat infections caused by bacteria and other microorganisms.

anxiety: Feelings of fear, dread, and uneasiness that may occur as a reaction to stress. A person with anxiety may sweat, feel restless and tense, and have a rapid heartbeat.

aspiration: The removal of fluid or tissue through a needle. Also, the accidental breathing in of food or fluid into the lungs.

assessment: The process of gathering evidence and documentation of a student's learning.

assisted living facility: Residential living arrangement that provides individualized personal care, assistance with Activities of Daily Living, help with medications, and services, such as laundry and housekeeping. Facilities may also provide health and medical care, but care is not as intensive as care offered at a nursing home.

assistive device: Tools that enable individuals with disabilities to perform essential job functions, e.g., telephone headsets, adapted computer keyboards, and enhanced computer monitors.

assistive technology: Products, devices, or equipment that help maintain, increase, or improve the functional capabilities of people with disabilities.

bacteria: A large group of single-cell microorganisms. Some cause infections and disease in animals and humans.

balance: A performance-related component of physical fitness that involves the maintenance of the body's equilibrium while stationary or moving.

biomarker: A specific physical trait or a measurable biologically produced change in the body connected with a disease or health condition.

bladder: The organ in the human body that stores urine. It is found in the lower part of the abdomen.

board and care home: Residential private homes designed to provide housing, meals, housekeeping, personal care services, and supports to frail or disabled residents. At least one caregiver is on the premises at all times. In many states, board and care homes are licensed or certified and must meet criteria for facility safety, types of services provided, and the number and type of residents they can care for.

brain tumor: The growth of abnormal cells in the tissues of the brain. Brain tumors can be benign (not cancer) or malignant (cancer).

breast cancer: Cancer that forms in tissues of the breast. The most common type of breast cancer is ductal carcinoma, which begins in the lining of the milk ducts (thin tubes that carry milk from the lobules of the breast to the nipple).

calcium: A mineral that is an essential nutrient for bone health. It is also needed for the heart, muscles, and nerves to function properly and for blood to clot.

calorie: A unit of energy in food. Carbohydrates, fats, protein, and alcohol in the foods and drinks we eat provide food energy or "calories."

carbohydrate: A major source of energy in the diet. There are two kinds of carbohydrates—simple carbohydrates and complex carbohydrates: simple carbohydrates are sugars and complex carbohydrates include both starches and fiber.

cardiopulmonary resuscitation (CPR): Combination of rescue breathing (mouth-to-mouth resuscitation) and chest compressions used if someone is not breathing or circulating blood adequately. CPR can restore circulation of oxygen-rich blood to the brain.

caregiver: A caregiver is anyone who helps care for an elderly individual or person with a disability who lives at home. Caregivers usually provide assistance with activities of daily living and other essential activities like shopping, meal preparation, and housework.

central nervous system (CNS): Comprised of the nerves in the brain and spinal cord. These nerves are used to send electrical impulses throughout the body, resulting in voluntary and reflexive movement. Information about the environment is received by the senses and sent to the central nervous system, which causes the body to respond appropriately.

charitable remainder trust (CRT): Special tax-exempt irrevocable trust written to comply with federal tax laws and regulations. You transfer cash or assets into the trust and may receive some income from it for life or a specified number of years (not to exceed 20).

chemotherapy: Treatment with anticancer drugs.

cholesterol: A fatty substance present in all parts of the body. It is a component of cell membranes and is used to make vitamin D and some hormones. Some cholesterol in the body is produced by the liver and some is derived from food, particularly animal products.

chronic disease: A disease that has one or more of the following characteristics: is permanent; leaves residual disability; is caused by nonreversible pathological alteration; requires special training of the patient for rehabilitation; or may be expected to require a long period of supervision, observation, or care.

chronic pain: Pain that can range from mild to severe, and persists or progresses over a long period of time.

chronically ill: Having a long-lasting or recurrent illness or condition that causes you to need help with Activities of Daily Living and often other health and support services. The condition is expected to last for at least 90 consecutive days.

cigarette: A tube-shaped tobacco product that is made of finely cut, cured tobacco leaves wrapped in thin paper. It may also have other ingredients, including substances to add different flavors.

clinical trial: A research study in which one or more human subjects are prospectively assigned to one or more interventions (which may include placebo or other control) to evaluate the effects of those interventions on health-related biomedical or behavioral outcomes.

cognitive impairment: Deficiency in short- or long-term memory, orientation to person, place and time, deductive or abstract reasoning, or judgment as it relates to safety awareness. Alzheimer disease is an example of a cognitive impairment.

community-based services: Services and service settings in the community, such as adult day services, home-delivered meals, or transportation services. Often referred to as home- and community-based services, they are designed to help older people and people with disabilities stay in their homes as independently as possible.

computed tomography (CT): A procedure for taking x-ray images from many different angles and then assembling them into a cross-section of the body. This technique is generally used to visualize bone.

constipation: A decrease in frequency of stools or bowel movements with hardening of the stool. Some forms of osteogenesis imperfecta are associated with increased risk for constipation caused by increased perspiration, growth impairment, pelvic malformation, and diminished physical activity.

continuing care retirement communities (CCRC): Retirement complex that offers a range of services and levels of care. Residents may move first into an independent living unit, a private apartment, or a house on the campus. The CCRC provides social and housing-related services and often also has an assisted living unit and an on-site or affiliated nursing home. If and when residents can no longer live independently in their apartment or home, they move into assisted living or the CCRC's nursing home.

dehydration: Excessive loss of body water that the body needs to carry on normal functions at an optimal level.

deoxyribonucleic acid (DNA): The double-helix molecule that provides the basis of genetic heredity, about two nanometers in diameter but often several millimeters in length.

depression: A mental condition marked by ongoing feelings of sadness, despair, loss of energy, and difficulty dealing with normal daily life. Other symptoms of depression include feelings of worthlessness and hopelessness, loss of pleasure in activities, changes in eating or sleeping habits, and thoughts of death or suicide.

diabetes: A disease in which blood glucose (blood sugar) levels are above normal. There are two main types of diabetes. Type 1 diabetes is caused by a problem with the body's defense system, called the "immune system." This form of diabetes usually starts in childhood or adolescence. Type 2 diabetes is the most common form of diabetes. It starts most often in adulthood.

diagnosis: The process of identifying a disease by the signs and symptoms.

diet: What a person eats and drinks. Any type of eating plan.

disorder: In medicine, a disturbance of normal functioning of the mind or body. Disorders may be caused by genetic factors, disease, or trauma.

durable power of attorney: Legal document that gives someone else the authority to act on your behalf on matters that you specify. The power can be specific to a certain task or broad to cover many financial duties. You can specify if you want the power to start immediately or upon mental incapacity. For the document to be valid, you must sign it before you become disabled.

duration: The length of time in which an activity or exercise is performed. Duration is generally expressed in minutes.

enzyme: A protein that speeds up chemical reactions in the body.

exercise: A type of physical activity that involves planned, structured, and repetitive bodily movement done to maintain or improve one or more components of physical fitness.

fat: A major source of energy in the diet. All food fats have nine calories per gram. Fat helps the body absorb fat-soluble vitamins, such as vitamins A, D, E, and K, and carotenoids. Some kinds of fats, especially saturated fats and trans fats, may raise blood cholesterol and increase the risk for heart disease. Other fats, such as unsaturated fats, do not raise blood cholesterol.

flexibility: A health- and performance-related component of physical fitness that is the range of motion possible at a joint. Flexibility is specific to each joint and depends on a number of specific variables, including but not limited to the tightness of specific ligaments and tendons.

fracture: Broken bone. People with osteoporosis, osteogenesis imperfecta, and Paget disease are at greater risk for bone fracture.

frequency: The number of times an exercise or activity is performed. Frequency is generally expressed in sessions, episodes, or bouts per week.

glucose: A major source of energy for our bodies and a building block for many carbohydrates. The food digestion process breaks down carbohydrates in foods and drinks into glucose. After digestion, glucose is carried in the blood and goes to body cells where it is used for energy or stored.

group home: Residential private homes designed to provide housing, meals, housekeeping, personal care services, and supports to frail or disabled residents. At least one caregiver is onsite at all times. In many states, group homes are licensed or certified and must meet criteria for facility safety, types of services provided, and the number and type of residents they can care for.

health: A human condition with physical, social, and psychological dimensions, each characterized on a continuum with positive and negative poles. Positive health is associated with a capacity to enjoy life and to withstand challenges; it is not merely the absence of disease. Negative health is associated with illness, and in the extreme, with premature death.

healthy weight: Compared to overweight or obese, a bodyweight that is less likely to be linked with any weight-related health problems, such as type 2 diabetes, heart disease, high blood pressure, and high blood cholesterol. A body mass index (BMI) of 18.5 to 24.9 is considered a healthy weight, though not all individuals with a BMI in this range may be at a healthy level of body fat; they may have more body fat tissue and less muscle. A person with a BMI of 25 to 29.9 is considered overweight, and a person with a BMI of 30 or more is considered obese.

hearing aid: An electronic device that brings amplified sound to the ear; it usually consists of a microphone, amplifier, and receiver.

heart disease: A number of abnormal conditions affecting the heart and the blood vessels in the heart. The most common type of heart disease is coronary artery disease, which is the gradual buildup of plaques in the coronary arteries, the blood vessels that bring blood to the heart. This disease develops slowly and silently, over decades. It can go virtually unnoticed until it produces a heart attack.

high blood pressure: Your blood pressure rises and falls throughout the day. An optimal blood pressure is less than 120/80 mmHg. When blood pressure stays high—greater than or equal to 140/90 mmHg—you have high blood pressure, also called "hypertension." With high blood pressure, the heart works harder, your arteries take a beating, and your chances of a stroke, heart attack, and kidney problems are greater.

hormone: Substance produced by one tissue and conveyed by the bloodstream to another to affect a function of the body, such as growth or metabolism.

hospice care: Short-term, supportive care for individuals who are terminally ill (have a life expectancy of six months or less). Hospice care focuses on pain management and emotional, physical, and spiritual support for the patient and family. It can be provided at home or in a hospital, nursing home, or hospice facility. Medicare typically pays for hospice care. Hospice care is not usually considered long-term care.

human immunodeficiency virus (HIV): A virus that infects and destroys the body's immune cells and causes a disease called "AIDS," or "acquired immunodeficiency syndrome."

hydration: The amount of fluid in your body. It is important to replace any fluid your body loses during physical activity.

immune system: A complex system of cellular and molecular components having the primary function of distinguishing self from not self and defense against foreign organisms or substances.

informal caregiver: Any person who provides long-term-care services without pay.

intensity: Intensity refers to how much work is being performed or the magnitude of the effort required to perform an activity or exercise.

intestines: Also known as the bowels, or the long, tube-like organ in the human body that completes digestion or the breaking down of food. They consist of the small intestine and the large intestine.

living will: Legal document that specifies whether you would like to be kept on artificial life support if you become permanently unconscious or are otherwise dying and unable to speak for yourself. It also specifies other aspects of healthcare you would like under those circumstances.

long-term care: Services and supports necessary to meet health or personal care needs over an extended period of time.

long-term-care facility: Licensed facility that provides general nursing care to those who are chronically ill or unable to take care of daily living needs.

long-term-care insurance: Insurance policy designed to offer financial support to pay for long-term-care services.

magnetic resonance imaging (MRI): A noninvasive procedure that uses magnetic fields and radio waves to produce three-dimensional computerized images of areas inside the body.

Medicaid: Joint federal and state public assistance program for financing healthcare for low-income people. It pays for healthcare services for those with low incomes or very high medical bills relative to income and assets. It is the largest public payer of long-term-care services.

Medicare: Federal program that provides hospital and medical expense benefits for people over age 65, or those meeting specific disability standards. Benefits for nursing home and home health services are limited.

nursing home: Licensed facility that provides general nursing care to those who are chronically ill or unable to take care of daily living needs.

nutrition: The taking in and use of food and other nourishing material by the body. Nutrition is a 3-part process. First, food or drink is consumed. Second, the body breaks down the food or drink into nutrients.

obesity: Obesity refers to excess body fat. Because body fat is usually not measured directly, a ratio of bodyweight to height is often used instead.

oils: Fats that are liquid at room temperature, oils come from many different plants and from seafood. Some common oils include canola, corn, olive, peanut, safflower, soybean, and sunflower oils. A number of foods are naturally high in oils, such as avocados, olives, nuts, and some fish.

organ: A part of the body that performs a specific function. For example, the heart is an organ.

over-the-counter (OTC): Diseases, including ulcerative colitis (UC) and Crohn disease, that cause swelling in the intestine and/or digestive tract, which may result in diarrhea, abdominal pain, fever, and weight loss. People with inflammatory bowel disease (IBD) are at an increased risk for osteoporosis.

overweight: Overweight refers to an excessive amount of bodyweight that includes muscle, bone, fat, and water. A person who has a body mass index (BMI) of 25 to 29.9 is considered overweight.

pedometer: A step counter that is worn at the waist or on a person's waistband. It tallies the number of steps a person takes each day. Walking 2,000 steps is equal to about one mile and roughly 100 calories are burned over and above calories for resting metabolism.

personal care: Nonskilled service or care, such as help with bathing, dressing, eating, getting in and out of bed or chair, moving around, and using the bathroom.

physical activity: Any bodily movement that is produced by the contraction of skeletal muscle and that substantially increases energy expenditure.

prevention: Actions that reduce exposure or other risks, keep people from getting sick, or keep disease from getting worse.

prognosis: The likely outcome or course of a disease; the chance of recovery or recurrence.

progression: The process of increasing the intensity, duration, frequency, or amount of activity or exercise as the body adapts to a given activity pattern.

protein: A molecule made up of amino acids. Proteins are needed for the body to function properly. They are the basis of body structures, such as skin and hair, and of other substances such as enzymes, cytokines, and antibodies.

radiation: Energy moving in the form of particles or waves. Familiar radiations are heat, light, radio, and microwaves.

respite care: Temporary care which is intended to provide time off for those who care for someone on a regular basis. Respite care is typically 14 to 21 days of care per year and can be provided in a nursing home, adult day service center, or at home by a private party.

side effect: A problem that occurs when treatment affects healthy tissues or organs. Some common side effects of cancer treatment are fatigue, pain, nausea, vomiting, decreased blood cell counts, hair loss, and mouth sores.

steroid: Any of a group of lipids (fats) that have a certain chemical structure. Steroids occur naturally in plants and animals or they may be made in the laboratory.

strength: A health and performance component of physical fitness that is the ability of a muscle or muscle group to exert force.

stretching: Stretching includes movements that lengthen muscles to their maximum extension and move joints to the limits of their extension.

stroke: Caused by a lack of blood to the brain, resulting in the sudden loss of speech, language, or the ability to move a body part, and, if severe enough, death.

supplemental security income (SSI): Program administered by the Social Security Administration (SSA) that provides financial assistance to needy persons who are disabled or aged 65 or older. Many states provide Medicaid without further application to persons who are eligible for SSI.

tai chi: A form of traditional Chinese mind/body exercise and meditation that uses slow sets of body movements and controlled breathing. Tai chi is done to improve balance, flexibility, muscle strength, and overall health.

tobacco: A plant with leaves that have high levels of the addictive chemical nicotine. After harvesting, tobacco leaves are cured, aged, and processed in various ways. The resulting products may be smoked (in cigarettes, cigars, and pipes), applied to the gums (as dipping and chewing tobacco), or inhaled (as snuff).

toxic: Causing temporary or permanent effects detrimental to the functioning of a body organ or group of organs.

transfer of assets: Giving away property for less than it is worth or for the sole purpose of becoming eligible for Medicaid. Transferring assets during the lookback period results in disqualification for Medicaid payment of long-term-care services for a penalty period.

urinary tract infection (UTI): An infection anywhere in the urinary tract, or organs that collect and store urine and release it from your body (the kidneys, ureters, bladder, and urethra).

x-ray: A type of high-energy radiation. In low doses, x-rays are used to diagnose diseases by making pictures of the inside of the body.

yoga: An ancient system of practices used to balance the mind and body through exercise, meditation (focusing thoughts), and control of breathing and emotions.

Chapter 67

Support Groups for End-of-Life Issues

American Association of Suicidology (AAS)
5221 Wisconsin Ave., N.W.
Second Fl.
Washington, DC 20015
Phone: 202-237-2280
Fax: 202-237-2282
Website: suicidology.org
E-mail: info@suicidology.org

American Cancer Society (ACS)
P.O. Box 22478
Oklahoma City, OK 73123
Toll-Free: 800-227-2345
Phone: 404-320-3333
Website: www.cancer.org

The Compassionate Friends (TCF)
National Office
P.O. Box 3696
Oak Brook, IL 60522
Toll-Free: 877-969-0010
Phone: 630-990-0010
Fax: 630-990-0246
Website: www.
compassionatefriends.org
E-mail: nationaloffice@
compassionatefriends.org

First Candle / SIDS Alliance
49 Locust Ave.
Ste. 104
New Canaan, CT 06840
Toll-Free: 800-221-7437
Phone: 203-966-1300
Website: www.firstcandle.org
E-mail: info@firstcandle.org

Resources in this chapter were compiled from several sources deemed reliable; all contact information was verified and updated in September 2019.

GriefShare
P.O. Box 1739
Wake Forest, NC 27588-1739
Toll-Free: 800-395-5755
Fax: 919-562-2114
Website: www.griefshare.org
E-mail: info@griefshare.org

Leukemia & Lymphoma Society (LLS)
Three International Dr.
Ste. 200
Rye Brook, NY 10573
Toll-Free: 888-557-7177
Website: www.lls.org
E-mail: infocenter@lls.org

National Hospice and Palliative Care Organization (NHPCO)
1731 King St.
Alexandria, VA 22314
Toll-Free: 800-658-8898
Phone: 703-837-1500
Fax: 703-837-1233
Website: www.nhpco.org

Share
National Share Office
402 Jackson St.
St. Charles, MO 63301-3468
Toll-Free: 800-821-6819
Phone: 636-947-6164
Fax: 636-947-7486
Website: nationalshare.org
E-mail: info@nationalshare.org

Suicide Prevention Resource Center (SPRC)
Education Development Center, Inc.
43 Foundry Ave.
Waltham, MA 02453
Toll-Free: 800-273-TALK (800-273-8255)
Website: www.sprc.org

Tragedy Assistance Program for Survivors, Inc. (TAPS)
3033 Wilson Blvd.
Third Fl.
Arlington, VA 22201
Toll-Free: 800-959-TAPS (800-959-8277)
Phone: 202-588-8277
Fax: 571-385-2524
Website: www.taps.org
E-mail: info@taps.org

Well Spouse® Association (WSA)
63 W. Main St.
Ste. H
Freehold, NJ 07728
Toll-Free: 800-838-0879
Phone: 732-577-8899
Website: wellspouse.org
E-mail: info@wellspouse.org

Yellow Ribbon Suicide Prevention Program® / The Light for Life Foundation Int'l
P.O. Box 644
Westminster, CO 80036
Phone: 303-429-3530
Website: yellowribbon.org
E-mail: ask4help@yellowribbon.org

Chapter 68

Resources for Information about Death and Dying

Government Agencies That Provide Information about Death and Dying

Administration for Community Living (ACL)
330 C. St., S.W.
Washington, DC 20201
Phone: 202-401-4634
Website: www.acl.gov
E-mail: aclinfo@acl.hhs.gov

Agency for Healthcare Research and Quality (AHRQ)
Office of Communications
5600 Fishers Ln.
Seventh Fl.
Rockville, MD 20847
Phone: 301-427-1104
Website: www.ahrq.gov

AIDSinfo
P.O. Box 4780
Rockville, MD 20849-6303
Toll-Free: 800-HIV-0440
(800-448-0440)
Toll-Free TTY: 888-480-3739
Fax: 301-315-2818
Website: aidsinfo.nih.gov
E-mail: ContactUs@aidsinfo.nih.gov

Resources in this chapter were compiled from several sources deemed reliable; all contact information was verified and updated in September 2019.

*Alzheimer's Disease
Education and Referral
Center (ADEAR)*
National Institute on Aging (NIA)
P.O. Box 8250
Silver Spring, MD 20907-8250
Toll-Free: 800-438-4380
Website: www.nia.nih.gov/
alzheimers
E-mail: adear@nia.nih.gov

Benefits.gov
Toll-Free: 800-FED-INFO
(800-333-4636)
Website: www.benefits.gov

*Centers for Disease Control
and Prevention (CDC)*
1600 Clifton Rd.
Atlanta, GA 30329-4027
Toll-Free: 800-CDC-INFO
(800-232-4636)
Toll-Free TTY: 888-232-6348
Website: www.cdc.gov

*Centers for Medicare &
Medicaid Services (CMS)*
7500 Security Blvd.
Baltimore, MD 21244
Toll-Free: 877-267-2323
Phone: 410-786-3000
TTY: 410-786-0727
Toll-Free TTY: 866-226-1819
Website: www.cms.gov

Eldercare Locator
Administration for Community
Living (ACL)
Toll-Free: 800-677-1116
Website: www.eldercare.gov
E-mail: eldercarelocator@n4a.
org

Eunice Kennedy Shriver
*National Institute of
Child Health and Human
Development (NICHD)*
NICHD Information Resource
Center (IRC)
P.O. Box 3006
Rockville, MD 20847
Toll-Free: 800-370-2943
Phone: 301-496-5133
Toll-Free Fax: 866-760-5947
Website: www.nichd.nih.gov
E-mail: NICHDInformation
ResourceCenter@mail.nih.gov

*Federal Trade Commission
(FTC)*
600 Pennsylvania Ave., N.W.
Washington, DC 20580
Toll-Free: 877-FTC-HELP
(877-382-4357)
Phone: 202-326-2222
Website: www.ftc.gov

*Internal Revenue Service
(IRS)*
Joint Board for the Enrollment
of Actuaries (JBEA)
1111 Constitution Ave., N.W.
SE:RPO, Rm. 3422
Washington, DC 20224
Toll-Free: 800-829-1040
Toll-Free TTY/TDD:
800-829-4059
Website: www.irs.gov
E-mail: nhqjbea@irs.gov

National Cancer Institute (NCI)
9609 Medical Center Dr.
BG 9609, MSC 9760
Bethesda, MD 20892-9760
Toll-Free: 800-4-CANCER
(800-422-6237)
Website: www.cancer.gov
E-mail: NCIinfo@nih.gov

National Heart, Lung, and Blood Institute (NHLBI)
NHLBI Center for Health Information
P.O. Box 30105
Bethesda, MD 20824-0105
Phone: 301-592-8573
Website: www.nhlbi.nih.gov
E-mail: nhlbiinfo@nhlbi.nih.gov

National Institute on Aging (NIA)
Bldg. 31, Rm. 5C27
31 Center Dr., MSC 2292
Bethesda, MD 20892
Toll-Free: 800-222-2225
Toll-Free TTY: 800-222-4225
Website: www.nia.nih.gov
E-mail: niaic@nia.nih.gov

National Institutes of Health (NIH)
9000 Rockville Pike
Bethesda, MD 20892
Phone: 301-496-4000
TTY: 301-402-9612
Website: www.nih.gov

NIH News in Health
NIH Office of Communications and Public Liaison (OCPL)
Bldg. 31, Rm. 5B52
Bethesda, MD 20892-2094
Phone: 301-451-8224
Website: newsinhealth.nih.gov
E-mail: nihnewsinhealth@od.nih.gov

Substance Abuse and Mental Health Services Administration (SAMHSA)
5600 Fishers Ln.
Rockville, MD 20857
Toll-Free: 877-SAMHSA-7
(877-726-4727)
Toll-Free TTY: 800-487-4889
Website: www.samhsa.gov
E-mail: SAMHSAInfo@samhsa.hhs.gov

U.S. Bureau of Labor Statistics (BLS)
2 Massachusetts Ave., N.E.
Postal Square Bldg.
Washington, DC 20212-0001
Phone: 202-691-5200
Toll-Free TDD: 800-877-8339
Website: www.bls.gov

U.S. Department of Health and Human Services (HHS)
200 Independence Ave., S.W.
Washington, DC 20201
Toll-Free: 877-696-6775
Website: www.hhs.gov

U.S. Department of Labor (DOL)
200 Constitution Ave., N.W.
Washington, DC 20210
Toll-Free: 866-4-USA-DOL
(866-487-2365)
Website: www.dol.gov

U.S. Department of Veterans Affairs (VA)
810 Vermont Ave., N.W.
Washington, DC 20420
Toll-Free: 844-698-2311
Toll-Free TTY: 711-698-2311
Website: www.va.gov

U.S. Environmental Protection Agency (EPA)
1200 Pennsylvania Ave., N.W.
Washington, DC 20460
Phone: 202-564-4700
TTY: 202-272-0165
Fax: 202-501-1450
Website: www.epa.gov

U.S. Food and Drug Administration (FDA)
10903 New Hampshire Ave.
Silver Spring, MD 20993-0002
Toll-Free: 888-INFO-FDA
(888-463-6332)
Website: www.fda.gov

U.S. Social Security Administration (SSA)
Office of Earnings &
International Operations (OEIO)
P.O. Box 17769
Baltimore, MD 21235-7769
Toll-Free: 800-772-1213
Toll-Free TTY: 800-325-0778
Website: www.ssa.gov

Private Agencies That Provide Information about Death and Dying

ADvancing States
241 18th St., S.
Ste. 403
Arlington, VA 22202
Phone: 202-898-2578
Fax: 202-898-2583
Website: www.advancingstates.
org
E-mail: info@advancingstates.
org

ALS Association
1275 K. St., N.W.
Ste. 250
Washington, DC 20005
Toll-Free: 800-782-4747
Phone: 202-407-8580
Fax: 202-464-8869
Website: www.alsa.org
E-mail: alsinfo@alsa-national.
org

Alzheimer's Association®
225 N. Michigan Ave.
17th Fl.
Chicago, IL 60601
Toll-Free: 800-272-3900
Website: www.alz.org

American Academy of Hospice and Palliative Medicine (AAHPM)
8735 W. Higgins Rd.
Ste. 300
Chicago, IL 60631
Phone: 847-375-4712
Fax: 847-375-6475
Website: aahpm.org
E-mail: info@aahpm.org

American Association of Retired People (AARP)
601 E. St., N.W.
Washington, DC 20049
Toll-Free: 888-OUR-AARP
(888-687-2277)
Toll-Free TTY: 877-434-7598
Website: www.aarp.org

American Association of Suicidology (AAS)
5221 Wisconsin Ave., N.W.
Second Fl.
Washington, DC 20015
Phone: 202-237-2280
Fax: 202-237-2282
Website: suicidology.org
E-mail: info@suicidology.org

American Chronic Pain Association (ACPA)
P.O. Box 850
Rocklin, CA 95677
Toll-Free: 800-533-3231
Fax: 916-652-8190
Website: www.theacpa.org
E-mail: ACPA@theacpa.org

American Pain Society (APS)
8735 W. Higgins Rd.
Ste. 300
Chicago, IL 60631
Website: americanpainsociety.
org
E-mail: info@
americanpainsociety.org

Americans for Better Care of the Dying (ABCD)
5568 General Washington Dr.
Alexandria, VA 22314-2866
Phone: 703-333-6960
Website: www.abcd-caring.org

Association for Death Education and Counseling (ADEC)
400 S. Fourth St.
Ste. 754E
Minneapolis, MN 55415
Phone: 612-337-1808
Fax: 612-337-1808
Website: www.adec.org
E-mail: adec@adec.org

549

Association of Professional Chaplains® (APC)
2800 W. Higgins Rd.
Ste. 295
Hoffman Estates, IL 60169
Phone: 847-240-1014
Fax: 847-240-1015
Website: www. professionalchaplains.org
E-mail: info@ professionalchaplains.org

Bereaved Parents of the USA (BPUSA)
National Office, c/o Katherine Corrigan
Five Vanek Rd.
Poughkeepsie, NY 12603-5403
Website: bereavedparentsusa. org

CancerCare®
National Office
275 Seventh Ave.
22nd Fl.
New York, NY 10001
Toll-Free: 800-813-HOPE
(800-813-4673)
Phone: 212-712-8400
Fax: 212-712-8495
Website: www.cancercare.org
E-mail: info@cancercare.org

Caregiver Action Network (CAN)
1150 Connecticut Ave., N.W.
Ste. 501
Washington, DC 20036-3904
Toll-Free: 855-CARE-640
(855-227-3640)
Phone: 202-454-3970
Website: caregiveraction.org
E-mail: info@caregiveraction.org

CARF (Commission on Accreditation of Rehabilitation Facilities) International
6951 E. Southpoint Rd.
Tucson, AZ 85756-9407
Toll-Free: 888-281-6531
TTY: 520-495-7077
Fax: 520-318-1129
Website: www.carf.org

Children's Hospice International (CHI)
1800 Diagonal Rd.
Ste. 600
Alexandria, VA 22314
Phone: 703-684-0330
Website: www.chionline.org
E-mail: Info@CHIonline.org

Compassion & Choices
101 S.W. Madison St.
Ste. 8009
Portland, OR 97207
Toll-Free: 800-247-7421
Website: compassionandchoices. org

The Compassionate Friends (TCF)
National Office
P.O. Box 3696
Oak Brook, IL 60522
Toll-Free: 877-969-0010
Phone: 630-990-0010
Fax: 630-990-0246
Website: www.
compassionatefriends.org
E-mail: nationaloffice@
compassionatefriends.org

The Dougy Center
The National Center for
Grieving Children and Families
P.O. Box 86852
Portland, OR 97286
Toll-Free: 866-775-5683
Phone: 503-775-5683
Fax: 503-777-3097
Website: www.dougy.org
E-mail: help@dougy.org

*Family Caregiver Alliance®
(FCA)*
National Center on Caregiving
(NCC)
101 Montgomery St.
Ste. 2150
San Francisco, CA 94104
Toll-Free: 800-445-8106
Phone: 415-434-3388
Website: www.caregiver.org
E-mail: info@caregiver.org

First Candle / SIDS Alliance
49 Locust Ave.
Ste. 104
New Canaan, CT 06840
Toll-Free: 800-221-7437
Phone: 203-966-1300
Website: www.firstcandle.org
E-mail: info@firstcandle.org

*Funeral Consumers Alliance
(FCA)*
33 Patchen Rd.
South Burlington, VT 05403
Phone: 802-865-8300
Website: funerals.org

*The George Washington
Institute for Spirituality and
Health (GWish)*
2600 Virginia Ave., N.W.
Ste. 300
Washington, DC 20037
Phone: 202-994-6220
Fax: 202-994-6413
Website: smhs.gwu.edu/gwish
E-mail: caring@gwish.org

Health in Aging Foundation
40 Fulton St.
18th Fl.
New York, NY 10038
Phone: 212-308-1414
Fax: 212-832-8646
Website: www.healthinaging.org
E-mail: info@healthinaging.org

Hospice Foundation of America (HFA)
1707 L. St., N.W.
Ste. 220
Washington, DC 20036
Toll-Free: 800-854-3402
Phone: 202-457-5811
Website: hospicefoundation.org
E-mail: info@hospicefoundation.org

International Cemetery, Cremation & Funeral Association (ICCFA)
107 Carpenter Dr.
Ste. 100
Sterling, VA 20164
Toll-Free: 800-645-7700
Phone: 703-391-8400
Fax: 703-391-8416
Website: iccfa.com

Joint Commission Resources (JCR)
1515 W. 22nd St.
Ste. 1300W
Oak Brook, IL 60523
Phone: 630-268-7400
Website: www.jcrinc.com
E-mail: info@jcrinc.com

National Association for Home Care & Hospice (NAHC)
228 Seventh St., S.E.
Washington, DC 20003
Phone: 202-547-7424
Fax: 202-547-3540
Website: www.nahc.org

National Association of Area Agencies on Aging (N4A)
1100 New Jersey Ave., S.E.
Ste. 350
Washington, DC 20003
Phone: 202-872-0888
Fax: 202-872-0057
Website: www.n4a.org
E-mail: info@n4a.org

National Association of Catholic Chaplains (NACC)
4915 S. Howell Ave.
Ste. 501
Milwaukee, WI 53207
Phone: 414-483-4898
Fax: 414-483-6712
Website: www.nacc.org
E-mail: info@nacc.org

National Funeral Directors Association (NFDA)
13625 Bishop's Dr.
Brookfield, WI 53005
Toll-Free: 800-228-6332
Phone: 262-789-1880
Fax: 262-789-6977
Website: www.nfda.org
E-mail: nfda@nfda.org

National Hospice and Palliative Care Organization (NHPCO)
1731 King St.
Alexandria, VA 22314
Toll-Free: 800-658-8898
Phone: 703-837-1500
Fax: 703-837-1233
Website: www.nhpco.org

Safe Kids Worldwide
1255 23rd St., N.W.
Ste. 400
Washington, DC 20037-1151
Phone: 202-662-0600
Fax: 202-393-2072
Website: www.safekids.org
E-mail: info@safekids.org

Share
National Share Office
402 Jackson St.
St. Charles, MO 63301-3468
Toll-Free: 800-821-6819
Phone: 636-947-6164
Fax: 636-947-7486
Website: nationalshare.org
E-mail: info@nationalshare.org

Society of Critical Care Medicine (SCCM)
500 Midway Dr.
Mount Prospect, IL 60056
Phone: 847-827-6888
Fax: 847-439-7226
Website: www.sccm.org
E-mail: support@sccm.org

Suicide Prevention Resource Center (SPRC)
Education Development Center, Inc.
43 Foundry Ave.
Waltham, MA 02453
Toll-Free: 800-273-TALK
(800-273-8255)
Website: www.sprc.org

Visiting Nurse Associations of America (VNAA)
2519 Connecticut Ave., N.W.
Washington, DC 20008
Phone: 202-508-9458
Website: www.vnaa.org
E-mail: vnaa@vnaa.org

Yellow Ribbon Suicide Prevention Program® / The Light for Life Foundation Int'l
P.O. Box 644
Westminster, CO 80036
Phone: 303-429-3530
Website: yellowribbon.org
E-mail: ask4help@yellowribbon.org

Index

Index

Page numbers followed by 'n' indicate a footnote. Page numbers in *italics* indicate a table or illustration.

A

AAA *see* Area Agency on Aging
abuse
  alcohol 90
  euthanasia 222
  pain 4
accelerated death benefit
  defined 531
  life insurance policies 411
accessory dwelling unit (ADU),
  long-term care 233
acetaminophen
  over-the-counter (OTC) drugs 86
  pain medications 78
  pain treatment for children 331
  palliative care 64
acquired immune deficiency syndrome
  (AIDS)
  end-of-life issues 181
  palliative care 191
activities of daily living (ADL)
  caregivers 240
  chronic diseases 38, 159
  defined 531
  group living arrangements 234

activities of daily living (ADL),
  continued
  home healthcare 251
  long-term care 228
  long-term-care insurance 270
acupuncture
  pain management 79
  palliative care 67
acute care, defined 531
acute pain, described 76
acute respiratory distress syndrome
  (ARDS), overview 117–24
"Acute Respiratory Distress
  Syndrome" (NHLBI) 117n
AD *see* Alzheimer disease
ADL *see* activities of daily living
Administration for Community Living
  (ACL)
  contact 545
  publications
    home healthcare 251n
    long-term-care insurance 270n
adolescents
  health-related behaviors 40
  suicide rate 519
ADU *see* accessory dwelling unit
adult day services
  defined 531
  respite care 298
adult daycare, long-term care 228

557

Adult Protective Services, Medicaid
  hospice program 268
advance care planning
  healthcare directives 398
  organ and tissue donation 403
  research 160
"Advance Care Planning: Healthcare
  Directives" (NIA) 397n
"Advance Care Planning, Preferences
  for Care at the End of Life"
  (AHRQ) 159n
advance directives
  defined 531
  healthcare directives 398
  organ and tissue donation 403
  research 160
  see also advance care planning;
    durable power of attorney; living
    wills
"Advance Directives" (NIH) 397n
advance planning
  end-of-life care decisions 176
  end-of-life care preferences 159
ADvancing States, contact 548
AED *see* automated external
  defibrillator
African Americans
  ethnicity and spirituality 26
  injury death risk 514
  transplant waiting list 218
Agency for Healthcare Research and
  Quality (AHRQ)
  contact 545
  publications
    advance care planning 159n
    chronic illness 73n
aging
  delirium 150
  long-distance caregiving 291
  older adult caregiver 246
  pain 77
  Resources for enhancing
    Alzheimer's Caregiver Health
    (REACH) 303
AIDS *see* acquired immune deficiency
  syndrome
AIDS*info*, contact 545
air sacs, acute respiratory distress
  syndrome (ARDS) 117

alcohol
  age-adjusted death rate 496
  cancer treatment 130
  death 521
  fatigue 99
  over-the-counter (OTC) drugs 86
  pain medication 78
  pregnancy 524
"Alcohol Facts and Statistics"
  (NIAAA) 521n
alcohol-use disorder (AUD),
  statistics 521
Allow Natural Death (AND)
  end-of-life medical issues 402
  healthcare decisions 14
ALS Association, contact 548
Alzheimer disease (AD)
  causes of death 491
  defined 532
  end-of-life care 167
  long-term care 235
  Program of All-Inclusive Care for
    the Elderly (PACE) 409
Alzheimer's Association®, contact 549
Alzheimer's Disease Education
  and Referral Center (ADEAR),
  contact 546
American Academy of Hospice and
  Palliative Medicine (AAHPM),
  contact 549
American Association of Retired
  People (AARP), contact 549
American Association of Suicidology
  (AAS), contact 543
American Cancer Society (ACS),
  contact 543
American Chronic Pain Association
  (ACPA), contact 549
American Pain Society (APS),
  contact 549
Americans for Better Care of the
  Dying (ABCD), contact 549
amino acid
  defined 532
  oral glutamine 147
analgesics, cancer pain 86
AND *see* Allow Natural Death
anemia
  advanced cancer 208

anemia, *continued*
blood tests 108
defined 532
fatigue 105
treatment 109
anesthetics
defined 532
pain management 66
pediatric critical care 365
anger
brief measure of religious coping
(RCOPE) 28
grief reactions 357, 463
spiritual distress 206
annuities
defined 532
described 412
private payment options 410
anorexia
cancer patients 136
end-of-life symptoms 145
malnutrition 130
antibiotics
acute respiratory distress syndrome
(ARDS) 123
defined 532
infection 65
pain management 67
uses 16
anticipatory grief, coping with
loss 462
antidepressants
cancer pain management 88
fatigue 107
pain medicines 78
antiretroviral therapy (ART),
human immunodeficiency virus
(HIV) 482
antiseizure medicines
(anticonvulsants), pain medicines 88
anxiety
acute respiratory distress syndrome
(ARDS) 124
cancer survivorship 302
defined 532
fatigue 105
grief reactions 462
guided imagery 79
withdrawal symptoms 90

appetite
changes 306
digestive problems 6
exercise 100
malnutrition 130
medicines 144
palliative care 60
trouble swallowing 200
APS *see* Adult Protective Services
ARDS *see* acute respiratory distress
syndrome
"Are There Ways to Reduce the Risk
of Infant Mortality?" (NICHD) 349n
Area Agency on Aging (AAA)
emergency response systems 230
healthcare directives 404
ART *see* antiretroviral therapy
arthritis
caregivers' health risks 302
chronic pain 76
artificial hydration
described 125
see also artificial nutrition
"Artificial Hydration and Nutrition"
(Omnigraphics) 125n
artificial nutrition, overview 125–7
aspiration
defined 532
nutrition support 145
supplemental nutrition 200
assessment
caregiver 249
defined 532
fatigue 107
nutrition in cancer care 134
pain 66
assisted living
hospice care 266
long-term care 230
Medicare 408
assisted living facility
defined 532
hospice care 258
long-distance caregivers 298
Medicare 408
assisted oral feeding *see* hand-feeding
assistive device
defined 532
described 254

assistive technology, defined 532
Association for Death Education and
    Counseling (ADEC), contact 549
Association of Professional Chaplains®
    (APC), contact 550
AUD *see* alcohol-use disorder
automated external defibrillator
    (AED), death onboard 457
autonomy, physician-assisted
    suicide 222
autopsy, cause of death 311

B

bacteria
    antibiotics 16
    defined 532
    infection 65
    sepsis 118
balance
    defined 533
    exercises 100
beneficence, ethical obligations 193
benefits
    antibiotics 208
    communication with doctor 285
    exercise 111
    hospice services 266
    long-term-care insurance 271
    Social Security 413
BenefitsCheckUp®, described 410
Benefits.gov
    contact 546
    publication
        Social Security benefits 413n
benzydamine, topical anesthetics 66
Bereaved Parents of the USA
    (BPUSA), contact 550
bereavement
    described 462
    see also grief
binge drinking, statistics 521
biofeedback
    alternative pain control methods 67
    coping with emotions 320
    pain management 79
biologic therapy
    cancer treatments 101
    fatigue 104

biomarker
    defined 533
    delirium 153
biopsy, cancer pain 81
birth defects, causes of infant
    mortality 349
bladder
    defined 533
    delirium 156
bleeding
    acute respiratory distress syndrome
        (ARDS) 118
    intestines 123
    local wound care 65
    nonsteroidal anti-inflammatory
        drugs (NSAIDs) 78
    pregnancy loss 344
    tracheotomy 14
blood pressure
    acute respiratory distress syndrome
        (ARDS) 119
    stillbirth 341
    stroke 528
blood tests
    acute respiratory distress syndrome
        (ARDS) 121
    anemia 108
blood transfusions
    advanced cancer 208
    indirect lung injury 119
BLS *see* U.S. Bureau of Labor
    Statistics
board and care home
    defined 533
    long-term-care services 230
brain tumor
    defined 533
    delirium 155
breast cancer
    cancer-related fatigue 104
    defined 533
    support groups 34
breathing machine
    do-not-resuscitate (DNR)
        order 402
    living will 177, 397
burial
    versus cremation 449
    fund 415

burial container, described 435
burial flag, military funeral 447
burial fund
  described 415
  see also prepaid burial arrangement
burial vaults
  described 435
  see also burial container

C

cachexia, cancer care 131
caffeine
  fatigue 99
  miscarriage 346
  pain 80
calcium, defined 533
calorie, defined 533
CAM *see* complementary and
  alternative medicine
cancer
  caregiving 302
  causes of death 491
  child 315
  communication 283
  coping with loss 461
  delirium 155
  end-of-life care 171
  ethics and legal issues 191
  family caregivers 247
  fatigue 97
  home care 240
  hospice care 258
  life expectancy 482
  nutrition, overview 129–47
  pain control, overview 80–92
  palliative care 69
  spirituality 26
  telephone-based rehab,
    overview 52–5
cancer treatment
  caregiving 302
  communication 288
  end of life 202
  fatigue 103
  life-sustaining treatment 206
  nutrition 130
  palliative care 70
Cancer*Care*®, contact 550

carbohydrates
  defined 533
  nutrition 129
cardiopulmonary resuscitation (CPR)
  advance directives 399
  advance planning 177
  collaborative pediatric 368
  defined 533
  healthcare decisions 14
  life-sustaining treatments 209
  preferences for care 162
  traveling 457
care goals
  dementia 168
  end-of-life care 174
Caregiver Action Network (CAN),
  contact 550
caregivers
  communication 283
  coping with caregiving,
    overview 302–7
  death approaches 306
  defined 533
  end-of-life care 172
  financial assistance 408
  home care, overview 240–50
  hospice care 259
  infant death 353
  life-sustaining treatments 210
  long-distance caregiving 289
  responsibilities with family
    members 298
  self-care 299
  sudden infant death syndrome
    (SIDS) 335
"Caregiving for Family and
  Friends—A Public Health Issue"
  (CDC) 73n
CARF (Commission on Accreditation
  of Rehabilitation Facilities)
  International, contact 550
caskets
  described 434–5
  funeral services 431
  planning a funeral 442
causes of death
  chronic illness 37
  disparities 506
  life expectancy 480

causes of death, *continued*
  medical certification 451
  overview 491–5
CBT *see* cognitive-behavioral therapy
CCRCs *see* continuing care retirement
  communities
CCU *see* coronary care unit
CDC *see* Centers for Disease Control
  and Prevention
"CDC Childhood Injury Report"
  (CDC) 513n
Census of Fatal Occupational Injuries
  (CFOI), work-related fatalities 510
Centers for Disease Control and
  Prevention (CDC)
  contact 546
  publications
    causes of death statistics 491n
    childhood injury-related
      deaths 513n
    chronic illness and old age 37n
    death certification 451n
    death during travel 457n
    dementia and pain
      assessment 2004 93n
    end-of-life care 73n
    infant and maternal mortality
      trends 503n
    infant mortality 349n
    life expectancy statistics 499n
    mortality statistics 483n
    stillbirth 340n
    stroke 527n
    suicide statistics 517n
Centers for Medicare & Medicaid
  Services (CMS)
  contact 546
  publications
    hospice care insurance 266n
    long-term care 228n
central nervous system (CNS)
  defined 534
  tabulated *454*
central venous access catheter,
  nutrition support 144
cerebrovascular diseases, causes of
  death 491
CFOI *see* Census of Fatal
  Occupational Injuries

CFS *see* chronic fatigue syndrome
CGT *see* complicated grief treatment
chaplains
  end-of-life care 173
  life-sustaining treatments 210
  pediatric palliative care 329
  spirituality in end-of-life care 33
charitable remainder trust
  defined 534
  financial assistance 412
chemotherapy
  cancer and fatigue 103
  cancer pain 88
  defined 534
  end of life 203
  healthcare decisions 17
  hospice care 259
  nutrition 131
  patient's rights 386
  probiotics 147
Cheyne-Stokes breathing, death 310
children
  cancer, overview 315–24
  caregiver 250
  collaborative pediatric critical
    care 370
  developmental stages,
    overview 356–60
  family consequences 523
  fatigue 104
  grief expressions 363
  home care 240
  nonfatal injuries 515
  providing care 8
  role of parents 286
  spirituality 22
Children's Hospice International
  (CHI), contact 550
choking
  cancer treatment 133
  end of life 196
  sudden infant death syndrome
    (SIDS) 337
cholesterol
  defined 534
  delirium 198
  stroke 528
"Choosing a Funeral Provider"
  (FTC) 441n

"Choosing a Nursing Home" (NIA) 236n
chromosomes, miscarriage 345
chronic condition *see* multiple chronic
  conditions
chronic disease
  advance planning 160
  chronic illness 73
  defined 534
  delirium 153
  miscarriage 346
  older adults 37
  pain management 90
chronic fatigue syndrome (CFS),
  described 101
chronic illness
  advance directives 399
  end of life 159
  end-of-life care, overview 73–4
  healthcare decisions 14
  old age 39
  palliative care 191, 258
  spirituality 25
chronic pain
  defined 534
  overview 76–7
  pain control 81
chronically ill
  defined 534
  palliative care 65
  primary caregiver 298
cigarette
  defined 534
  stillbirth 341
  sudden infant death syndrome
    (SIDS) 335
clergy *see* chaplain
"A Clinical Guide to Supportive and
  Palliative Care for HIV/AIDS"
  (HRSA) 181n
clinical trials
  collaborative pediatric critical
    care 366
  coping with loss 467
  defined 534
  delirium 153
  informed consent 391
  nutrition 146
CMS *see* Centers for Medicare &
  Medicaid Services

CNS *see* central nervous system
cognitive-behavioral therapy (CBT)
  coping with loss 466
  fatigue 99
  pain 79
cognitive impairment
  coping with loss 466
  defined 534
  fatigue 99
"Collaborative Pediatric Critical Care
  Research Network (CPCCRN)"
  (NICHD) 365n
collapsed lung
  acute respiratory distress syndrome
    (ARDS) 120
  healthcare decisions 14
coma
  advance directives 400
  end of life 165
  HIV/AIDS 185
comfort care
  advance directives 400
  end-of-life care 179
  healthcare decisions 16
  palliative care 258
  providing care 3
communication
  advanced cancer 174
  death of a spouse 471
  effective care 280
  end of life 44
  ethics and legal issues 192
  family caregivers 285
  grief 360
  healthcare team 323
  home care 245
  insurance coverage 266
  nutrition 145
  palliative care 61
"Communication in Cancer Care
  (PDQ®)—Patient Version"
  (NCI) 283n
community-based services
  defined 535
  financial assistance 408
  long-term care 232
community care, periodic palliative
  care 331

compassion
  end of life 45
  ethics and legal issues 192
  financial assistance 410
  mourning 470
Compassion & Choices, contact 550
The Compassionate Friends (TCF),
  contact 543
complementary and alternative
  medicine (CAM), end-of-life
  care 23
complicated grief
  described 464–7
  pediatric critical care 366
complicated grief treatment (CGT),
  coping with loss 466
computed tomography (CT) scan
  acute respiratory distress syndrome
    (ARDS) 121
  defined 535
confusion
  acute respiratory distress syndrome
    (ARDS) 119
  advance directives 397
  caregiving 303
  death 310
  delirium, overview 150–2
  effective care 280
  end of life 160
  healthcare decision 18
  hospital culture 51
  life-sustaining treatments 205
constipation
  advance directives 400
  cancer care 132
  defined 535
  described 91–2
  end of life 6
consular mortuary certificate *see*
  death certificate
continuing care retirement
  communities (CCRCs)
  defined 535
  described 233
  long-term care 230
COPD *see* chronic obstructive
  pulmonary disease
"Coping with Caregiving" (*NIH News
  in Health*) 301n

"Coping with the Death of a
  Student or Staff Member"
  (ED) 361n
coronary care unit (CCU), end-of-life
  care 262
coroner
  cremation 459
  death 311
  described 456
  medical certification 451
"Costs and How to Pay" (ACL) 270n
counseling
  advance care planning 400
  coping with loss 467
  death 364
  end-of-life care 173
  hospice care 267
  mourning 470
  nutrition 135
  spirituality 32
  talk therapy 113
counselors
  acute respiratory distress syndrome
    (ARDS) 124
  death 311
  end of life 7
  grief counseling 470
  life-sustaining treatments 211
  long-term care 231
  mental-health providers 364
  palliative care 62
  pediatric palliative care 329
CPR *see* cardiopulmonary
  resuscitation
cremains, cremation 450
cremation
  death onboard 459
  described 435–6
  funeral services 431
  military funeral planning 447
  overview 449–50
critically ill patients
  home care
    overview 239–55
CT scan *see* computed tomography
  scan
cultural beliefs
  home care 246
  family caregivers 285

cultural traditions, healthcare
  decisions 13
culture
  death, overview 19–20
  diagnostic tests 121
  end-of-life care 50
  family caregivers 285
  healthcare decisions 17
  HIV/AIDS 186
  home care 249
  spirituality 23
cystic fibrosis, palliative care 62

D

D&C *see* dilation and curettage
death
  advance directives 402
  alcohol use 522
  chronic illness 39
  cultural response 20
  end-of-life care 6
  financial assistance 410
  funeral services 438
  grief and developmental
    stages 356
  grief counseling 470
  leading causes 491
  life expectancy 499
  medical certification 451
  stillbirth 340
  sudden infant death syndrome
    (SIDS) 333
  suicide 515
  traveling 459
  see also death certificate; infant
    mortality; stillbirth
death certificates
  cause of death 488
  cremation 459
  funeral costs 432
  see also medical certification of
    death
death rattle
  breathing problems 5
  described 201
  end-of-life care 51
  HIV/AIDS 187
debriding, palliative care 66

"The Deceased Donation Process"
  (HRSA) 213n
"Deceased Taxpayers—
  Understanding the General Duties
  as an Estate Administrator"
  (IRS) 417n
decision making, home care 245
deep breathing, pediatric palliative
  care 331
defibrillation, cardiopulmonary
  resuscitation (CPR) 14, 399
dehydration
  artificial hydration and
    nutrition 126
  cancer-related fatigue 102
  defined 535
  delirium 155, 198
  tabulated *454*
delirium
  described 197
  HIV/AIDS 185
  hospital culture 51
  overview 150–6
"Delirium and Cancer Treatment"
  (NCI) 155n
"Delirium or Sudden Confusion in
  Elderly Adults" (VA) 150n
dementia
  artificial nutrition and
    hydration 399
  delirium 150
  dementia 167
  digestive problems 6
  insurance 272
  life expectancy 478
  long-term care 230
  pain assessment 93
  palliative care 258
  tabulated *454*
deoxyribonucleic acid (DNA)
  death 457
  defined 535
Department of Health and Human
  Services (DHHS; HHS) *see* U.S.
  Department of Health and Human
  Services
Department of Labor (DOL) *see* U.S.
  Department of Labor

depression
  acute respiratory distress syndrome
    (ARDS) 123
  cancer 320
  cancer treatment 103
  caregiver needs 249
  defined 535
  delirium 152
  end-of-life care 7
  grief 462
  HIV/AIDS 182
  life-sustaining treatments 207
  pain management 88
  palliative care 70
dexamethasone, fatigue 111
DHHS *see* U.S. Department of Health
  and Human Services
diabetes
  caregiving 302
  defined 535
  enteral nutrition 144
  financial assistance 409
  life expectancy 477
  mortality trends 485
  stillbirth 341
  transplants 218
diagnosis
  cancer care 284
  caregiver 240
  death 311
  defined 535
  dementia 93
  end-of-life care 22
  fatigue 103
  life insurance 411
  palliative care 71
  sudden infant death syndrome
    (SIDS) 333
diagnostic test
  acute respiratory distress syndrome
    (ARDS) 121
  death certification 451
dialysis
  advance directives 397
  healthcare decisions 13
  life-sustaining treatments 205
  preference patterns 165
diarrhea
  artificial hydration and
    nutrition 125

diarrhea, *continued*
  cancer-related fatigue 102
  chronic illness 37
  tabulated *454*
diet
  alcohol-related deaths 522
  cancer care 129
  chronic illness 39
  defined 536
  fatigue 109
  home care 247
  life expectancy 477
dietary supplements
  cancer 146
  fatigue 111
  pain 78
dietitian, cancer care 129
dilation and curettage (D&C),
  pregnancy 347
"The Dilemma of Delirium in Older
  Patients" (NIA) 150n
direct burial, described 438
direct cremation
  described 438
  see also cremation
disability
  alcohol-related deaths 523
  chronic illness 38
  financial assistance 410
  infant death 353
  life expectancy 478
  long-term care 228
  rehabilitative technologies 255
disabled
  caregiver 298
  long-term care 235
  military funeral planning 447
  Social Security 410
disorder
  defined 536
  fatigue 100
  hemorrhage 202
  infant death 506
distraction
  caregiving 291
  pain 79
  self-care 300
DNAR *see* do not attempt to
  resuscitate

DNI *see* do not intubate
DNR orders *see* do-not-resuscitate
  (DNR) orders
do not attempt to resuscitate (DNAR)
  advance directives 402
  healthcare decisions 14
do not intubate (DNI)
  advance directives 402
  cancer 178
  healthcare decisions 14
do-not-resuscitate (DNR) orders
  defined 178
  described 402
  life-sustaining treatments 209
DOL *see* U.S. Department of Labor
The Dougy Center, contact 551
drowsiness
  fatigue 103
  pain 86
  sleep changes 306
drug use
  alcohol use 521
  death 495
  delirium 152
dry mouth
  cancer 131
  tabulated *187*
durable power of attorney
  advance directives 401
  caregiving 294
  defined 536
  healthcare proxy (HCP) 178
  see also advance directives; living
    wills
duration
  defined 536
  patients' rights 383
  sudden infant death syndrome
    (SIDS) 336
dying process
  described 307
  end-of-life comfort 10
  tabulated *187*
dyspnea
  death 309
  end-of-life issues 183

E

economic growth, life expectancy 478

"Economic Impact Analysis of
  Proposed Other Solid Waste
  Incinerator Regulation" (EPA) 449n
ED *see* U.S. Department of Education
"Effective Communication in Caring
  for Older Adults" (NIA) 280n
"8 Tips for Long-Distance Caregiving"
  (NIA) 289n
Eldercare Locator, contact 546
electric shocks *see* defibrillation
electrical nerve stimulation
  pain 79
  palliative care 67
embalming, funeral rule 430
emergency medical technician (EMT),
  healthcare decisions 15
emergency response system, long-
  term care 229
emotional stress
  cancer 177
  fatigue 99
emotional support
  cancer 240
  chronic illness 74
  long-distance caregiving 290
  palliative care 61
  stillbirth 341
employer
  death 457
  estate administrator 420
  health information privacy
    rights 390
  insurance 275
EMT *see* emergency medical
  technician
end-of-life
  cancer 171
  death 305
  delirium 197
  dementia 167
  economic issues 373
  healthcare decisions 11
  home care 243
  nutrition 145
  spiritual concerns 29
"End-of-Life" (NIH) 43n
end-of-life care, BEACON study 48
"End-of-Life Care for People Who
  Have Cancer" (NCI) 305n

"End-of-Life Care for People with
Dementia" (NIA) 167n
"End of Life: Helping with Comfort
and Care" (NIA) 281n
end-of-life issues
    cancer 173
    mental and emotional needs 7
    palliative care 191
enteral nutrition
    life-sustaining treatments 208
    nutrition in cancer care 143
enzyme
    defined 536
    lung injury 119
EPA *see* U.S. Environmental
    Protection Agency
erythropoietin, fatigue 109
estate administrator, duties of a
    personal representative 417
"Ethical Practices in End-of-Life Care"
    (VA) 191n
ethics
    palliative care 191
    suicide 223
Eunice Kennedy Shriver National
    Institute of Child Health and
    Human Development (NICHD)
    contact 546
    publications
        assistive devices 254n
        infant mortality 349n
        pediatric critical care 365n
        pregnancy loss 344n
        sudden infant death syndrome
            (SIDS) 333n
euthanasia
    end-of-life healthcare decisions 17
    see also physician-assisted suicide
executor
    duties
        overview 417–20
exercise
    defined 536
    Family and Medical Leave Act
        (FMLA) 425
    fatigue 98
    grief counseling 470
    home care 247
    support groups 34

exudate, palliative wound care 65

F

"Facing Forward—Life after Cancer
    Treatment" (NCI) 114n
faith
    funeral services 433
    home care 247
    life-sustaining treatments 206
    palliative care 70
    spiritual needs 8
    see also religion; spirituality
Family and Medical Leave Act
    (FMLA)
    home care 248
    overview 421–6
"Family and Medical Leave Act"
    (DOL) 421n
family caregiver
    cancer 240
    dementia 169
    end-of-life care 21
Family Caregiver Alliance® (FCA),
    contact 551
"Family Caregivers in Cancer
    (PDQ®)—Patient Version"
    (NCI) 240n
"Family Involvement Improves End-
    of-Life-Care" (RR&D) 56n
FAS *see* fetal alcohol syndrome
FASD *see* fetal alcohol spectrum
    disorders
fat
    cancer 146
    fatigue 99
fat embolism, acute respiratory
    distress syndrome (ARDS) 119
fatal injury rate, work-related
    fatalities 509
fatalities
    alcohol-related deaths 522
    work-related, overview 509–12
fatigue
    death 306
    defined 198
    dementia 169
    end of life 7
    home care 247

fatigue, *continued*
overview 98–101
palliative care 60
tabulated *182*
"Fatigue (PDQ®)—Patient Version" (NCI) 101n
"Fatigue in Older Adults" (NIA) 98n
FDA *see* U.S. Food and Drug Administration
FD&C Act *see* Federal Food, Drug, and Cosmetic Act
Federal Food, Drug, and Cosmetic Act (FD&C Act), informed consent 387
federal food, patients' rights 387
Federal Trade Commission (FTC)
contact 546
publications
funeral planning 441n
feeding tubes
funeral services 429n
end-of-life care 51
enteral nutrition 143
life-sustaining treatments 207
fentanyl
pain management 89
palliative care 67
pediatric critical care 369
fetal alcohol spectrum disorders (FASD), alcohol and pregnancy 524
fetal alcohol syndrome (FAS), alcohol and pregnancy 524
fever
cancer care 134
end of life 45
fatigue 104
myoclonic jerking 202
pain management 87
pregnancy loss 345
First Candle/SIDS Alliance, contact 543
flexibility
defined 536
insurance benefits 272
pain management 79
palliative care 329
fluid intake
dying process 307
end-of-life issues 185

FMLA *see* Family and Medical Leave Act
Foley catheter, intensive care unit (ICU) 262
fracture
defined 536
delirium 152
medical certification 455
frequency
defined 536
informed consent 392
spirituality definitions 24
FTC *see* Federal Trade Commission
FTC's Funeral Rule, funeral services 430
funeral *see* funeral fee; funeral home; funeral provider; traditional funeral
funeral arrangements, federal trade commission (FTC) 430
Funeral Consumers Alliance (FCA), contact 551
funeral cost
checklist 432
organ donation 216
funeral fees, funeral services 432
funeral home
death 311
funeral planning tips 429
imminent death 186
planning a funeral 441
funeral provider
funeral services 429
planning a funeral 441

G

gastrostomy (G) tube, artificial hydration and nutrition 126
The George Washington Institute for Spirituality and Health (GWish), contact 551
"Getting Started with Long-Distance Caregiving" (NIA) 289n
"Getting Your Affairs in Order" (NIA) 375n
ginseng, dietary supplements 111
"Global Health and Aging" (NIA) 477n
glucose
cancer 146
defined 536

grave liners, funeral services 435
grief
  coping 461
  death 19
  dementia 169
  developmental stages 355
  fatigue 99
  pediatric critical care 366
"Grief, Bereavement, and
  Coping with Loss (PDQ®)—
  Health Professional Version"
  (NCI) 356n, 361n
"Grief, Bereavement, and Coping
  with Loss (PDQ®)—Patient Version"
  (NCI) 19n, 461n
GriefShare, contact 544
group home
  defined 537
  long-term care 230
"Guidance: Personal Representatives"
  (HHS) 417n
guided imagery
  cancer 320
  pain 79

H

hair loss, cancer 319
hallucinations, distress 198
hand-feeding, advance
  directives 399
handicap, nursing home 237
hCG *see* human chorionic
  gonadotropin
HCP *see* healthcare proxy
health, defined 537
Health in Aging Foundation,
  contact 551
health information privacy rights,
  overview 389–91
health insurance
  advance directives 400
  Family and Medical Leave Act
    (FMLA) 425
  home healthcare 263
  long-term care 236
  long-term-care insurance 270
  palliative care 72
  personal representative 417

Health Insurance Portability and
  Accountability Act (HIPAA)
  informed consent 387
  long-distance caregiving 291
health plan, personal
  representative 417
Health Resources and Services
  Administration (HRSA)
  publications
    organ donation 213n
    supportive and palliative care
      for HIV/AIDS 181n
healthcare proxy (HCP)
  advance directive 397
  described 177
  see also medical power of attorney
healthcare team
  acute respiratory distress syndrome
    (ARDS) 124
  cancer pain 82
  effective communication 283
  end-of-life care decisions 13
  exercise 112
  family caregivers 240
  nutrition in cancer care 134
healthy eating
  long-term care 235
  nutrition in cancer care 129
healthy weight
  defined 537
  infant death 352
  pain treatment 79
hearing aid
  defined 537
  delirium 152
  home healthcare 253
heart disease
  causes of death 491
  chronic illness 37
  defined 537
  fatigue 98
  infant mortality 352
  palliative care 62
heart rate
  end-of-life care 262
  pain management 79
  sudden infant death syndrome
    (SIDS) 335

hemorrhage
  described 202
  tabulated *454*
HHS *see* U.S. Department of Health
  and Human Services
high blood pressure
  advance directives 400
  defined 537
  hospice care 259
  organ donation and
    transplantation 218
  pain treatment 78
  stillbirth 341
  stroke 528
HIPAA *see* Health Insurance
  Portability and Accountability Act
Hispanics
  suicide statistics 519
  transplants 218
HIV *see* human immunodeficiency
  virus
home care
  cancer 240
  financial assistance 411
  long-distance caregiver 289
  long-term care 233
  palliative care 62
  see also nursing home care
"Home Health Care" (ACL) 251n
home healthcare
  overview 251–4
  see also home care
homemaker, home-based long-term
  care 229
homicide
  causes of death 493
  work-related fatalities 510
hormone
  acute respiratory distress syndrome
    (ARDS) 119
  cancer-related fatigue 102
  defined 537
  pregnancy loss 346
hospice care
  cancer care 135
  defined 538
  described 176
  long-term-care insurance 271
  overview 258–60

hospice care, *continued*
  versus palliative care 60
  see also end-of-life palliative care;
    palliative care
Hospice Foundation of America
  (HFA), contact 552
"Hospice Toolkit—An Overview of
  the Medicaid Hospice Benefit"
  (CMS) 266n
"How Social Security Can Help You
  When a Family Member Dies"
  (SSA) 413n
"How to Share Caregiving
  Responsibilities with Family
  Members" (NIA) 296n
human chorionic gonadotropin (hCG),
  pregnancy loss 346
human immunodeficiency virus (HIV)
  causes of death 494
  defined 538
  organ transplantation 214
hydration
  advance directives 399
  defined 538
hypertension
  causes of death 492
  see also high blood pressure
hypnosis
  pain management 79
  palliative care 67
hypoxemia, shortness of breath 199

I

ibuprofen
  pain treatment 78
  palliative care 64
  pediatric palliative care 331
ICU *see* intensive care unit
imagery, pain management 79
immune system
  defined 538
  fatigue 103
  miscarriage 346
  palliative care 65
IMR *see* infant mortality rate
income tax return
  estate administrator
    responsibility 419
  financial records 376

infant death
   medical certification 453
   overview 349–53
"Infant Mortality" (CDC) 349n
infants
   death certification 453
   life expectancy 499
   mortality rates 503
infections
   acute respiratory distress syndrome
      (ARDS) 117
   cancer-related fatigue 102
   cancer treatment 88
   delirium 153
   infant mortality 352
   life-sustaining treatments 208
   palliative care 65
   pregnancy 346
   see also human immunodeficiency
      virus
informal caregiver, defined 301, 538
informed consent
   clinical trials, overview 391–5
   overview 382–9
"Informed Consent" (FDA) 382n
"Informed Consent" (NCI) 382n
"Informed Consent for Clinical Trials"
      (FDA) 391n
in-home care, long-distance
   caregiving 289
Institute of Medicine (IOM), alcohol-
   attributable deaths 524
insurance coverage
   Family and Medical Leave Act
      (FMLA) 421
   hospice, overview 266–9
intensity, defined 538
intensive care unit (ICU)
   delirium 154
   end-of-life care 262
   life-sustaining treatments 209
   palliative care 191
   tabulated *188*
Internal Revenue Service (IRS)
   contact 546
   publication
      estate administrator
         duties 417n

International Cemetery, Cremation
   & Funeral Association (ICCFA),
   contact 552
intestines, defined 538
intravenous (IV), acute respiratory
   distress syndrome (ARDS) 122
intravenous fluids, tabulated *187*
intubation
   advance care planning 399
   medical orders for life-sustaining
      treatment (MOLST) 178
   respiratory arrest 14
IOM *see* Institute of Medicine
IRS *see* Internal Revenue Service
IV *see* intravenous

J

JCAHO *see* Joint Commission
   on Accreditation of Healthcare
   Organization
Joint Commission on Accreditation of
   Healthcare Organization (JCAHO),
   home care 252
Joint Commission Resources (JCR),
   contact 552
junk food, fatigue 99

K

kidney dialysis, advance
   directives 402
kidney failure
   Medicare 408
   palliative care 62
kidneys
   acute respiratory distress syndrome
      (ARDS) 117
   organ donation 217

L

"Last Days of Life (PDQ®)—Patient
   Version" (NCI) 195n, 205n
law
   advance care planning 161
   ethics and legal issues 193
   Family and Medical Leave Act
      (FMLA) 426

law, *continued*
  funeral planning 442
  health information privacy
    rights 389
  organ donation 217
legal documents
  advance directives 397
  advance planning 177
  long-distance caregiving 294
Leukemia & Lymphoma Society
  (LLS), contact 544
lidocaine, palliative care 67
life expectancy
  birth, overview 499–502
  ethics and legal issues 191
  mortality trends 483
  trends, overview 477–82
life insurance
  financial assistance 411
  funeral planning 443
  long-distance caregiving 294
  see also insurance coverage
life settlement, financial
  assistance 411
life-sustaining treatments
  advance care planning 178
  overview 205–11
life-threatening
  acute respiratory distress syndrome
    (ARDS) 117
  advance directives 399
  artificial hydration and
    nutrition 125
  communication in cancer care 283
  palliative care 60
  private financing options 411
living will
  advance planning 177
  communication in cancer care 284
  defined 538
  life-sustaining treatments 206
  see also advance directives; durable
    power of attorney
long-term care
  defined 538
  financial assistance 409
  hospice care 266
  insurance 270
  life expectancy 478

long-term care, *continued*
  overview 228–38
  palliative care 69
long-term-care facility
  defined 538
  financial assistance 409
  hospice care 266
  palliative care 69
long-term-care insurance
  defined 538
  overview 270–6
  private financing options 410
LSDP *see* Lump-Sum Death Payment
Lump-Sum Death Payment (LSDP),
  Social Security benefits 415
lung scarring, acute respiratory
  distress syndrome (ARDS) 120

M

magnetic resonance imaging (MRI)
  defined 538
  informed consent 385
"Make Yourself a Priority, Too: Tips
  for Caregivers" (NIA) 299n
malnutrition
  cancer care 130
  supportive care 123
massage therapy, pain
  management 79
maternal health, stillbirth 341
mausoleum
  cremation 450
  funeral services 437
MCC *see* multiple chronic conditions
Medicaid
  defined 538
  end-of-life care planning 161
  financial assistance for long-term/
    end-of-life care 408
  insurance coverage for hospice 266
  long-term care 232
  long-term-care insurance 274
  palliative care 72, 258
Medicaid Fraud Control Unit
  (MFCU), hospice care 269
medical equipment
  caregiving 247
  Medicaid hospice program 266

medical examiner
  death 311
  death certificate 455
Medical Orders for Life-Sustaining
  Treatment (MOLST)
  advance directives 403
  end-of-life care for advanced
    cancer 178
medical power of attorney (MPOA),
  end-of-life care for advanced
  cancer 178
Medicare
  chronic illness in old age 39
  defined 539
  end-of-life care planning 161
  financial assistance for long-term/
    end-of-life care 408
  hospice care 259, 268
  legal documents 377
  long-term care 229
  mortality trends 489
  palliative care 72
medications
  advance directives 400
  chronic illness in old age 42
  delirium 152
  end-of-life care for dementia 167
  financial assistance for long-term/
    end-of-life care 409
  HIV/AIDS and end-of-life issues 183
  informed consent 384
  long-term care 231
  pain management 77
  palliative wound care 67
  pediatric palliative care 331
  pregnancy loss 347
meditation
  fatigue 99
  pain management 79
  spirituality in end-of-life care 35
memorial services
  funeral services 430
  guiding children through grief 362
  HIV/AIDS and end-of-life issues 184
memories
  assistive devices and rehabilitative
    technologies 254
  chronic fatigue syndrome 101
  death 311

memories, *continued*
  delirium 152
  end-of-life care for dementia 168
  end-of-life healthcare decisions 12
  end-of-life spiritual needs 8
  grief and developmental
    stages 357
  long-distance caregiving 291
  mourning death of spouse 470
men, alcohol-attributable deaths 521
mental health
  caregiver self-care 299
  coping with loss 461
  spirituality in end-of-life care 25
meperidine, palliative wound care 67
MFCU *see* Medicaid Fraud Control
  Unit
miscarriage
  overview 344–8
  see also pregnancy loss
mobility
  assistive devices and rehabilitative
    technologies 254
  chronic illness in old age 38
MOLST *see* Medical Orders for Life-
  Sustaining Treatment
morphine
  end-of-life physical comfort 5
  medicines to treat cancer pain 89
  palliative wound care 67
  tabulated *189*
"Mortality in the United States, 2017"
  (CDC) 483n
motion analysis, rehabilitative
  technologies 255
mourning
  bereavement 462
  cultural response to death 20
  grief and developmental stages 356
  guiding children through grief 362
  see also grief
"Mourning the Death of a Spouse"
  (NIA) 469n
mouth sores, nutrition in cancer
  care 134
MPOA *see* medical power of attorney
mucositis
  end of life 202
  nutrition in cancer care 147

multidisciplinary
  ethics and legal issues 192
  palliative care 69, 258
multiple chronic conditions (MCC),
  chronic illnesses and end-of-life
  care 73
"Multiple Chronic Conditions
  Chartbook" (AHRQ) 73n

N

NACC *see* National Association of
  Catholic Chaplains
NAHC *see* National Association for
  Home Care & Hospice
narcotic
  pain management 78
  palliative wound care 67
nasogastric (NG) tube
  artificial hydration and
    nutrition 126
  end-of-life healthcare decisions 15
  nutrition support 143
National Association for Home Care &
  Hospice (NAHC), contact 552
National Association of Area Agencies
  on Aging (N4A), contact 552
National Association of Catholic
  Chaplains (NACC), contact 552
National Cancer Institute (NCI)
  contact 547
  publications
    cancer care
      communication 283n
    cancer pain management 80n
    cancer treatment and
      fatigue 114n
    caregiver self-care 299n
    coping with loss 356n
    delirium and cancer
      treatment 155n
    end-of-life cancer care 171n,
      305n
    fatigue 101n
    grief management 19n
    home care for cancer
      patients 240n
    informed consent 382n
    last days of life 195n, 205n

National Cancer Institute (NCI)
  publications, *continued*
    nutrition and cancer care 129n
    palliative care in cancer 69n
    spirituality 21n
    supporting families 315n
    telephone-based rehab
      program 52n
"National Census of Fatal
  Occupational Injuries in 2017"
  (BLS) 509n
National Funeral Directors
  Association (NFDA), contact 552
National Heart, Lung, and Blood
  Institute (NHLBI)
  contact 547
  publication
    acute respiratory distress
      syndrome (ARDS) 117n
National Hospice and Palliative Care
  Organization (NHPCO), contact 544
National Institute of Nursing
  Research (NINR)
  publications
    palliative care 60n
    pediatric palliative care 325n
National Institute on Aging (NIA)
  contact 547
  publications
    advance care planning 397n
    caregivers self-care 299n
    caregiving responsibilities 296n
    choosing a nursing home 236n
    chronic illness 37n
    comfort care 3n
    delirium 150n
    effective communication 280n
    end-of-life care for people with
      dementia 167n
    end-of-life care settings 261n
    end-of-life healthcare
      decisions 11n
    end-of-life wishes 281n
    fatigue in older adults 98n
    financial assistance 407n
    legal documentation 375n
    life expectancy 477n
    long-distance caregiving 289n
    long-term care 228n

National Institute on Aging (NIA)
publications, *continued*
    long-term-care plans 235n
    mourning death of
      spouse 469n
    pain management 76n
    palliative care and hospice
      care 257n
    when death occurs 309n
National Institute on Alcohol Abuse
  and Alcoholism (NIAAA)
  publication
    alcohol-attributed death
      statistics 521n
National Institutes of Health (NIH)
  contact 547
  publications
    advance directives 397n
    end of life 43n
    quality of life (QOL) 191n
National Survey on Drug Use
  and Health (NSDUH), alcohol-
  attributed deaths 521
National Violent Death Reporting
  System (NVDRS), suicide facts and
  statistics 517
National Vital Statistics Report
  (NVSR), causes of death 495
"National Vital Statistics Reports"
  (CDC) 491n, 499n, 503n
National Vital Statistics System
  (NVSS)
  injury-related death 513
  mortality trends 489
  stillbirth 341
nausea
  advance directives 400
  miscarriage 345
  nutrition in cancer care 134
  pain management 92
  palliative care 60
NCI *see* National Cancer Institute
nerve block, pain management 78
neurologic disorders, pediatric
  palliative care 328
neurologic dysfunction, HIV/AIDS and
  end-of-life issues 185
NFDA *see* National Funeral Directors
  Association

N4A *see* National Association of Area
  Agencies on Aging
NG tube *see* nasogastric tube
NHLBI *see* National Heart, Lung, and
  Blood Institute
NHPCO *see* National Hospice and
  Palliative Care Organization
NIA *see* National Institute on Aging
NIAAA *see* National Institute on
  Alcohol Abuse and Alcoholism
NICHD *see Eunice Kennedy Shriver
  National Institute of Child Health
  and Human Development*
nightmares
  fatigue 110
  pain medicine side effects 91
NIH *see* National Institutes of Health
NIH News in Health
  contact 547
  publication
    coping with caregiving 301n
NINR *see* National Institute of
  Nursing Research
nonfatal injuries, injury-related
  deaths 513
nonmaleficence, ethics and legal
  issues 193
nonsteroidal anti-inflammatory drugs
  (NSAIDs), pain management 78
NSDUH *see* National Survey on Drug
  Use and Health
nursing care
  long-term care 231
  long-term-care insurance 271
  Medicaid hospice program 266
nursing homes
  defined 539
  dementia 169
  end-of-life care for advanced
    cancer 176
  end-of-life care settings 262
  financial assistance for long-term/
    end-of-life care 408
  hospice care 258
  long-distance caregiving 291
  long-term care 228
  overview 236–8
  pain management in dementia 93
nursing service, long-term care 234

nutrition
  acute respiratory distress syndrome
    (ARDS) 123
  advance directives 399
  cancer care 129
  defined 539
  delirium among cancer patients 156
  fatigue 115
  HIV/AIDS and end-of-life issues 185
  life-sustaining treatments 205
  "Nutrition in Cancer Care (PDQ®)—
    Patient Version" (NCI) 129n
nutrition therapy
  cancer care 129
  life-sustaining treatments 207
nutritionists
  cancer care 129
  fatigue 115
  palliative care 63, 258
  pediatric palliative care 329
NVDRS *see* National Violent Death
  Reporting System
NVSR *see* National Vital Statistics
  Report
NVSS *see* National Vital Statistics
  System

O

OAA *see* Older Americans Act
obesity
  defined 539
  nutrition in cancer care 30
  stillbirth 341
  stroke 528
obituary notice, funeral services 433
occupational injuries, statistics 510
Office on Women's Health (OWH)
  publication
    organ donation and
      transplantation 213n
oils
  defined 539
  funeral services 436
  work-related fatalities 512
older adults
  chronic illness in old age 39
  delirium 150
  end-of-life healthcare decisions 14

older adults, *continued*
  financial assistance for long-term/
    end-of-life care 407
  home care 250
Older Americans Act (OAA)
  home healthcare 254
  long-term care 236
Omnigraphics
  publications
    artificial hydration and
      nutrition 125n
    palliative wound care 64n
    physician-assisted suicide and
      euthanasia 221n
opioid
  end of life 200
  pain management 90
  palliative care 67
OPM *see* U.S. Office of Personnel
  Management
OPO *see* Organ Procurement
  Organization
organ, defined 539
organ donation
  advance directives 403
  overview 213–20
  "Organ Donation and Transplantation
    Fact Sheet" (OWH) 213n
  "Organ Donation FAQs" (HRSA) 213n
  "Organ Donation Statistics"
    (HRSA) 213n
organ donor
  legal documents 379
  transplantation 214
Organ Procurement Organization
  (OPO), organ donation and
  transplantation 219
OTC *see* over-the-counter
over-the-counter (OTC)
  defined 539
  end of life 200
  pain management 78
overweight
  defined 539
  stillbirth 342
oxygen levels
  acute respiratory distress syndrome
    (ARDS) 117
  end-of-life care settings 262

577

oxygen therapy, acute respiratory
   distress syndrome (ARDS) 122

P

PACE *see* Program of All-Inclusive
   Care for the Elderly
pacemakers
   dementia 168
   healthcare decisions 15
pain
   advance directives 400
   advanced cancer 171
   assessment 93
   communication 281
   delirium 153
   end of life 43
   end-of-life care 4
   ethics and legal issues 192
   miscarriage 344
   mourning 469
   overview 76–80
   palliative care and hospice care 257
   patients' rights 385
   pediatric palliative care 325
   physician-assisted suicide 222
   radiation therapy 132
   spirituality 29
   suicide 517
   treatment 110
   withdrawal 306
"Pain: You Can Get Help" (NIA) 76n
palliative care
   comforting the terminally ill 257
   dementia 168
   end of life 44
   euthanasia and palliative
      sedation 222
   healthcare decisions 17
   HIV/AIDS 187
   nutrition therapy 135
   overview 60–4
   pain 306
   pain management and
      assessment 86
   personal awareness 35
"Palliative Care for Children"
   (NINR) 325n
"Palliative Care in Cancer" (NCI) 69n

"Palliative Care: The Relief You Need
   When You Have a Serious Illness"
   (NINR) 60n
"Palliative Wound Care"
   (Omnigraphics) 64n
pancreatitis, acute respiratory
   distress syndrome (ARDS) 119
paranoia, depression 110
parents
   advance directives 405
   chronic illness 74
   end-of-life wishes 282
   family consequences 523
   grief 362
   grief counseling 470
   organ donation 214
   pediatric palliative care 328
   personal representative 418
   pregnancy loss 345
Parkinson disease (PD)
   causes of death 492
   long-term-care insurance 272
   palliative care 258
PAS *see* physician-assisted suicide
patients' rights, overview 381–95
"Paying for Care" (NIA) 407n
PCOS *see* polycystic ovary syndrome
PD *see* Parkinson disease
pediatric intensive care unit (PICU),
   bereavement and grief 368
pediatrician, cancer 324
pedometer, defined 539
PEEP *see* positive-end expiratory
   pressure
PEG *see* percutaneous endoscopic
   gastronomy
pension
   financial assistance 407
   financial records 376
   insurance for end-of-life care 275
   long-term care 236
percutaneous endoscopic gastronomy
   (PEG)
   artificial hydration and
      nutrition 126
   end-of-life healthcare decisions 16
personal care
   defined 539
   financial assistance 407

personal care, *continued*
  insurance for end-of-life care 271
  long-term care 228
  weakness 306
personal representative *see* estate
  administrator; executor
"Personal Representatives"
  (HHS) 417n
PHN *see* postherpetic neuralgia
physical activity
  caregivers 302
  defined 540
  drugs 111
  fatigue 99
  long-term care 235
physical comfort
  care and comfort 4
  HIV/AIDS 181
physical therapy
  fatigue 114
  home healthcare 251
  insurance for end-of-life care 267
  long-term care 232
  pain management and
    assessment 79
  telephone-based rehab program 53
physician-assisted suicide (PAS),
  overview 221–3
"Physician-Assisted Suicide and
  Euthanasia" (Omnigraphics) 221n
Physician Orders for Life-Sustaining
  Treatment (POLST)
  advance directives 403
  advanced cancer 178
  end of life 45
PICU *see* pediatric intensive care
  unit
"Plan a Burial for a Veteran, Spouse,
  or Dependent Family Member"
  (VA) 445n
plan of care (POC)
  advanced cancer 173
  Medicaid hospice program 266
"Planning for Long-Term Care"
  (NIA) 235n
"Planning the Transition to End-
  of-Life Care in Advanced Cancer
  (PDQ®)—Patient Version"
  (NCI) 171n

"Planning Your Own Funeral"
  (FTC) 441n
PMC *see* Presidential Memorial
  Certificate
pneumonia
  acute respiratory distress syndrome
    (ARDS) 118
  advance directives 401
  artificial hydration and
    nutrition 126
  causes of death 485
  chronic illness 38
  end of life 199
  feeding tube 16
  HIV/AIDS 188
  infection and sepsis 370
  tabulated *454*
pneumothorax (collapsed lung), acute
  respiratory distress syndrome
  (ARDS) 120
POC *see* plan of care
pollution, pregnancy 348
POLST *see* Physician Orders for Life-
  Sustaining Treatment
polycystic ovary syndrome (PCOS),
  pregnancy 346
positive-end expiratory pressure
  (PEEP), tabulated *189*
"Possible Solutions to Common
  Problems in Death Certification"
  (CDC) 451n
postherpetic neuralgia (PHN),
  pain 76
power of attorney
  advance care 401
  end-of-life care 162
  legal and financial paperwork 473
  long-distance caregiving 294
  personal representative 417
  see also durable power of attorney
prayer
  spirituality 24
  support groups 34
pregnancy
  infant death 352
  miscarriage 344
  sudden infant death syndrome
    (SIDS) 334
  pregnancy loss, stillbirth 340

"Pregnancy Loss (Before 20
Weeks of Pregnancy)" (NICHD) 344n
prepaid burial arrangement, burial
fund 415
Presidential Memorial Certificate
(PMC), military funeral 447
pressure ulcer
dementia 94
palliative care 65
preterm birth
infant mortality trends 508
sudden infant death syndrome
(SIDS) 334
"Prevalence and Management of
Pain, by Race and Dementia among
Nursing Home Residents: United
States, 2004" (CDC) 93n
privacy rule *see* Health Insurance
Portability and Accountability Act
probate proceeding, personal
representative 419
probiotics, described 147
prognosis
care and comfort 3
caregiver 240
defined 540
end-of-life care 165
hospital culture 50
Program of All-Inclusive Care for the
Elderly (PACE)
defined 234
government programs 409
progression
defined 540
dementia 168
protein
complete blood count (CBC) 108
defined 540
infection and sepsis 371
nutrition 136
"Providing Care and Comfort at the
End of Life" (NIA) 3n
psychologist
advanced cancer 175
cancer 320
grief 363
life-sustaining treatments 207
nutrition 135
palliative care 69

psychologist, *continued*
social issues 247
psychotherapy, grief 466

Q

QOL *see* quality of life
quality of life (QOL)
acute respiratory distress syndrome
(ARDS) 124
advance care planning 400
cancer and fatigue 101
care and comfort 3
caregiving 284
chronic illnesses 74
HIV/AIDS 183
home care 243
pediatric palliative care 327
physician-assisted suicide 223
telerehabilitation 54
"Quality of Life for Individuals at the
End-of-Life" (NIH) 191n

R

RA *see* rheumatoid arthritis
race
cancer therapies 55
dementia 93
emergency response systems 230
healthcare decisions 17
infant and maternal mortality 504
infant death 350
mortality trends 483
organ donation 217
quality care 267
stroke 528
sudden infant death syndrome
(SIDS) 334
radiation
cancer 81, 101
cancer treatment 132
defined 540
hemorrhage 202
patients' rights 385
pregnancy 348
rehabilitation
acute respiratory distress syndrome
(ARDS) 124

rehabilitation, *continued*
  insurance cover 266
  long-term care 231
  telephone-based rehab program 52
Rehabilitation Research &
  Development Service (RR&D)
  publications
    end-of-life care 56n
    research on end-of-life
      care 48n
rehabilitative technologies,
  overview 255–6
religion
  after death 311
  grief reactions 465
  healthcare decisions 17
  HIV/AIDS 185
  physician-assisted suicide 223
  quality care 267
  see also spirituality
"Residential Facilities, Assisted
  Living, and Nursing Homes"
  (NIA) 228n
respiratory arrest, healthcare
  decisions 14
respiratory therapy, fatigue 114
respite care
  defined 540
  end of life 204
  insurance covers 271
  long-term care 232
  palliative care and hospice
    care 259
  pediatric palliative care 327
resuscitation
  advance care planning 398
  advanced cancer 172
  cancer care 285
  end of life 203
  healthcare decisions 14
  intensive care 368
  preferences for care 162
  traveling 457
  see also cardiopulmonary
    resuscitation; do-not-resuscitate
    orders
reverse mortgage, described 411
rheumatoid arthritis (RA), fatigue 98
rigor mortis, stiffness after death 310

risk factors
  acute respiratory distress syndrome
    (ARDS) 118
  delirium 151
  sudden infant death syndrome
    (SIDS) 334
rituals
  cultural response 19
  end of life 197
  HIV/AIDS 186
  intervention 31, 362
  physician-assisted suicide 223
robotics, rehabilitative
  technologies 255

S

safe deposit box
  financial records 376
  funeral planning tips 443
Safe Kids Worldwide, contact 553
SCCM *see* Society of Critical Care
  Medicine
sedation
  delirium 156
  emergency treatment 399
  euthanasia 222
  intensive care 210
  ventilator withdrawal *189*
sedatives
  delirium 153
  end-of-life healthcare 16
  palliative sedation 210
  ventilator withdrawal *189*
seizures
  ambiguity avoidance *454*
  neurologic dysfunction 186
self-care
  caregivers 299
  dementia 169
  fatigue 113
senior center, long-term care 233
seniors *see* older adults
sepsis
  acute respiratory distress syndrome
    (ARDS) 118
  nutrition support 145
  pediatric critical care 370
  tabulated *454*

serotonin, sudden infant death
  syndrome (SIDS) 335
Share, contact 544
shingles, pain management 76
SHIP *see* State Health Insurance
  Assistance Program
shock, grief 463
shock lung *see* acute respiratory
  distress syndrome (ARDS)
"Shopping for Funeral Services"
  (FTC) 429n
shortness of breath
  acute respiratory distress syndrome
    (ARDS) 118
  breathing problems 5
  end-of-life care 400
  final days 198
  HIV/AIDS 182
  palliative care 61
  pediatric palliative care 327
side effects
  antibiotics 16
  artificial hydration 126
  cancer treatment 288
  chronic illness 42
  defined 540
  delirium 197
  dementia 168
  home care 245
  medication 144
  nutrition 106
  over-the-counter (OTC) drugs 86
  pain management 77
  palliative care 60
  supportive care 175
SIDS *see* sudden infant death
  syndrome
skilled nursing facility *see* nursing
  homes
sleep
  caregiver's health 302
  chemotherapy 104
  children 323
  chronic cough 200
  delirium 152
  drowsiness 91
  fatigue 98
  oxygen therapy 122
  pain 76

sleep, *continued*
  palliative care 60
  sedation 16
  sudden infant death syndrome
    (SIDS) 334, 353
  systemic analgesics 67
sleep problems, fatigue 106, 198
sleep–wake cycle, cancer
  treatment 103
Social Security, benefits 413
Social Security Disability Income
  (SSDI), Medicare 408
"Social Security Lump Sum Death
  Payment" (Benefits.gov) 413n
Social Security Number (SSN)
  benefits 413
  hospice services 268
  personal records 375
social support
  bereavement 465
  home care 243
  palliative care 70, 325
  spirituality 26
  talk therapy 113
social worker
  advance directives 162
  caregiving 291
  community 364
  end-of-life spiritual needs 8
  long-term care 231
  nutrition counseling 135
  palliative care 62, 258
  pediatric palliative care 329
  spiritual health 207
  spiritual support 173
Society of Critical Care Medicine
  (SCCM), contact 553
spiritual support
  cancer 173
  caregiver 240
  hospice care 259
  quality of life (QOL) 207
spirituality
  end-of-life care, overview 21–36
  euthanasia 223
  HIV/AIDS patients 185
  see also religion; spiritual support
"Spirituality in Cancer Care (PDQ®)—
  Health Professional Version"
  (NCI) 21n

"Spotlight on Burial Funds—2019
   Edition" (SSA) 413n
SPRC *see* Suicide Prevention Resource
   Center
"Spreading Best Practices for End-of-
   Life Care" (RR&D) 48n
sputum culture, acute respiratory
   distress syndrome (ARDS) 121
SSA *see* U.S. Social Security
   Administration
SSDI *see* Social Security Disability
   Income
SSI *see* Supplemental Security Income
SSN *see* Social Security Number
State Health Insurance Assistance
   Program (SHIP), described 409
"The State of Aging and Health in
   America 2013" (CDC) 37n
statistics
   alcohol deaths 521
   birth 499
   causes of death 491
   infant and maternal mortality 503
   life expectancy 477
   maternal mortality rates
   mortality trends 483
   stroke 527
   suicide 517
   work-related fatalities 509
stem cell transplant, cancer 130
steroid
   defined 540
   exudates 65
   infants 352
   nonsteroidal anti-inflammatory
      drugs (NSAIDs) 87
stiff lung *see* acute respiratory
   distress syndrome (ARDS)
stillbirths
   overview 340–3
   see also miscarriage
strength
   cancer-related fatigue 102
   caregiving 296
   chronic illness 41
   defined 540
   hydration 186
   nutrition 129
   spirituality 30

strength, *continued*
   sudden infant death syndrome
      (SIDS) 338
stretching
   defined 540
   exercise 112
stroke
   advance care planning 400
   chronic illness 37, 160
   defined 540
   end of life 282
   home care 255
   insurance 272
   life expectancy 478
   long-term care 228
   organ donation 218
   palliative care 191
"Stroke Facts" (CDC) 527n
Substance Abuse and Mental Health
   Services Administration (SAMHSA),
   contact 547
sucralfate, topical anesthetics 67
sudden infant death syndrome
   (SIDS)
   death certificate 453
   infant death statistics 487
   infant mortality 349
   overview 333–8
"Sudden Infant Death Syndrome
   (SIDS)" (NICHD) 333n
suffocation
   childhood injury-related deaths 513
   infant death 349
   sudden infant death syndrome
      (SIDS) 336
suicide
   bereavement 363
   end of life 17
   statistics 517
   see also physician-assisted suicide
"Suicide—Facts at a Glance"
   (CDC) 517n
Suicide Prevention Resource Center
   (SPRC), contact 544
Supplemental Security Income (SSI)
   burial fund 416
   defined 540
"Support for Families When a Child
   Has Cancer" (NCI) 315n

"Support for People with Cancer—Cancer Pain Control" (NCI) 80n

support groups
  chronic illness 41
  grief counseling 470
  intervention 31
  palliative care 327

"Supporting Older Patients with Chronic Conditions" (NIA) 37n

supportive care
  acute respiratory distress syndrome (ARDS) 122
  dementia 167
  cancer 52, 283
  fatigue 109

surgery
  acute pain 76
  care preference 165
  fatigue 105
  hydration 125
  nonsteroidal anti-inflammatory drugs (NSAIDs) 88

surgical procedures
  patient's rights 385
  pregnancy loss 347

symptom management
  children 329
  palliative care 72

T

tai chi
  defined 541
  fatigue 100

talk therapy
  described 113
  grief 466

tax
  estate administrator 419
  financial records 376
  reverse mortgage 411
  see also income tax return

taxable
  estate administrator 419
  insurance 412

tDCS *see* transcranial direct current stimulation

telephone-based rehab program, overview 52–5

"Telephone-Based Rehab Program Helps People with Advanced Cancer Maintain Independence" (NCI) 52n

TENS *see* transcutaneous electrical nerve stimulation

terminal sedation, euthanasia 222

terminally ill
  end of life 195
  euthanasia 222
  life insurance 411
  palliative wound care 64

"3 Tips for Caregiver Self-Care" (NCI) 299n

tissue donation, advance directive 397

TMS *see* transcranial magnetic stimulation

tobacco
  chronic illness 39
  defined 541
  nutrition 139
  pain management 80

total parenteral nutrition (TPN), defined 126

toxic
  cancer 103
  defined 541

toxins
  nutrition 145
  pregnancy 345

TPN *see* total parenteral nutrition

traditional funeral, cremation 449

Tragedy Assistance Program for Survivors, Inc. (TAPS), contact 544

transcranial direct current stimulation (tDCS), rehabilitative technologies 255

transcranial magnetic stimulation (TMS), rehabilitative technologies 255

transcutaneous electrical nerve stimulation (TENS), palliative care 67

transfer of assets
  defined 541
  estate administrator 420

transfusions
  anemia 109
  described 209

transplantation, organs 213

"Travelers' Health—Death during Travel" (CDC) 457n
trusts
    legal documents 377
    private financing 410
tube feeding
    advanced directives 399
    cancer care 137
    end-of-life healthcare 15
    see also enteral nutrition; feeding tubes
Tylenol® (acetaminophen), pain 86

U

"Understanding Healthcare Decisions at the End of Life" (NIA) 11n
Uniformed Services Employment and Reemployment Rights Act (USERRA), Family and Medical Leave Act (FMLA) 423
urinary tract infection (UTI)
    antibiotics 16
    defined 541
U.S. Bureau of Labor Statistics (BLS)
    contact 547
    publication
        fatal occupational injuries statistics 509n
U.S. Department of Education (ED)
    publication
        coping through grief 361n
U.S. Department of Health and Human Services (HHS)
    contact 547
    publications
        health information privacy rights 389n
        personal representatives 417n
U.S. Department of Labor (DOL)
    contact 548
    publication
        Family and Medical Leave Act (FMLA) 421n
U.S. Department of Veterans Affairs (VA)
    contact 548
    publications
        delirium 150n

U.S. Department of Veterans Affairs (VA)
    publications, *continued*
        end-of-life care 191n
        military funeral 445n
U.S. Environmental Protection Agency (EPA)
    contact 548
    publication
        cremation 449n
U.S. Food and Drug Administration (FDA)
    contact 548
    publications
        clinical trials consent 391n
        informed consent 382n
U.S. Office of Personnel Management (OPM), Family and Medical Leave Act (FMLA) 426
U.S. Social Security Administration (SSA)
    contact 548
    publications
        burial funds 413n
        Social Security benefits 413n
USERRA *see* Uniformed Services Employment and Reemployment Rights Act
UTI *see* urinary tract infection

V

VA *see* U.S. Department of Veterans Affairs
"VA Study Leads to Improved End-of-Life Care" (RR&D) 48n
vaccine
    chronic illness 38
    sudden infant death syndrome (SIDS) 338
vasoconstrictors, wound care 65
ventilators, birth defects 352
veteran
    end-of-life care 48
    government programs 409
    military funeral 445
veterans' benefits, government programs 410
viatical settlement, life insurance 412

Visiting Nurse Associations of
America (VNAA), contact 553
VNAA *see* Visiting Nurse Associations
of America
vomiting
artificial hydration 125
cancer-related fatigue 102
digestive problems 6
pain management 90
palliative care 70
pregnancy loss 346

W

Wage and Hour Division (WHD),
Family and Medical Leave Act
(FMLA) 426
weight loss
cancer care 131
grief 357
nutrition therapy 144
Well Spouse® Association (WSA),
contact 544
wet lung *see* acute respiratory distress
syndrome
"What Are My Other Long-Term Care
Choices?" (CMS) 228n
"What Are Palliative Care and
Hospice Care?" (NIA) 257n
"What Are Some Types of Assistive
Devices and How Are They Used?"
(NICHD) 254n
"What Happens When Someone
Dies?" (NIA) 309n
"What Is Long-Term Care?"
(NIA) 228n
"What Is Stillbirth?" (CDC) 340n
"What to Do after Someone Dies"
(NIA) 309n
WHD *see* Wage and Hour Division
"Where Can I Find Care for a Dying
Relative?" (NIA) 261n
wills, paperwork 294
withdrawal, pain management 90
women
alcohol-abuse statistics 521
caregiving 301

women, *continued*
fatigue and radiation therapy 104
grief 465
infant death 351
maternal mortality 504
remotely delivered care 53
spirituality 25
stillbirth 341
sudden infant death syndrome
(SIDS) 337
support groups 34
workplace
acute respiratory distress syndrome
(ARDS) 124
assistive technologies 255
work-related fatalities 510
see also Family and Medical Leave
Act (FMLA)
wound care, pain management 66
WSA *see* Well Spouse® Association

X

x-rays
acute respiratory distress syndrome
(ARDS) 121
defined 541

Y

Yellow Ribbon Suicide Prevention
Program®/The Light for Life
Foundation Int'l, contact 544
yoga
defined 541
exercise 112
fatigue management 100
pain management 79
stress management 323
see also meditation
"Your Health Information"
(HHS) 389n

Z

Zika, pregnancy loss 346

1/20

For Reference

Not to be taken from this room